CA   W
Pediatric imaging

Series Editor
David M. Yousem, MD, MBA
Professor of Radiology
Director of Neuroradiology
The Russell H. Morgan Department of Radiology and Radiological Science
Johns Hopkins Medical Institutions
Baltimore, Maryland

Other Volumes in the CASE REVIEW Series
Brain Imaging
Breast Imaging
Cardiac Imaging
Emergency Radiology
Gastrointestinal Imaging
General and Vascular Ultrasound
Genitourinary Imaging
Head and Neck Imaging
Musculoskeletal Imaging
Nuclear Medicine
OB/GYN Ultrasound
Spine Imaging
Thoracic Imaging
Vascular and Interventional Imaging

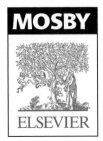

Thierry A.G.M. Huisman, MD, EQNR, FICIS
Medical Director
Division of Pediatric Radiology;
Professor of Radiology
The Russell H. Morgan Department of Radiology
    and Radiological Science
Johns Hopkins Hospital
Baltimore, Maryland

Jane Benson, MD
Assistant Professor of Radiology and Pediatrics
Division of Pediatric Radiology
The Russell H. Morgan Department of Radiology
    and Radiological Science
Johns Hopkins Hospital
Baltimore, Maryland

Melissa Spevak, MD
Assistant Professor of Radiology
Division of Pediatric Radiology
The Russell H. Morgan Department of Radiology
    and Radiological Science
Johns Hopkins Hospital
Baltimore, Maryland

Renee Flax-Goldenberg, MD
Clinical Associate
Division of Pediatric Radiology
The Russell H. Morgan Department of Radiology
    and Radiological Science
Johns Hopkins Hospital
Baltimore, Maryland

Aylin Tekes, MD
Assistant Professor of Radiology
Division of Pediatric Radiology
The Russell H. Morgan Department of Radiology
    and Radiological Science
Johns Hopkins Hospital
Baltimore, Maryland

CASE REVIEW

Pediatric Imaging

SECOND EDITION

CASE REVIEW SERIES

MOSBY
ELSEVIER

1600 John F. Kennedy Blvd.
Ste 1800
Philadelphia, PA 19103-2899

PEDIATRIC IMAGING: CASE REVIEW   ISBN: 978-0-323-06698-3

Library of Congress Cataloging-in-Publication Data
Case review : pediatric imaging. – 2nd ed. / Thierry A.G.M. Huisman . . . [et al.].
    p. ; cm. – (Case review series)
   Other title: Pediatric imaging
   Rev. ed. of: Pediatric imaging : case review / Robert J. Ward, Hans Blickman. c2007.
   Includes bibliographical references and index.
   ISBN: 978-0-323-06698-3 (pbk. : alk. paper)   1. Pediatric diagnostic imaging–Case studies.
I. Huisman, Thierry A.G.M.   II. Ward, Robert J., MD. Pediatric imaging.   III. Title: Pediatric imaging.
IV. Series: Case review series.
   [DNLM: 1. Diagnostic Imaging–methods–Case Reports.   2. Diagnostic Imaging–methods–Problems and Exercises.   3. Child.   4. Infant.   5. Pediatrics–methods–Case Reports.   6. Pediatrics–methods–Problems and Exercises.   WN 18.2 C337 2011]
  RJ51.R3W37 2011
  618.92'00754–dc22

                                2010021008

Acquisitions Editor: Rebecca Gaertner
Editorial Assistant: David Mack
Publishing Services Manager: Anne Altepeter
Senior Project Manager: Doug Turner
Designer: Steve Stave

Printed in the United States of America

Last digit is the print number: 9   8   7   6   5   4   3   2   1

This is a new collection of cases for the pediatric radiology *Case Review Series*. I was pleased to collect and arrange these cases upon the friendly invitation by Dr. David Yousem. The collection will be part of the second edition of the *Requisite Series of Pediatric Radiology*. The purpose of the *Case Review Series* is a didactic one. It allows readers to explore, deepen, and further develop their knowledge in a most fascinating area of imaging—pediatric radiology. The cases match the daily routine practice and will stimulate readers to further diagnostic investigation using textbooks, journals, and the Internet. Studying these cases should be fun.

The creation of an attractive collection of cases was only possible with the help of my gifted and dedicated colleagues from the pediatric radiology medical staff: Drs. Jane Benson, Renee Flax-Goldenberg, Melissa Spevak, and Aylin Tekes. They all contributed from their fields of interest and expertise. We tried to cover the spectrum of pediatric radiology to the best of our abilities. I thank all my staff pediatric radiologists for their contributions, help, and patience.

Another essential factor in completing this case review is the fact that we are supported and intellectually challenged by brilliant pediatric physicians at the Johns Hopkins Hospital and University, with their professional requests and stimulating discussions at our daily joint conferences. This interdisciplinary culture has its roots in Johns Hopkins' four core values: (1) excellence and discovery, (2) leadership and integrity, (3) diversity and inclusion, and (4) respect and collegiality. These are as valid today as they were at the founding of our hospital and our school of medicine in the late nineteenth century. Our clinical colleagues are aware of the value and expert use of our imaging tools in the diagnosis and treatment of their patients. Our thanks goes to both: to our colleagues and to their patients who sought help at our institution and provided us with their imaging data.

I am thankful to my most supportive and dedicated secretary, Iris Bellamy, for her effort in arranging all the text and illustration material.

Last but not least, I would like to express my gratitude to my wife Charlotte, especially for her patience, support, and encouragement. And to our wonderful children, Max, Laura, and Emily, who are the source of my daily inspiration. They remind me that the goal of our professional work with children is to strive for the betterment of our common future.

I hope that studying this case collection will be as enjoyable for readers as its preparation was for its authors.

Thierry A.G.M. Huisman
May 2010

Opening Round

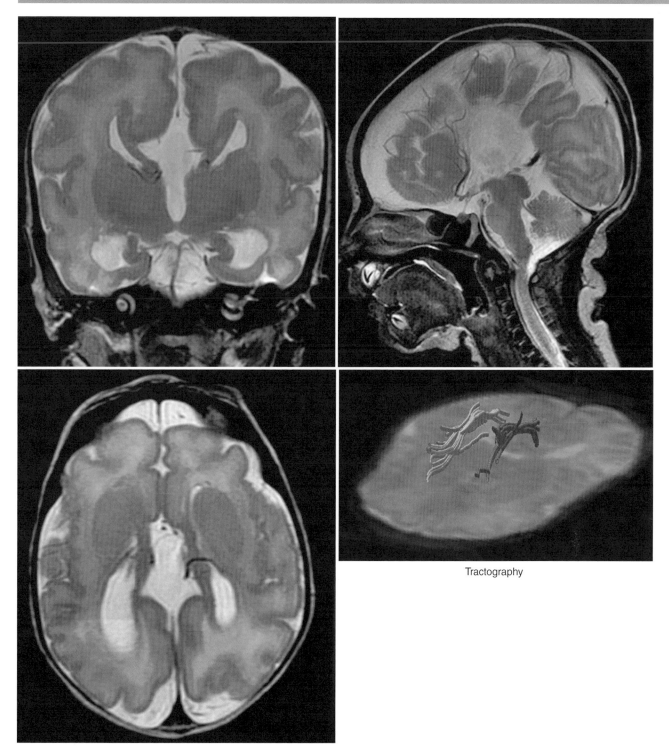

Tractography

1. Summarize all imaging findings seen on this neonatal magnetic resonance image (MRI).

2. What is your diagnosis?

3. In which order does the corpus callosum (CC) develop?

4. In which malformation is the posterior CC developed without an anterior part?

Diagnosis: Corpus Callosum Agenesis

1. Complete lack of the CC, radiating appearance of the medial brain sulci, no inversion of the cingulate gyrus, trident shape of the ventricles on coronal imaging, malrotated hippocampi, high-riding third ventricle, prominent adhesion interthalamica, colpocephaly, parallel course of the lateral ventricles on axial images, Probst bundle (tractography) that runs in the anteroposterior (AP) direction without left-right crossing, mild ventriculomegaly.

2. Complete agenesis of the CC.

3. Genu, truncus, splenium, and rostrum.

4. Lobar and semilobar holoprosencephaly.

Reference

Hetts SW, et al: Anomalies of the corpus callosum: an MR analysis of the phenotypic spectrum of associated malformations, *AJR Am J Roentgenol* 187:1343–1348, 2006.

Cross-Reference

Blickman JG, Parker BR, Barnes PD: *Pediatric radiology—the requisites*, ed 3, Philadelphia, 2009, Mosby, p 222.

Comment

The CC is the largest commissure (bundle of white matter tracts) connecting both cerebral hemispheres. Additional hemispheric connections are the anterior commissure and the hippocampal commissure. The CC has a complex, programmed anterior-to-posterior development starting with the genu and followed by the truncus and splenium. The rostrum of the CC is the final segment to develop. Agenesis of the CC is observed on imaging with multiple, characteristic anatomic sequelae. Most of the classical sequelae are demonstrated in this case. The lack of the CC is usually evident in the midline, sagittal slice. In addition, the sulci along the medial surface of both cerebral hemispheres show a typical radiating appearance converging to the third ventricle. The third ventricle may be enlarged and extend interhemispherically. In rare cases the third ventricle may reach the vertex, or an associated interhemispheric cyst may be revealed. On axial imaging the lateral ventricles reveal a parallel course because the CC is lacking. In addition, frequently the occipital horns of the ventricles are enlarged (colpocephaly). The fibers that cannot cross the midline usually realign along the medial contour of the lateral ventricles and run in an anterior-to-posterior direction. These fibers are known as Probst bundles and can easily be recognized on tractography reconstructions using diffusion tensor imaging data. On coronal imaging the combination of the separated lateral ventricles, the medial impression of these ventricles by the Probst bundles, and the shape of the adjacent third ventricle mimic a trident or Texas longhorn cow. Because the CC is one part of the commissures connecting both hemispheres, the remainder of the commissures should be studied for additional malformations. The hippocampi may be malrotated; the anterior commissure may be lacking. In 50% of children a CC agenesis is part of a more extensive malformation (e.g., Dandy-Walker malformation, Arnold-Chiari II malformation, septooptic dysplasia). In addition, migrational abnormalities are frequently encountered. Ruling out additional malformations is essential; doing so will determine a functional and cognitive prognosis. Clinically, an isolated CC agenesis may be an incidental finding on an MRI. If additional malformations are present, then seizures, a developmental delay, and a hypothalamic-pituitary dysfunction may result. CC agenesis should be differentiated from secondary injury of the CC. For example, a severe atrophy of the CC resulting from an extensive periventricular leukomalacia should not be confused with a primary CC agenesis. In addition, it is important to remember that the only exception to the anterior-to-posterior rule of development is a semilobar or lobar holoprosencephaly. In these malformations the posterior CC may be present without the genu or anterior trunk of the CC.

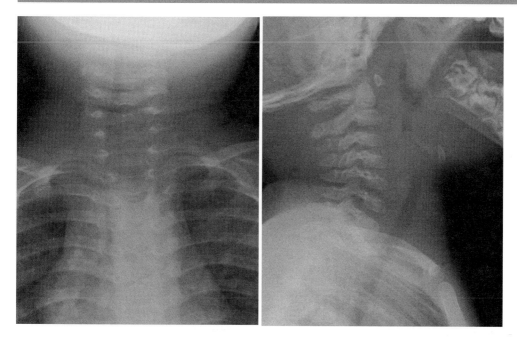

1. What are the imaging findings in this 13-month-old child with a "barking" cough?

2. If you watched this child breathe under fluoroscopy, what would you notice?

3. What other things would the fluoroscopy help you to exclude if the plain films were not conclusive?

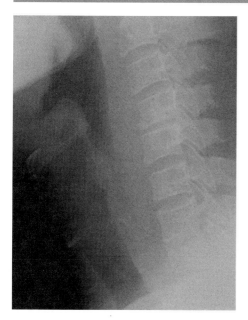

1. What are the findings in this young adult?

2. How will the patient present?

3. What age group is most likely to be affected?

4. Are there any special considerations in the imaging of this kind of patient?

CASE 2

Diagnosis: Croup

1. Subglottic narrowing, normal epiglottis, and aryepiglottic folds.

2. Pharynx overdistends on inspiration; subglottic narrowing more obvious on expiration (as normal lower trachea distends against the obstruction); narrowed segment appears rigid.

3. Congenital subglottic stenosis or subglottic hemangioma (narrowing might be more rigid or asymmetric); airway or esophageal foreign body (subtle radiodensity or tracheal shift may be evident on an oblique or magnified view); false-positive plain films (forceful inspiration can cause subglottic collapse; observation of respiratory cycles shows normal tracheal wall mobility).

Reference

Kuhn JP, Slovis TL, Haller JO: *Caffey's pediatric diagnostic imaging*, ed 10, Philadelphia, 2004, Mosby, p 814.

Cross-Reference

Blickman JG, Parker BR, Barnes PD: *Pediatric radiology—the requisites*, ed 3, Philadelphia, 2009, Mosby.

Comment

Symptoms connected with viral laryngotracheobronchitis peak in the 3-month to 3-year age range. Usually intercurrent upper respiratory infection exists. Since the advent of vaccines against *Haemophilus influenzae*, epiglottitis has ceased to be the main clinical masquerader. Pulmonary edema is a rare acute complication.

CASE 3

Diagnosis: Epiglottitis

1. The epiglottis is enlarged; the swelling extends to the aryepiglottic folds. The vallecular airspace is not seen because of the extensive pharyngeal swelling.

2. Usually high fever, drooling, dysphasia, and respiratory distress.

3. Between 3 and 6 years old.

4. If epiglottitis is present, a possibility exists that the patient will need urgent intubation or tracheostomy. A radiograph should be obtained (ideally by personnel nearby who can do so portably in the patient care area).

Reference

Kuhn JP, Slovis TL, Haller JO: *Caffey's pediatric diagnostic imaging*, ed 10, Philadelphia, 2004, Mosby, p 811.

Cross-Reference

Blickman JG, Parker BR, Barnes PD: *Pediatric radiology—the requisites*, ed 3, Philadelphia, 2009, Mosby, pp 10-12.

Comment

Common infectious causes of upper respiratory symptoms in childhood include epiglottitis, croup and/or tracheitis, and retropharyngeal abscess. Epiglottitis is usually caused by *Haemophilus influenzae* type B (HIB), which is much less common now that immunization against HIB is routine. Differentiation from the other causes of upper respiratory infection in part is determined by the clinical setting. Croup is often seen in a younger patient, 6 months to 3 years old; it is a viral illness and fever is usually not as high as in epiglottitis. Tracheitis is less common and has more extensive involvement of the trachea compared with croup. It is usually of bacterial origin and is seen in the same age group as croup. Retropharyngeal abscess may be a complication of bacterial tonsillitis, and clinical findings of tonsillar infection may be present. This illness can be seen in infants younger than 6 months old.

If imaging is needed, anteroposterior (AP) and lateral views of the neck are necessary. The AP view is most important in the identification of the subglottic narrowing seen in croup. If findings point toward retropharyngeal abscess, contrast-enhanced computerized tomography is usually performed.

In 25% of patients with epiglottitis, subglottic narrowing consistent with edema is also present. Causes of epiglottic enlargement other than infection are angioneurotic edema, aryepiglottic or epiglottic cyst, hemophilia (hemorrhage), and thermal injury sometimes seen in child abuse.

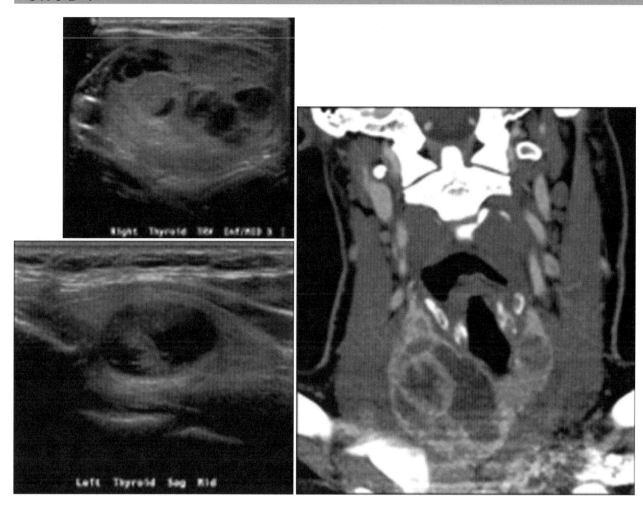

1. What are the findings in this teenage boy?

2. How would the patient likely present?

3. What would be the reason or reasons to intervene?

4. What additional imaging test may be useful?

Diagnosis: Goiter

1. Masses in the enlarged thyroid, many of which appear cystic; right lobe much larger than the left.

2. Neck swelling; thyroid function variable.

3. If patient has symptoms of impingement on adjacent structures (in this case, trachea is significantly deviated to the left).

4. I-123 nuclear scan.

Reference

Hegedus L, Bonnema SJ, Bennedbaek FN: Management of simple nodular goiter: current status and future perspectives, *Endocr Rev* 24(1):102, 2003.

Cross-Reference

Blickman JG, Parker BR, Barnes PD: *Pediatric radiology—the requisites*, ed 3, Philadelphia, 2009, Mosby, pp 8 and 324.

Comment

A *goiter* is a clinically recognizable enlargement of the thyroid gland that is often nodular. Goiters are endemic in areas of the world with iodine-deficient diets but also occur sporadically. Both endemic and sporadic goiters develop because of genetic predisposition and environmental factors such as iodine intake and cigarette smoking.

Most patients with nodular goiter are euthyroid, but they may become hyperthyroid or, less commonly, hypothyroid. This dysfunction occurs after the goiter has been present for many years. Clinically unapparent hyperthyroidism with low serum thyroid-stimulating hormone (TSH) and normal T_4 and T_3 is often present. As the TSH decreases, the size and nodularity of the gland may increase.

Ultrasound evaluation of the enlarged thyroid allows the detection and characterization of nodules, as well as guidance for fine needle aspiration and cytologic evaluation. Widespread use of this modality is due to its ready availability, low cost, minimal discomfort to the patient, and nonionizing nature. Cystic lesions are usually benign. When solid in appearance, lesions that are hypoechogenic have microcalcification and increased vascular flow; they are more likely to be malignant. Fine needle aspiration is the most direct technique to determine the makeup of a nodule and is widely used. I-123 nuclear studies are less sensitive to small nodules but in larger nodules can differentiate cold versus hot nodules (i.e., those that are not functioning versus those that have radioisotope uptake). Those nodules that function are highly unlikely to be malignant. In practice, this examination is not widely used in the setting of goiter evaluation. Computerized tomography and magnetic resonance image examinations offer reliable volume measurement and show the goiter extent, as well as its effect on adjacent structures.

In the absence of a malignant component and with normal thyroid function, the determination to treat a patient with goiter is mostly based on the symptoms from its mass effect and the cosmetic concerns. Total surgical thyroidectomy is the most common treatment. Ablation of the gland with iodine (I-131) therapy and L-thyroxine (L-T_4) administration are other options.

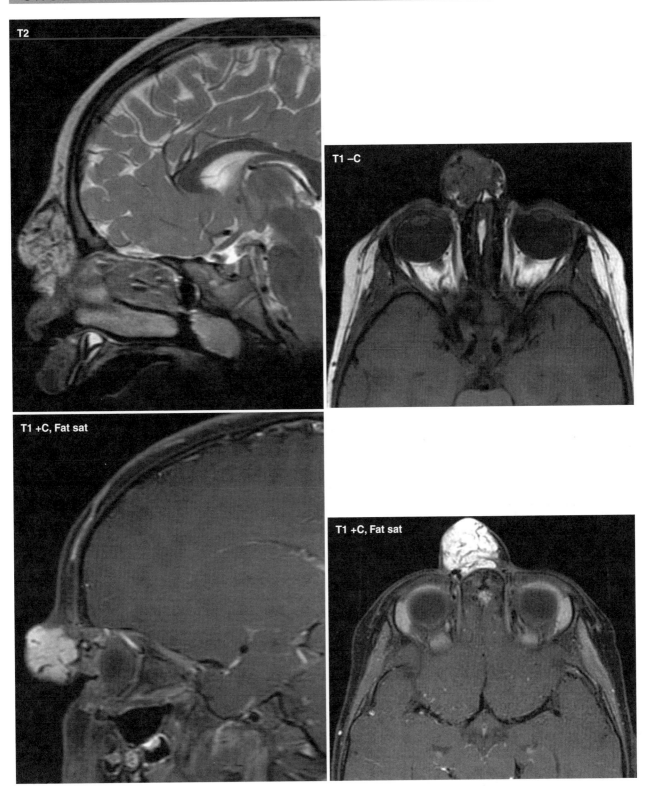

1. What are the imaging findings in this 1-year-old girl?

2. What is your diagnosis?

3. What is the differential diagnosis?

4. Are there any malformative anomalies associated with this entity?

C A S E 5

Diagnosis: Nasal Hemangioma

1. The image shows a well-circumscribed lobular mass, with increased T_2 signal and avid contrast enhancement noted in the subcutaneous fat of the nasal bridge. There are vascular flow voids within the mass seen best on T_2-weighted image. No evidence of intracranial extension exists.

2. The patient has nasal hemangioma.

3. In general, vascular malformations such as venous malformations, lymphatic malformations, and arteriovenous malformation (AVM) can be considered. Differential diagnosis would be affected by the location as well. In this case encephalocele, nasal dermoid, and nasal glioma could also be considered, but the previously defined imaging features lead to a correct diagnosis.

4. Yes, the malformative anomalies include PHACES syndrome (posterior fossa malformations, hemangiomas, arterial abnormalities, coarctation of the aorta, and eye abnormalities); Dandy-Walker malformation; spine anomalies if located in the lumbar region; and Kasabach-Merritt syndrome.

Reference

Mulliken JB, Glowacki J: Hemangiomas and vascular malformations in infants and children: a classification based on endothelial characteristics, *Plast Reconstr Surg* 69(3):412–422, 1982.

Cross-Reference

Blickman JG, Parker BR, Barnes PD: *Pediatric radiology—the requisites*, ed 3, Philadelphia, 2009, Mosby Elsevier, pp 314–316.

Comment

Hemangiomas are the most common tumors in infancy and childhood and account for 7% of benign soft tissue tumors. Hemangiomas are tumors that express a localized increase in angiogenic growth factors. Mulliken and Glowacki first described the classification of vascular anomalies based on clinical, histologic, and cytologic features. Vascular anomalies are divided into two major groups: (1) vascular tumors (hemangiomas), and (2) vascular malformations including venous malformations, lymphatic malformations, AVMs, and arteriovenous fistulas. The correct classification is important because treatment options differ significantly between the two groups. Hemangiomas have cellular proliferation of endothelial cells, and they are true neoplasms. Hemangiomas have subgroups consisting of infantile, congenital, noninvoluting, intramuscular, and kaposiform hemangioendothelioma types. The most common type is infantile hemangioma. Hemangiomas test positive for immunological markers such as glut1, FcrII, merosin, and Lewis Y antigen. A 3:1 female-to-male ratio exists.

Hemangiomas usually appear in the first week of life and can be located in the head and neck (60%), the trunk (25%), and the extremities. The patient displays a typical history of rapid neonatal growth (3 to 9 months) and slow involution characterized by hypercellularity during the proliferating phase, as well as fibrosis and diminished cellularity during the involuting phase (18 months to 10 years). This typical clinical history is oftentimes diagnostic; however, certain cases would require imaging confirmation.

Imaging findings would obviously depend on the phase of the hemangioma. In the rapid-growth phase, ultrasound would reveal a variable echogenicity mass with increased flow on color-coded Doppler sonography. Involuting hemangiomas are heterogeneous masses with less intense color flow and fibrofatty changes. A magnetic resonance image (MRI) is advised with T_1, T_2, and postcontrast T_1-weighted images. Fat suppression is of additional value in identifying this lesion. On MRI, typically a parenchymal, well-circumscribed mass with intermediate signal intensity on T_1 and increased signal intensity on T_2-weighted images is visualized. Avid contrast uptake is also noted, and the presence of flow voids within and around the soft tissue mass is an important feature.

In the majority of cases, no treatment is required because of spontaneous involution. Indications for treatment in the remainder of the cases are primarily functional, such as obscuration of vision or breathing or persistent cutaneous ulceration, high cardiac output failure. Systemic or intralesional steroid agents can be used for treatment. Promising results with systemic propranolol admission has been reported.

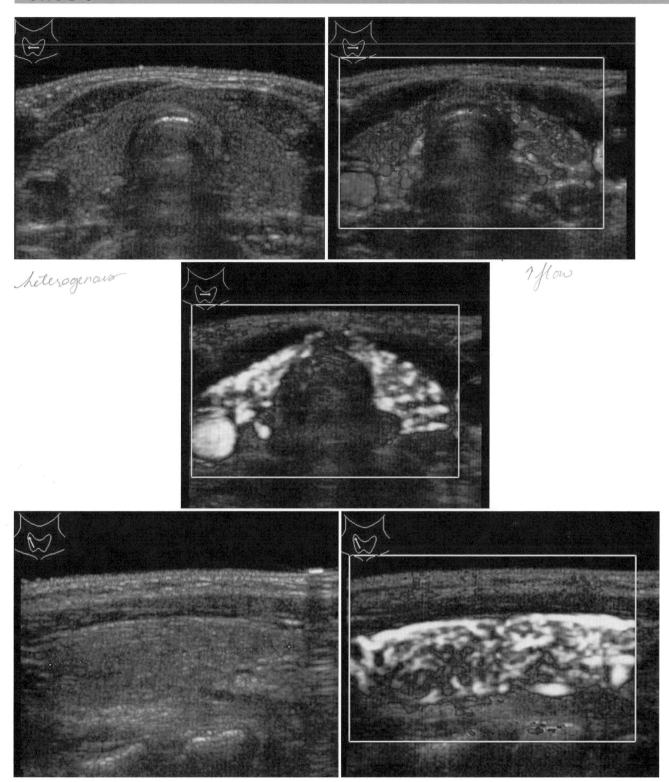

heterogenous

↑ flow

1. What are the imaging findings on the ultrasound examination?

2. What is the most likely diagnosis in this 14-year-old girl?

3. What is the next test that should be performed?

4. Which long-term complication develops frequently?

Diagnosis: Hashimoto Thyroiditis

1. Diffusely heterogeneous, hyperperfused thyroid gland

2. Hashimoto thyroiditis

3. Blood workup with determination of thyroid hormones and thyroid antibodies

4. Hypothyroidism

Reference

Lorini R, Gastaldi R, Traggiai C, et al: Hashimoto's thyroiditis, *Pediatr Endocrinol Rev* 1(Suppl 2):205, 2003.

Cross-Reference

Blickman JG, Parker BR, Barnes PD: *Pediatric radiology—the requisites*, ed 3, Philadelphia, 2009, Mosby, p 324.

Comment

Hashimoto thyroiditis, also known as autoimmune thyroiditis or chronic lymphocytic thyroiditis, is the most common acquired disorder of the thyroid gland in children and the most common cause of hypothyroidism in the United States. Dr. Hakaru Hashimoto first described this disorder in 1912. Hashimoto thyroiditis is an autoimmune disease of unknown cause and may finally destroy the thyroid gland with resultant hypothyroidism. Incidence is estimated to be 1.3%. Blood tests are mandatory to determine the thyroid function by detecting the levels of thyroid hormones in general and to identify antithyroid peroxidase antibodies or antithyroglobulin antibodies in particular. Currently no cure exists for Hashimoto thyroiditis; however, the hypothyroidism can be treated effectively by substituting the deficient thyroid hormones. Symptoms are usually related to the progressive drop in thyroid hormones and not specific for Hashimoto thyroiditis. Hashimoto thyroiditis is more frequent in females and increases in frequency over age during childhood and adolescence.

Ultrasound examination is the primary imaging modality of choice. On ultrasound, the thyroid gland is usually diffusely enlarged, hypoechoic, and reveals significant hyperperfusion on color-coded Doppler sonography and power Doppler sonography, especially in the acute phase. Micronodulation characterized by multiple, small hypoechoic micronodules ranging between 1 and 6 mm in diameter are considered to be indicative of Hashimoto thyroiditis. Occasionally, discrete focal nodules are identified and fine needle aspiration cytology is necessary to confirm diagnosis. Hashimoto thyroiditis appears to occur more frequently in diabetic patients. Ultrasonography is also helpful to rule out additional lesions. Scintigraphy is rarely necessary to confirm diagnosis.

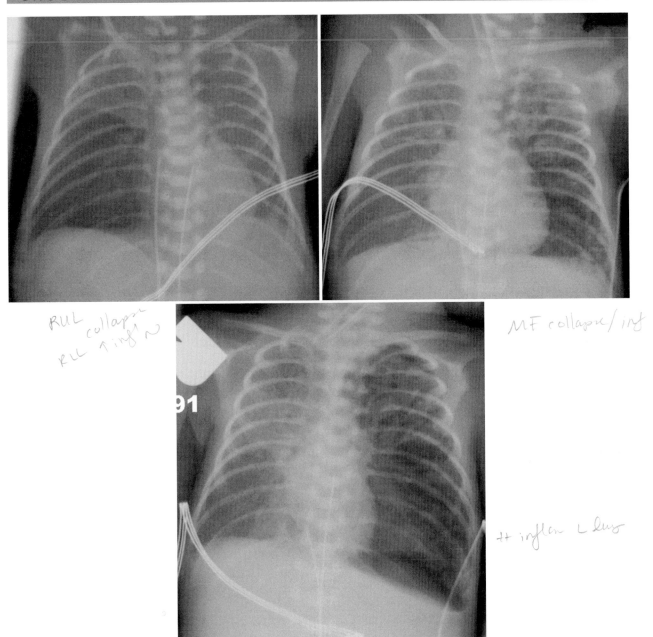

RUL collapse
RLL ↑ inf'n

MF collapse/inf

++ inflam L lung

91

1. This patient had these three sequential films (first, second, and third figures) within a 24-hour period. What patient group accounts for the largest proportion of these cases?

2. What plain film finding may precede the development of this abnormality?

3. What complications do you look for? pneumo thorax/mediastinum

4. What lung pathologic conditions promote this abnormality?

Diagnosis: Pulmonary Interstitial Emphysema

1. Premature infants (however, it can happen in any patient in whom airway pressures exceed the integrity of the airway epithelium).

2. Hyperinflation with endotracheal tube in place.

3. Pneumatoceles, pneumothorax, pneumomediastinum, pneumoperitoneum.

4. Surfactant deficiency, neonatal pneumonia, meconium aspiration, persistent pulmonary hypertension.

Reference

Kuhn JP, Slovis TL, Haller JO: *Caffey's pediatric diagnostic imaging*, ed 10, Philadelphia, 2004, Mosby, p 814.

Cross-Reference

Blickman JG, Parker BR, Barnes PD: *Pediatric radiology—the requisites*, ed 3, Philadelphia, 2009, Mosby, pp 28–29.

Comment

The lungs of a premature infant are stiff and noncompliant. This is due to lack of surfactant, normally produced by type II alveolar cells, beginning in week 24 of gestation and usually complete by week 32. Without this protein, alveolar distension and adequate oxygenation must be maintained by high-pressure ventilation with oxygen-rich air. This combination injures the already fragile alveolar walls and allows air to leak between the lining cells into the interstitial spaces and lymphatics. The air is first visible lying parallel to the bronchi, forming characteristic lucent lines and dots. Movement of the lungs with respiration causes the air to change configuration. It can dissect centrally or peripherally, causing pneumomediastinum and pneumothorax, or it can become centrally confluent, creating a pneumatocele. Air in the mediastinum can dissect downward through the inferior pulmonary ligaments and result in sterile pneumoperitoneum.

Aggressive treatment with exogenous surfactant in the delivery room can decrease the severity of the lung disease and avert this complication. Once present, it is treated by decreasing ventilatory pressures. Jet ventilation allows greater control of airway pressures. If unilateral, decubitus positioning onto the affected lung can effectively decrease pressure locally and hasten healing. Pneumatoceles occasionally must be surgically removed if they become intractably large.

Chest radiographs, which are a valuable monitor for this disease, can alert clinicians to dangerous levels of hyperinflation that could precipitate air leaks, enabling diagnosis of the emphysema and its complications and determining efficacy of therapeutic measures.

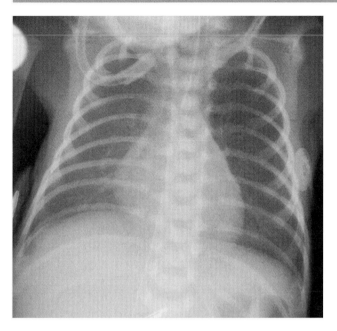

1. What are the findings in this neonate's radiograph?

2. Before what gestational age do you expect to find this entity?

3. Under what conditions might you find it outside the usual age group?

4. What condition can mimic this entity and has very different treatment?

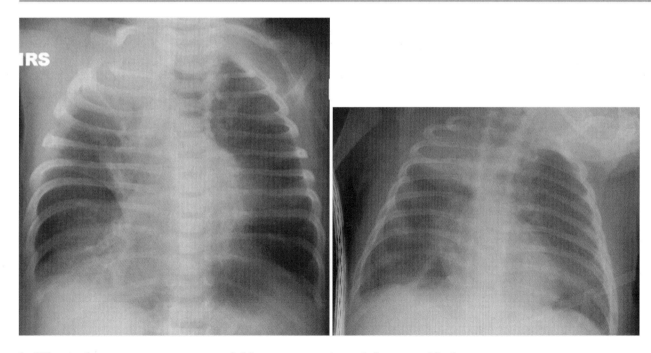

1. What is the most common cause of this appearance in an infant or toddler?

2. What organism (or organisms) commonly causes this illness?

3. In older children, this appearance is more likely from what?

4. What is the normal lung volume in a quiet infant?

CASE 8

Diagnosis: Surfactant Deficiency Disease

1. Moderate lung inflation better on the left, hazy granularity more evident on the right, normal heart size.

2. 32 weeks.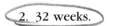

3. Seen more often in male patients (2:1). (The presence of maternal diabetes, maternal or fetal hemorrhage, sepsis, and multiple gestations further increases the likelihood of developing this condition.)

4. Group B streptococcal pneumonia.

References

Kuhn JP, Slovis TL, Haller JO: *Caffey's pediatric diagnostic imaging*, ed 10, Philadelphia, 2004, Mosby, pp 77-79.

Donoghue V: *Radiologic imaging of the neonatal chest*, ed 2, Berlin-Heidelberg-New York, 2008, Springer, pp 67-72.

Cross-Reference

Blickman JG, Parker BR, Barnes PD: *Pediatric radiology—the requisites*, ed 3, Philadelphia, 2009, Mosby, pp 26-30.

Comment

Surfactant is manufactured by type II alveolar cells, beginning around week 24 of gestation and peaking at about week 32. This compound lowers the surface tension of alveolar epithelium and prevents alveolar collapse. In its absence, the infant's lungs fail to aerate and appear uniformly white on radiography. The standard delivery room treatment is intubation and tracheally administered synthetic surfactant, which is then distributed throughout the lungs by hand bagging. If distribution is uniform, the lungs inflate and the radiographic appearance changes to one of diffuse granularity, which may look very fine, almost hazy in infants less severely affected, or more dense and coarse. Nonuniform distribution (e.g., if intubation was too deep and bypassed a lobe or an entire lung) would give a more uneven picture of hyperinflated areas and persistently dense areas. Additional doses of surfactant may be given over the first few days of life but with caution (because this can promote pulmonary hemorrhage). The surfactant is given in the hope that by the time it breaks down (in 24 to 72 hours), the infant will be producing sufficient endogenous surfactant to keep the alveoli open.

CASE 9

Diagnosis: Bronchiolitis

1. Bronchiolitis.

2. Respiratory syncytial virus and, much less commonly, adenoviruses. RSV

3. Reactive airway disease.

4. Tidal volume is the maximum volume during a normal inspiration. An infant, of course, cannot cooperate for a film taken in deep inspiration. Therefore the films of a normal infant breathing quietly will often appear to be of small volume.

Reference

Schuh S, Lalani A, Allen U, et al: Evaluation of the utility of radiography in acute bronchiolitis, *J Pediatr* 150 (4):429-433, 2007.

Cross-Reference

Blickman JG, Parker BR, Barnes PD: *Pediatric radiology—the requisites*, ed 3, Philadelphia, 2009, Mosby, pp 32-36.

Comments

Bronchiolitis is a viral respiratory illness that affects the smaller airways of infants and toddlers. It results in fever, congestion, wheezing, and diffuse lower respiratory tract signs. The disease is self-limited and usually managed on an outpatient basis.

Chest radiographs, as in this example, usually show hyperinflation and areas of atelectasis. During the illness, the location of atelectasis often changes rapidly. These findings are manifestations of the inflammatory changes in the small airways. The airways are quite flexible in this age group and can collapse partially or completely during expiration, resulting in air trapping and hyperinflation and/or atelectasis.

Similar radiographic findings are seen in reactive airway disease. In general, bronchiolitis is seen in the infant, and reactive airway disease is observed in the older child; however, an overlap occurs in their incidences.

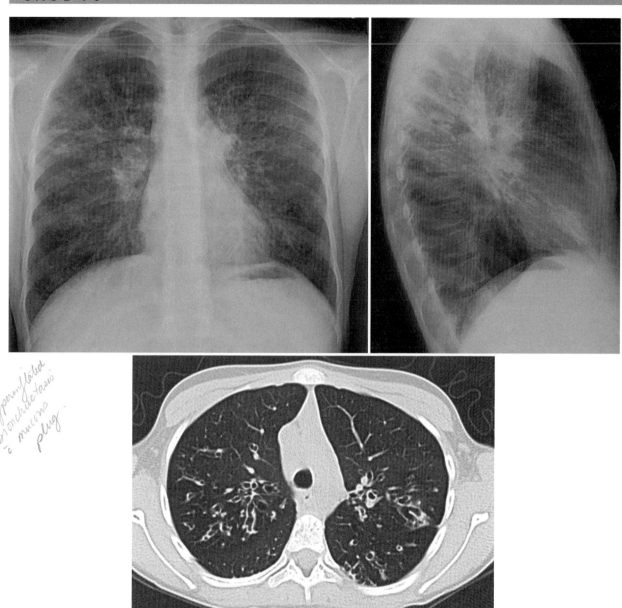

(handwritten annotation at left of CT image:) hyperinflated. Bronchiectasis ē mucous plug.

1. This example is an Aunt Minnie. What is the disease process in this 11-year-old girl?

2. What are some nonpulmonary manifestations of this disease? *pan. insufficiency, malabsorption, sterility*

3. What laboratory test is used to make the diagnosis? *Cl sweat test.*

4. What is the prognosis of this disease?

CASE 10

Diagnosis: Cystic Fibrosis

1. Cystic fibrosis (CF).

2. Pancreatic insufficiency, malabsorption, failure to thrive, liver cirrhosis, infertility in males.

3. A sweat chloride test.

4. Mild examples of the disease exist; however, the median age of survival is 36.8 years. Most patients die from respiratory failure.

Reference

Rowe SM, Miller S, Sorscher EJ: Cystic fibrosis, *N Engl J Med* 352(19):1992-2001, 2005.

Cross-Reference

Blickman JG, Parker BR, Barnes PD: *Pediatric radiology—the requisites*, ed 3, Philadelphia, 2009, Mosby, pp 36-37.

Comments

CF is an inherited, autosomal recessive disorder of exocrine gland function. The most common manifestations of CF are chronic respiratory infection and pancreatic enzyme insufficiency. CF is caused by defects in the gene for cystic fibrosis transmembrane conductance regulator (CFTR), which results in decreased secretions of chloride, increased reabsorption of sodium and water across epithelial cells, and ultimately to abnormal sticky mucous production. This viscous mucous is less effective in clearing secretions and results in a lung environment conducive to infection, as well as the other manifestations of this disease. CF is diagnosed by an abnormal sweat chloride test. The sweat is analyzed for its chloride content—the chloride will be high in CF. Specific gene typing is useful in further characterizing the disease, because more than 1400 types of mutations have been found in the CFTR gene.

The radiographs shown here reveal the typical findings of hyperinflation, diffuse interstitial thickening, tram tracking of bronchiectasis, and mucous plugging. Although diffuse disease is usual, focal infiltrates and/or focal areas of more severe disease are common. As in this case, hilar enlargement because of lymphadenopathy (a manifestation of chronic infection) often is seen. Computed tomography (CT) examination generally shows more involvement than evident on chest radiographs. CT findings include, but are not limited to, peribronchial thickening, centrilobular opacity, bronchiectasis, mucous plugging, hilar adenopathy, bullae formation, and lung abscess.

The radiographic findings are nearly pathognomic for CF; hence the use of the term *Aunt Minnie* in this case. Rarely, other causes of chronic inflammatory disease may resemble CR; these include asthma and immunodeficiency syndromes.

Hemoptysis is common in advanced cases, and arteriography and direct embolization of the bronchial arteries may be necessary to treat it.

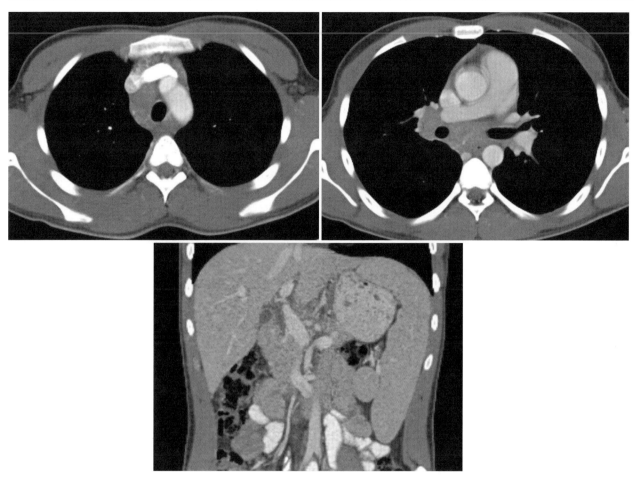

1. What are the findings in this teenage boy? ↑ Nodes

2. What is the differential diagnosis? lymphoma, sarcoid, TB

3. What is the classification system for Hodgkin disease? Ann Arbor.

4. Is 18F-fluorodeoxyglucose (18F-FDG)-positron emission tomography (PET) computed tomography (CT) imaging useful in lymphoma?

Diagnosis: Hodgkin Lymphoma

1. Lymphadenopathy in the mediastinum and the right hilum; splenomegaly with large hilar splenule; subsequent PET-CT showed uptake in multiple lymph node areas and in the bone.

2. Lymphoma, tuberculosis or other granulomatous infectious process, Langerhans histiocytosis, or metastatic disease.

3. Stage I: One lymph node region involved (e.g., the right neck or right axilla or mediastinum).
   Stage II: Involvement of two lymph nodes on same side of diaphragm (e.g., both sides of neck).
   Stage III: Lymph node involvement on both sides of diaphragm (e.g., groin and armpit).
   Stage IV: Involves the spread of cancer outside the lymph nodes (e.g., to bone marrow, lungs, liver).

4. PET scans may show more disease than recognized on CT alone and may allow distinction between residual fibrotic mass versus mass with viable tumor after treatment.

Reference
Olson MR, Donaldson SS: Treatment of pediatric Hodgkin lymphoma, *Curr Treat Options Oncol* 9:81–94, 2008.

Cross-Reference
Blickman JG, Parker BR, Barnes PD: *Pediatric radiology—the requisites*, ed 3, Philadelphia, 2009, Mosby, pp 41-43.

Comments
This 16-year-old boy, whose images are shown in this case, presented with a several-month history of fever, night sweats, fatigue, bone pain, and weight loss. He was found to have pancytopenia. Lymph node biopsy showed classical Hodgkin lymphoma, and he was staged as IV B because of apparent bone marrow involvement seen on PET scanning (bone scan and bone radiographs were negative).

Hodgkin disease is a common hematological malignancy that has two peaks of incidence: (1) between 15 and 35 years and (2) older than 55 years. The commonly used staging system (cited previously) is the Ann Arbor Staging System. In addition to the areas of involvement, bulky mediastinal disease involving more than one third of the intrathoracic diameter is also taken into consideration. Varying definitions of low, intermediate, and high-risk groups include all of these factors, as well as the histology.

The World Health Organization classification separates Hodgkin lymphoma into two groups: (1) classical (which includes lymphocyte-depleted, nodular-sclerosing, mixed cellularity, and classical lymphocyte-rich cell types) and (2) the lymphocyte-predominant type. Ninety percent of Hodgkin lymphoma is of the classical type, with Reed-Sternberg cells, and positive for CD15 and CD30 (*CD* stands for *cluster of differentiation* and is a protocol used to identify and investigate the cell surface molecules present on leukocytes). Immunohistological differences are seen between the subgroups of classical Hodgkin lymphoma, but the response to treatment is similar. Lymphocyte-predominant Hodgkin lymphoma expresses markers not usually seen in the classical type; those are B cell markers (CD20, CD79a, CD75) and epithelial membrane antigen and lymphocyte marker (CD45). This type of Hodgkin disease has a more indolent course and good prognosis with treatment, but the patient has a slightly higher risk of developing non-Hodgkin lymphoma.

Ann Arbor

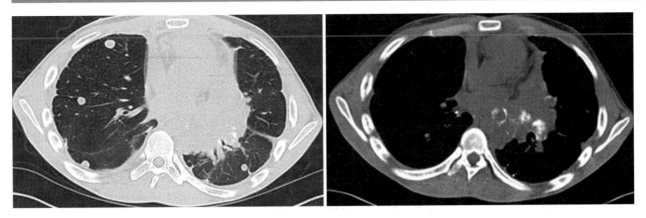

1. What are the findings in this teenage boy?

2. What is the differential?   TB   Metx   Tx Lymphoma

3. Does the calcification narrow the differential?

4. Is local therapy effective in this process?

Diagnosis: Pulmonary Nodules Due to Osteosarcoma

1. Multiple variable-sized discrete nodules appear in the lungs. A large mass on the left appears to invade the mediastinum, and it contains calcification.

2. Metastatic disease most likely; fungal infection, other multifocal infection, septic emboli, Wegener granulomatosis, and Langerhans histiocytosis much less likely.

3. Yes, it makes calcium-producing neoplasm such as osteosarcoma more likely.

4. After initial chemotherapy, resection of multiple lung metastatic lesions in a patient with osteosarcoma is effective and results in longer disease-free survival.

Reference

Antunes M, Benardo J, Salete M, et al: Excision of pulmonary metastases of osteogenic sarcoma of the limbs, *Eur J Cardiothorac Surg* 15(5):592–596, 1999.

Cross-Reference

Blickman JG, Parker BR, Barnes PD: *Pediatric radiology—the requisites*, ed 3, Philadelphia, 2009, Mosby, pp 37–38.

Comment

Nodular lung disease consists of multiple round opacities that can range from 1 mm to 1 cm or larger. The smaller lesions are only visible on computed tomography examination and are referred to as miliary. Further characterization of the nodules includes a description of their margins (smooth or irregular), presence or absence of cavitation, calcification, and their distribution. Multiple lesions of different sizes, especially in subpleural or peripheral locations, suggest metastatic disease. Multiple small smooth or irregularly marginated nodules in a perilymphatic distribution suggest sarcoidosis. Silicosis and coal workers' pneumoconiosis may also have this appearance. Upper lobe predominance is seen in coal workers' pneumoconiosis. Small nodules of ground-glass opacity can be seen in extrinsic allergic alveolitis or bronchiolitis. Miliary or larger nodules are seen in the hematogenous spread of tuberculosis, fungal infection, or metastatic disease. If the lesions include some with thin-walled cavities, Langerhans cell histiocytosis should be considered. Other lesions that cavitate include metastatic squamous cell carcinoma, Wegener granulomatosis, rheumatoid lung disease, septic emboli, and multifocal infection. Lymphoproliferative disorders, lymphoma, leukemia, and Kaposi sarcoma may cause irregular nodules in a bronchovascular distribution. Calcification can be seen in granulomatous disease, hamartomas, metastatic tumor such as osteosarcoma, rarely as a consequence of infection and in abnormal calcium metabolism, with so-called metastatic pulmonary calcifications.

The patient in this example had osteosarcoma of the proximal femur with lung metastases at presentation 5 years earlier. By the time of these images, the patient had multiple tiny lesions (>100 total) resected from each lung. Chemotherapy is the initial treatment of nonmetastatic and metastatic osteosarcoma. Surgical resection of the primary lesion generally follows chemotherapy. Experimental administration of the bone-seeking radioisotope samarium (if the lesions are calcified and avid on nuclear bone scan) has recently been used to treat metastatic disease in osteosarcoma. The outcome in patients with lung metastases from osteosarcoma is improved by the combination of chemotherapy and surgery. A strong correlation exists between the degree of necrosis of the aggregate metastatic disease and the need for reoperation. In one study, those that needed reoperation had less than 80% necrosis of metastases.

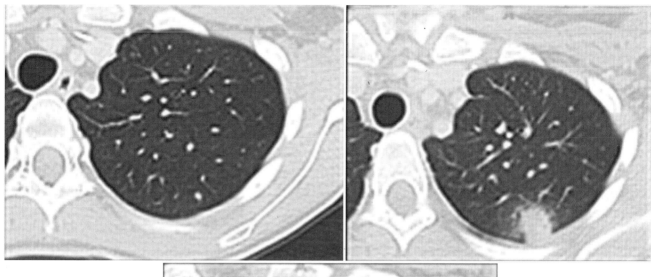

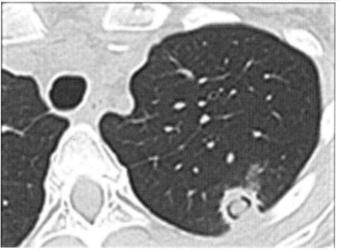

1. These three computerized tomography (CT) images represent the progression of a disease process in a teenager being treated for leukemia. What do they show?

2. What is the differential diagnosis?

3. What is the name of the finding seen on the last CT image?

4. In what sort of patient is this likely to occur?

Diagnosis: Fungal Disease Lungs

1. A small nodule progresses to a larger nodule with a hazy border; then cavitation is seen with a central soft tissue component.

2. Fungal mycetoma, abscess, metastatic disease, septic embolus, hematoma, and hydatid disease.

3. Air crescent sign.

4. This process is often seen in an immunocompromised patient.

Reference

Demirkazik FB, Akin A, Uzun O, et al: CT findings in immunocompromised patients with pulmonary infections, *Diagn Interv Radiol* 14:75–82, 2008.

Cross-Reference

Blickman JG, Parker BR, Barnes PD: *Pediatric radiology—the requisites*, ed 3, Philadelphia, 2009, Mosby, p 34.

Comment

CT of the lung is used to detect infection in the immunocompromised patient. It is considerably more sensitive to early infection than chest radiography. In patients with febrile neutropenia, it is reported that a CT will find 20% more pneumonias 5 days earlier than the chest radiograph. In addition to increasing the detection rate, a careful analysis of the CT features can help to determine the likely cause of the infection.

The patient in this example had invasive aspergillosis. The typical findings include single or multiple nodules, often with surrounding ground-glass opacity, the so-called halo sign. A lesion may cavitate and contain a solid nodule within it. This is called the air crescent sign. These features were all present in the patient.

The halo sign is seen in about half of patients with invasive aspergillosis and is caused by hemorrhage and necrosis around the necrotic nodule, which contains the fungal hyphae. This sign can also be seen in some bronchopneumonia, as well as tumors such as adenocarcinoma, alveolar cell carcinoma, Kaposi sarcoma, and metastasis. About 40% of nodules seen in fungal pneumonia are cavitary, and one half of them demonstrate the air crescent sign. This finding is not specific for invasive *Aspergillus* spp.; however, in the proper setting, it is highly suggestive for fungal disease (clinicians believe it to be caused by retracted and infarcted lung tissue within the cavity).

Although nodular disease is the most frequent manifestation of *Aspergillus* spp. infection on CT, ground-glass opacity and consolidation can also be seen.

Other fungal infections are less common; increasingly pulmonary candidiasis is the cause of fever in the immunocompromised patient and its appearance is similar to *Aspergillus* spp.

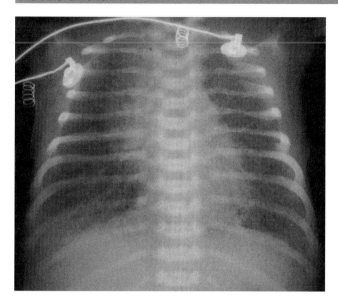

1. What are the imaging findings in this neonate with respiratory distress?

2. What is the differential diagnosis?

3. What are the possible complications?

4. What are the predisposing factors?

Diagnosis: Neonatal Pneumonia

1. Frontal radiograph of the chest demonstrates bilateral patchy interstitial markings in minimally hyperexpanded lungs. Of note, an umbilical artery catheter is seen, with the tip projecting over the $T_{3/4}$ interspace.

2. Differential diagnosis of these findings includes surfactant deficiency disease, neonatal pneumonia, transient tachypnea of the newborn, and meconium aspiration.

3. Complications of neonatal pneumonia include pleural effusion, empyema, abscess, and pneumatocele formation.

4. Factors that predispose to neonatal pneumonia include prolonged premature rupture of membranes, maternal ascending infection, placental infection, and perineal contamination.

Reference
Swischuk LE: *Imaging of the newborn, infant and young child*, ed 5, Philadelphia, 2004, Lippincott Williams & Wilkins, pp 43-46.

Cross-Reference
Blickman JG, Parker BR, Barnes PD: *Pediatric radiology—the requisites*, ed 3, Philadelphia, 2009, Mosby, pp 30-31.

Comments
Neonatal pneumonia is most often bacterial (*Streptococcus, Staphylococcus aureus,* and *Escherichia coli*) but may be viral (adenovirus, herpes simplex, influenza, and parainfluenza). Nonspecific findings are seen on chest radiograph, with hyperexpansion and diffuse increase in interstitial markings most common. Perihilar streaky densities and diffuse haziness favors viral infection. Coarse, patchy parenchymal infiltrates favor bacterial infection. Frank consolidation is rare in neonates. Pleural effusion may accompany bacterial pneumonia. Infection with group B streptococci may mimic surfactant deficiency disease with granularity, perhaps more prominent in the lower lobes.

Most commonly, the infant is infected in utero or during passage through the birth canal. Infants typically present with respiratory distress in the first 48 hours of life. Predisposing factors include prolonged premature rupture of the membranes, ascending infection from the vagina, placental infection, and contamination from a poorly prepared perineum or maternal fecal material. Long-term complications include chronic lung disease.

Delayed onset of right diaphragmatic hernia has been recognized as a complication, especially with group B streptococci infections. Other complications include empyema, abscess, and pneumatoceles.

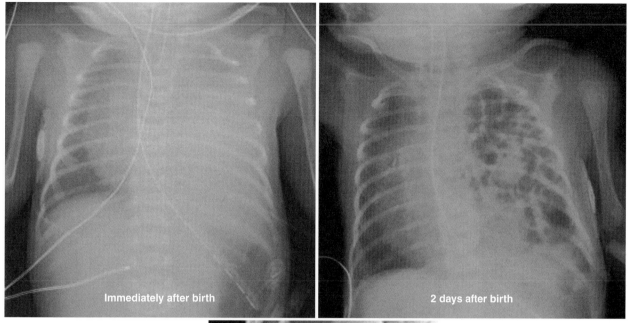

Immediately after birth

2 days after birth

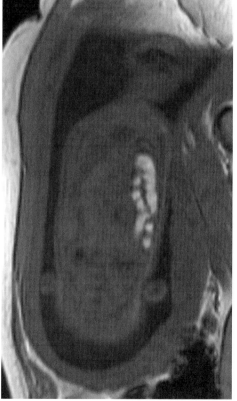

1. What are the imaging findings in this newborn on the first plain radiograph?

2. What is your diagnosis?

3. What is the differential diagnosis?

4. What are the predictors of morbidity and mortality?

Diagnosis: Congenital Diaphragmatic Hernia

1. The plain chest radiograph obtained immediately after birth shows complete opacification of the left hemithorax, mediastinal shift to the right, and nonvisualization of the left hemidiaphragm. The plain radiograph of the chest obtained on the second day of life shows interval aeration of the fluid-filled bowel loops in the left chest cavity. Bowel in the chest, mediastinal shift, nonvisualized diaphragm, position of nasogastric (NG) tube (in cases with herniation of the stomach) are all helpful plain radiograph findings for diagnosis. T_1-weighted coronal image of the same patient obtained during the third trimester shows herniation of the bowel loops. T_1 signal of the bowel lumen is from the meconium content.

2. Congenital diaphragmatic hernia (CDH): Bochdalek type.

3. Congenital cystic adenomatoid malformation, congenital lobar emphysema, and pneumonia complicated by cavitary necrosis.

4. Degree of pulmonary hypoplasia, pulmonary hypertension, size of the hernia, presence of liver and spleen in the chest.

prognostic factors!

Reference
Johnson AM: Congenital anomalies of the fetal/neonatal chest, *Semin Roentgenol* 39(2):197–214, 2004.

Cross-Reference
Blickman JG, Parker BR, Barnes PD: *Pediatric radiology—the requisites*, ed 3, Philadelphia, 2009, Mosby, pp 21–22.

Comment
CDH occurs in 1 of every 2000 to 3000 live births and accounts for 8% of all major congenital anomalies. CDH can be described as cases in which abdominal contents are herniated into the chest. The three basic types of CDH include (1) the posterolateral Bochdalek hernia (occurring at approximately 6 weeks gestation), (2) the anterior Morgagni hernia, and (3) the hiatus hernia. The left-sided Bochdalek hernia occurs in approximately 85% of cases. Bochdalek hernia is more common on the left than on the right (5:1). The hernia may have variable abdominal contents: stomach, small and/or large bowel, liver, and spleen. Most common signs and symptoms include severe respiratory distress. This type of hernia typically presents at or soon after birth and is often detected at prenatal imaging. Less severe cases may present later in life or incidentally on radiograph. Large CDH results in pulmonary hypoplasia and pulmonary

hypertension. Prognosis is primarily related to the degree of lung hypoplasia and pulmonary hypertension. Fetal magnetic resonance image (MRI) and fetal ultrasound have provided valuable information about lung volume, which is an important prognostic indicator in predicting pulmonary capacity after birth. Overall the survival rate is about 50%. Prenatal diagnosis, supportive care for pulmonary hypoplasia and respiratory failure, and use of extracorporeal membrane oxygenation (ECMO) resulted in improved survival rates. In utero surgical repair is an option when in utero diagnosis is made with ultrasound and MRI. Early diagnosis is crucial in guiding the mode of delivery (ex utero intrapartum treatment [EXIT] procedure) and immediate postnatal care. Surgical outcome is still variable. Up to one third of the cases have associated major malformations. Malrotation or stomach volvulus can be seen as a gastrointestinal tract abnormality, and 50% of the cases may have congenital heart disease.

"Baby Back"
Bochdalek — 85%, L > R
– presents soon after birth
– posterior/lateral

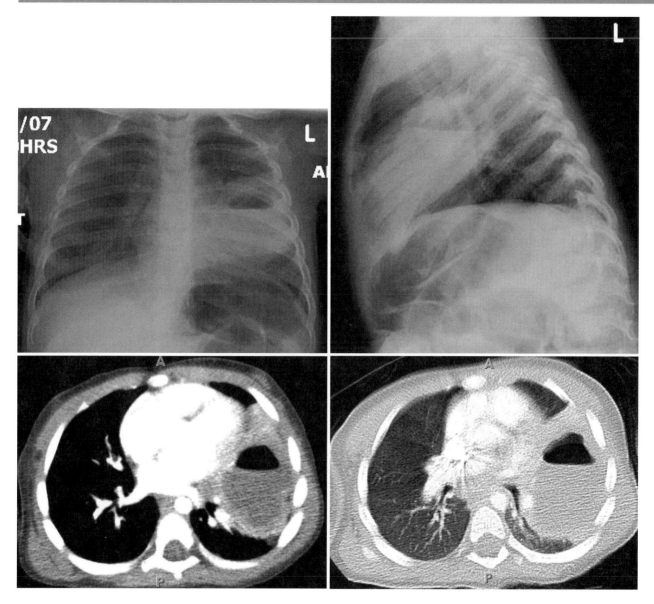

1. What are the imaging findings in this 3-year-old girl with persistent fever, cough, and malaise?

2. What is your diagnosis?

3. What is the differential diagnosis?

4. What is the most common microorganism?

Diagnosis: Lung Abscess

1. Round large mass with air fluid level in the left lower lobe, surrounded by normal lung parenchyma.

2. Lung abscess.

3. Primary versus secondary abscess: secondary to a congenital lesion such as a bronchogenic cyst, congenital cystic adenomatoid malformation, or pulmonary sequestration (in this particular case, the plain radiograph also includes diaphragmatic hernia [e.g., stomach in the chest cavity]).

4. The main causative organisms are usually streptococcal and anaerobic species, *Staphylococcus aureus* and *Klebsiella* spp.

Reference
Puligandla P, Laberge JM: Respiratory infections: pneumonia, lung abscess and empyema, *Semin Pediatr Surg* 17(1):42–52, 2008.

Cross-Reference
Blickman JG, Parker BR, Barnes PD: *Pediatric radiology—the requisites*, ed 3, Philadelphia, 2009, Mosby, pp 32–126.

Comment
A lung abscess develops when a localized area of parenchymal infection becomes necrotic and then cavitates. Primary lung abscesses occur in healthy children without lung abnormalities, whereas secondary abscesses occur in children with underlying lung disease that may be either congenital (e.g., cystic lung lesion) or acquired (e.g., cystic fibrosis, immunodeficiency). Aspiration may play a significant role, especially in children with neurodevelopmental delay or immune deficiency. Clinically, abscesses may develop indolently over a few weeks with tachypnea, cough, and fever being the most common symptoms.

Radiologic evaluation starts with plain films. Ultrasound has the benefit of avoiding radiation exposure; however, it may be less diagnostic in older children, especially in deeper locations. Computed tomography (CT) of the chest helps identifying underlying lung lesions predisposing to the development of the abscess such as a bronchogenic cyst, congenital cystic adenomatoid malformation, or pulmonary sequestration.

Up to 90% of patients with lung abscess may be adequately treated with intravenous antibiotic therapy. The duration of parenteral treatment varies from as little as 5 days to as long as 3 weeks; oral therapy may be required after intravenous medications have been stopped. Ultimately, antibiotic therapy should be tailored to the organisms present. Ultrasound- or CT-guided aspiration may be indicated for diagnosis and treatment. The overall outcome of children with a lung abscess is quite good, with mortality rates much lower than those of adults and mostly occurring in children with secondary lung abscesses or underlying medical problems.

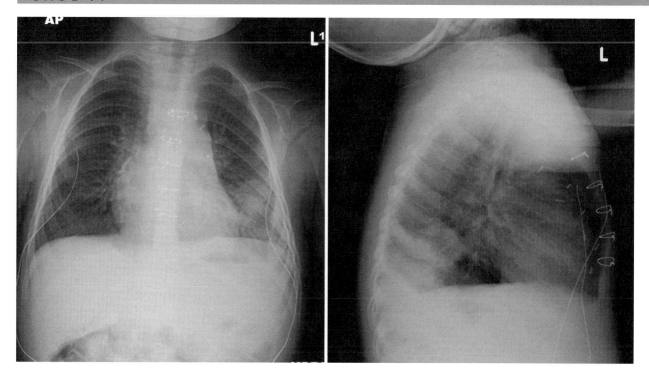

1. What are the imaging findings in this 3-year-old boy with cough and fever?

2. What is your diagnosis?

3. What is the differential diagnosis?

4. What is the cause?

Diagnosis: Round Pneumonia

1. Round well-demarcated opacity in the left lower lobe; patient had previous cardiac surgery and osteopenia.

2. Round pneumonia.

3. Bronchogenic cyst, neuroblastoma, congenital cystic adenomatoid malformation (CCAM), pulmonary sequestration.

4. Round pneumonia most commonly seen with *Streptococcus pneumoniae* infection.

Reference

Kim YW, Donnelly LF: Round pneumonia: imaging findings in a large series of children, *Pediatr Radiol* 37 (12):1235–1240, 2007.

Cross-Reference

Blickman JG, Parker BR, Barnes PD: *Pediatric radiology—the requisites*, ed 3, Philadelphia, 2009, Mosby, p 32.

Comment

Round pneumonia is bacterial in origin, with a very round, well-defined appearance on chest radiography, simulating a mass. It respects the lobar anatomy without crossing the fissures. Round pneumonia is seen in children younger than 8 years of age and is commonly seen in the lower lungs.

Clinical presentation is fever and cough, general malaise, and may present with abdominal pain. If a child has symptoms of pneumonia and round density is seen on the chest radiograph, additional imaging is not required. In children, collateral pathways or air circulation (channels of Lambert and pores of Kohn) are not well developed until 8 years old. This lack of well-developed collateral circulation is thought to hinder spread of bacterial infection and predispose to the round appearance.

If computed tomography is performed, air bronchograms can be seen. Magnetic resonance imaging is not necessary in the diagnostic workup of round pneumonia.

Treatment of choice is with antibiotic agents. Round pneumonia is one of the few indications in which a follow-up chest radiograph is required after the child becomes asymptomatic to exclude an underlying mass.

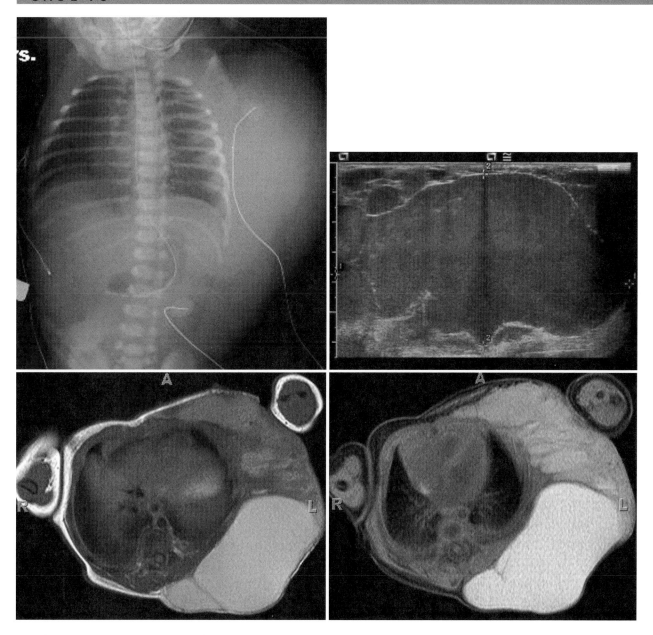

1. What are the imaging findings in this newborn with a large lateral chest wall and abdominal wall mass?

2. What is your diagnosis?

3. What is the differential diagnosis?

4. Does this entity regress spontaneously?

Diagnosis: Venolymphatic Malformation

1. Plain film reveals a large subcutaneous soft tissue mass extending from upper chest down to the pelvis. Ultrasound shows a large complex cystic mass with internal echoes. Magnetic resonance imaging (MRI) reveals a large lobular, septated mass in the left lateral chest wall, extending from the chest to the left lateral abdomen. The caudal part of the mass is precontrast T_1 bright (either from high-protein content or posthemorrhage), and the superior aspect of the mass is T_1 hypointense, revealing serpiginous areas on T_2 that show avid contrast enhancement. The caudal part represents the macrocystic lymphatic malformation component, and the cranial part represents the venous malformation component.

2. Venolymphatic malformation

3. Venous malformation or lymphatic malformation alone

4. No, vascular malformations never regress or involute spontaneously and may grow at a rate greater than normal somatic growth.

References

Legiehn GM, Heran MK: Classification, diagnosis, and interventional radiologic management of vascular malformations, *Orthop Clin North Am* 37(3):435–474, vii–viii, 2006.

Mulliken JB, Glowacki J: Hemangiomas and vascular malformations in infants and children: a classification based on endothelial characteristics, *Plast Reconstr Surg* 69(3):412–422, 1982.

Cross-Reference

Blickman JG, Parker BR, Barnes PD: *Pediatric radiology—the requisites*, ed 3, Philadelphia, 2009, Mosby, pp 314–315.

Comment

Few areas within medical diagnosis are fraught with as many persistent misconceptions and misnomers as within the group of vascular anomalies. In 1982 Mulliken and Glowacki published a landmark article proposing characterization of vascular anomalies based on biologic and pathologic differences. It is most important to make the differentiation between vascular tumors (hemangiomas) and vascular malformations, including venous malformations, lymphatic malformations, capillary malformation, mixed type of venolymphatic malformations, arteriovenous malformations (AVMs), arteriovenous fistulas, because the prognosis and treatment options differ significantly between the two groups.

Vascular malformations are described as lesions present at birth growing commensurately or pari passu with the child, composed of vascular channels lined with flat "mature" endothelium exhibiting normal rates of endothelial cell turnover. Vascular malformations are further subdivided based on their flow rate observed in angiograms: low-flow venous malformations and high-flow AVMs, with a separate group categorization for lymphatic malformations and hemangiomas. Vascular malformations are commonly seen in the head and neck region followed by trunk and extremities.

Lymphatic malformations have been called lymphangiomas in the past, which is a misnomer. They are multicystic (can be micro-macrocystic or mixed); vascular channels and spaces are separated by fibrous septa. The lumen may contain lymphatic fluid or proteinaceous material. Ultrasound is the first line of imaging in evaluation of vascular anomalies. Lymphatic malformations appear as cystic cavities with layering debris. They can have bleeding or inflammatory changes in these cysts. No flow is detectable within a lymphatic vascular malformation. MRI is very helpful in defining the extent of disease and further characterization. It may reveal increased T_1 signal secondary to bleeding, protein content and inflammatory changes, show increased T_2 signal, and may show peripheral contrast enhancement of the fibrous septa.

Vascular malformations may present as a combination of venous and lymphatic malformation (as in the presented case). It is important to clearly identify the parts of this lesion as lymphatic and venous because the used sclerotic agents differ.

Successful management requires an experienced multidisciplinary team allowing effective communication and integration of the most current clinical, pathologic, and image-based diagnosis and intervention.

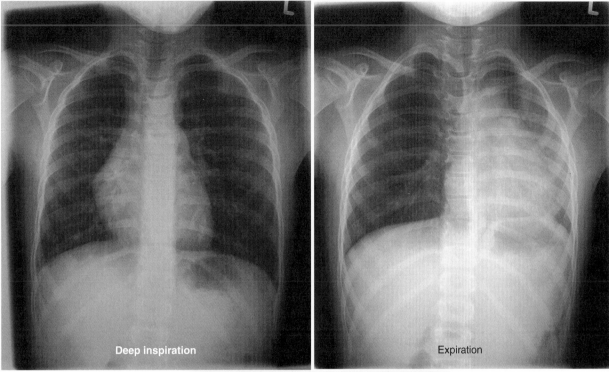

Deep inspiration   Expiration

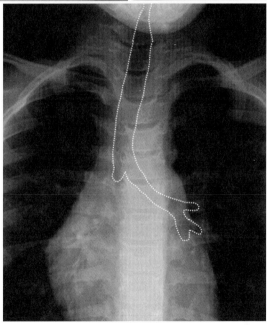

1. What is the principal finding comparing inspiration with expiration?

2. What is the most likely diagnosis?

3. Is this finding acute or chronic?

4. What to do next?

R ight

Diagnosis: Aspirated Carrot in the Left Main Bronchus

1. Air trapping in the right lung.

2. Nonradioopaque foreign body in the right main bronchus.

3. Acute. No signs of infection and/or fluid retention and/or chronic atelectasis is seen in the right lung.

4. Bronchoscopy with removal of the foreign body.

Cross-Reference

Blickman JG, Parker BR, Barnes PD: *Pediatric radiology—the requisites*, ed 3, Philadelphia, 2009, Mosby, p 15.

Comment

Children who suffer from acute, unexplained shortness of breath with wheezing should be suspected of a foreign body aspiration until proven otherwise. Especially small children and babies who explore their surroundings by putting many objects in their mouths are at risk for aspiration. Older children more frequently choke on food, especially hard candies and peanuts. It is important to be aware of the fact that most aspirated foreign bodies are not radioopaque and are consequently not visible on plain films.

By acquiring chest films in different degrees of inspiration (inspiration versus expiration), foreign bodies may indirectly be proven and located. Depending on the degree of obstruction, the lung distal to the foreign body may be partially or totally atelectatic. However, a ball valve effect may also result in a progressive hyperinflation of the lung distal to the obstruction increasing with every breath taken. The progressive air trapping may lead to a life-threatening mediastinal shift to the contralateral side compromising the ventilation of the contralateral lung. Imaging shows a hyperinflation of the air-trapped lung on inspiration, which persists on expiration. On expiration, however, the contralateral lung will deflate. The mediastinal structures will shift to the side of the nonobstructed lung.

The trachea and bronchi should also be studied in detail; air within the upper airways may serve as a natural contrast to a foreign body. In this particular case, the air column within the right bronchus was amputated just distal to the carina.

Aspirated foreign bodies are more frequently found in the right bronchus than in the left bronchus. The right bronchus is slightly larger than the left bronchus and in a more favorable orientation in relation to the trachea for aspiration than the left main bronchus.

If the patient's history and the clinical findings are highly suggestive for a foreign body aspiration, most children will go immediately into the bronchoscopy suite. In all other instances, plain chest films in inspiration and expiration should be performed. If the patient's compliance to follow instructions is limited, lateral decubitus should be considered. The air-trapped lung will not deflate in the dependent position (lateral decubitus).

Please do not forget that a foreign body may also have been expelled by an adequate coughing reflex but has been swallowed subsequently. Consequently, if a foreign body is not visible on chest films and the clinical history is highly suggestive of a foreign body aspiration, additional abdominal films should be acquired. The gastrointestinal tract should be examined from the mouth until the anus.

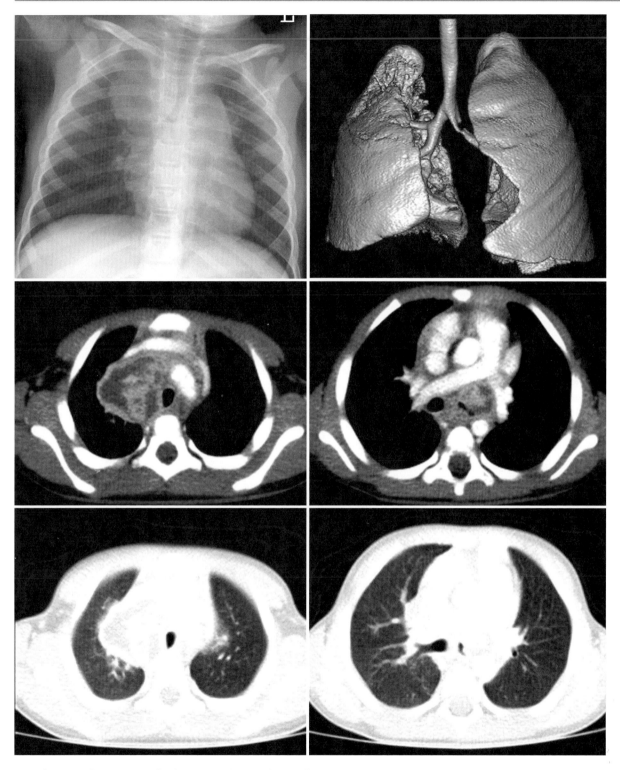

1. What are the imaging findings on plain radiography?

2. What are the imaging findings on chest computed tomography (CT)?

3. What is the most likely diagnosis?

4. Which patient population is more at risk for infection?

Diagnosis: Pulmonary Tuberculosis

1. Enlarged mediastinal contour, possibly the result of enlarged lymph nodes.

2. Necrotic paratracheal lymph nodes, deformed right upper lobe, and high-grade compression of left mainstem bronchus.

3. Pulmonary tuberculosis.

4. Immunocompromised patients and young children.

Reference

Santos JF: Tuberculosis in children, *Eur J Radiol* 55:202-208, 2005.

Cross-Reference

Blickman JG, Parker BR, Barnes PD: *Pediatric radiology—the requisites*, ed 3, Philadelphia, 2009, Mosby, pp 33-34.

Comment

Pulmonary tuberculosis (TBC) results from the inhalation of mycobacterium tuberculosis bacilli. A primary complex or Ghon complex results from the multiplication of TBC bacilli in one bronchiole or alveolus and the host's local inflammatory acute reaction. From this initial lesion, the bacilli may spread into the regional lymph nodes. Most frequently hilar lymph nodes are involved; depending on the location of the primary infection, paratracheal or subcarinal nodes may be affected. The combination of a primary focus and adjacent calcified hilar lymph nodes are known as Ranke complex. This primary complex may go undetected on plain radiography. In most cases the intrapulmonary lesion heals with frequently subtle signs of focal pulmonary scarring or fibrosis. Rarely, the primary focus may persist and evolve into a larger focal pneumonitis. The affected lymph nodes may develop fibrosis or calcifications during the healing phase. TBC bacilli may, however, survive within the lymph nodes for many years. In rare cases the lymph nodes may enlarge so significantly that they encroach or obstruct adjacent bronchi with resulting pulmonary atelectasis. Affected caseous lymph nodes may eventually erode bronchial walls with resultant endobronchial TBC and a fistulous tract. Depending on the location, fistulous tracts may extend into the pericardium or esophagus.

In addition, TBC bacilli may spread from the primary complex though the lymphatic system or bloodstream into almost any part of the body. Most frequently, the upper lung lobes are affected next to the liver, spleen, meninges, pleura, and bones. Massive lymphohematogenous dissemination may result in miliary or disseminated TBC. Young children are more at risk for miliary TBC than older children or adults.

On imaging, a primary complex may be difficult to detect. CT usually reveals enlarged lymph nodes with or without caseation and/or calcification. CT is extremely helpful to identify the degree of bronchial obstruction or other complications. The number of newly diagnosed TBC infections is unfortunately again on the rise. TBC should be included in the differential diagnosis when enlarged, possibly calcified lymph nodes are encountered.

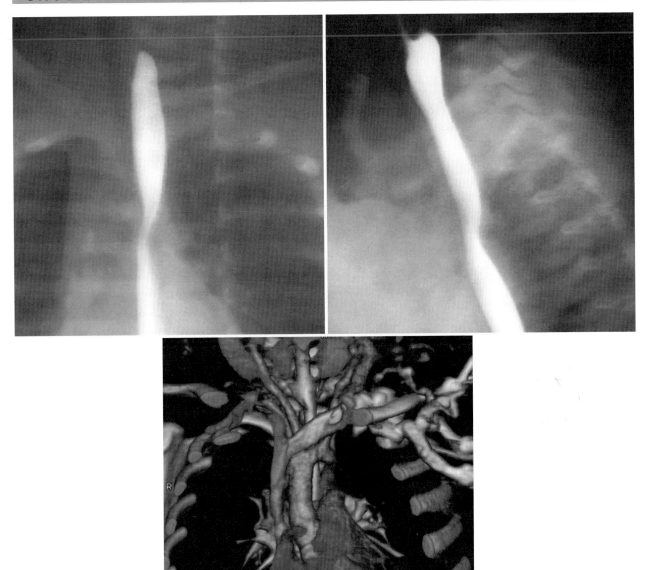

1. This 3-month-old infant presented with difficulty feeding. What other symptoms might the caregiver report?

2. What are the findings on upper gastrointestinal examination (first and second images)?

3. What examination should the clinician order next?

4. Why is one needed?

Diagnosis: Double Aortic Arch

1. Stridor; normal initially, then with progression of symptoms; choking on solid feeds but able to swallow liquids.

2. Lateral view: posterior compression on the esophagus, anterior compression on the trachea; anteroposterior view: "hourglass" compression of the esophagus.

3. Magnetic resonance image or magnetic resonance angiography has no radiation dose, but sedation may be dangerous if stridor is a prominent symptom. Computed tomographic angiography (third image) usually does not require sedation, but the radiation dose is large.

4. One arch is usually smaller than the other arch, and the surgeon generally will choose that side to divide.

Reference

Kirks DR, Griscom NT, editors: *Practical pediatric imaging*, ed 3, Philadelphia, 1998, Lippincott-Raven, pp 14-15 and pp 77-80.

Cross-Reference

Blickman JG, Parker BR, Barnes PD: *Pediatric radiology—the requisites*, ed 3, Philadelphia, 2009, Mosby, pp 14-15 and pp 78-79.

Comment

Although this is not the most common aortic arch anomaly (that would be left aortic arch and aberrant right subclavian artery), it is the most common vascular ring. Persistence of both fetal aortic arches occurs, and each gives off its own subclavian and carotid artery. The single ascending aorta divides around and encloses the trachea and esophagus, coming together posteriorly in a single descending aorta. If the ring is tight, the child might present with stridor at birth. Otherwise, symptoms may slowly develop as the child grows. Dysphagia is often the presenting symptom when the diet changes to include solid food. The right arch is usually larger, rises higher, and extends more posterior than the left arch.

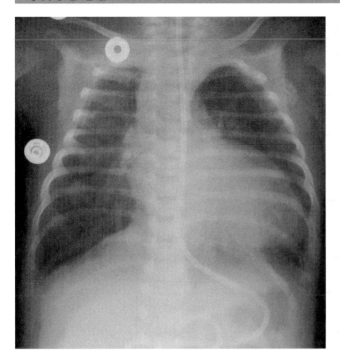

1. What are the radiographic findings in this 1-month-old cyanotic infant?

2. What aspect of the radiograph is potentially confusing? What causes this?

3. What proportion of these patients has a right-sided aortic arch?

CASE 22

Diagnosis: Tetralogy of Fallot

1. Cardiomegaly with broad, upturned silhouette; right-sided aortic arch, concave pulmonary arterial segment.

2. The appearance of increased pulmonary blood flow; large aorticopulmonary collaterals replace hypoplastic pulmonary artery system.

3. Twenty-five percent of patients with tetralogy of Fallot (TOF).

Reference
Park MK: *Pediatric cardiology for practitioners*, ed 4, St Louis, 2002, Mosby, pp 189-196.

Cross-Reference
Blickman JG, Parker BR, Barnes PD: *Pediatric radiology—the requisites*, ed 3, Philadelphia, 2009, Mosby, pp 55-56.

Comment
Clinicians postulate that a single intrauterine event in fetal life starts the chain of defects that causes TOF, the most common congenital cyanotic heart defect. This insult causes hypoplasia of the right ventricular (RV) outflow tract (1). This in turn causes malalignment of the membranous and muscular septa, leaving an opening, the ventricular septal defect (VSD) (2). In addition, the aorta is drawn medially by the lack of supporting tissue and ends up straddling the septum (3). As the RV is exposed to systemic pressures by the VSD and is forced to pump against the semiobstructed RV outflow tract, it hypertrophies (4). Ten percent of patients have an associated atrioventricular canal abnormality, whereas 15% to 20% have pulmonary atresia.

Palliation with shunts to improve pulmonary blood flow (the Blalock-Taussig shunt was the first of its kind) has given way to early definitive surgery to enlarge the outflow tract and close the VSD. This eliminates the complications of systemic shunting: excessive or uneven blood flow and the development of pulmonary hypertension. Complications of definitive repair include aneurysm of the outflow tract patch, restenosis with diminishing or asymmetric pulmonary blood flow, and stenosis of repaired valves.

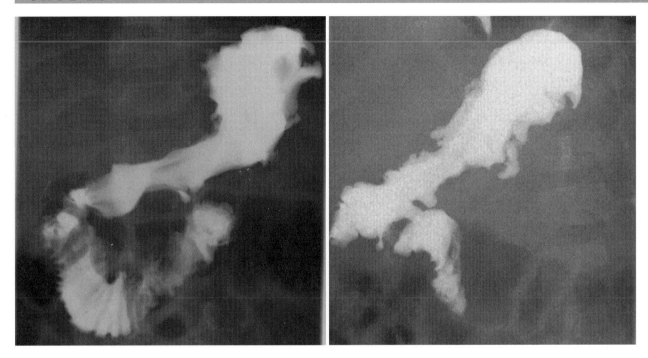

1. This 17-month old girl presented with a 5-day history of periorbital and pedal edema, not tolerating feeding. Two images from the upper gastrointestinal (GI) tract show what finding?

2. What eponym is associated with this finding?

3. What did the biopsy show?

4. How does the significance of this finding in children differ from that in adults?

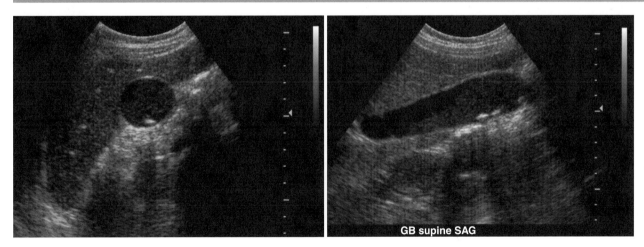

GB supine SAG

1. What are the imaging findings and most likely diagnosis?

2. List some predisposing factors.

3. What imaging studies should be performed with suspected gallbladder disease?

4. What are the possible complications of this disease?

CASE 23

Diagnosis: Ménétrier Disease (Giant Hypertrophic Gastritis)

1. Prominent, thickened gastric rugal folds.

2. Ménétrier disease—named for French pathologist Pierre Eugène Ménétrier (1859 to 1935).

3. Hyperplastic mucosa with eosinophilic and neutrophilic infiltration, occasional cells with cytomegalovirus (CMV) inclusion bodies.

4. In adults, the condition is chronic and increases the chance of gastric cancer, whereas in children it is most often self-limited and secondary to infection (CMV most often, *Campylobacter pylori* is also reported).

Reference

Stringer DA, Babyn PS: *Pediatric gastrointestinal imaging and intervention*, ed 2, Hamilton-London, 2000, BC Decker Inc, pp 286–287.

Cross-Reference

Blickman JG, Parker BR, Barnes PD: *Pediatric radiology—the requisites*, ed 3, Philadelphia, 2009, Mosby, p 85.

Comment

This condition causes protein-losing enteropathy that can result in hypoalbuminemia—helping to distinguish this disease from allergic gastritis, which can also cause enlarged rugal folds. The soft tissue edema secondary to the hypoalbuminemia may be subtle but should provide the alert practitioner with the differential diagnosis. Moreover, a viral prodrome often exists in the history.

CASE 24

Diagnosis: Cholelithiasis

1. Sonographic images of the gallbladder demonstrate mobile, shadowing, echogenic foci within the gallbladder consistent with gallstones.

2. Parenteral nutrition, sickle cell disease and other hemolytic anemias, malabsorption syndromes including short-gut syndrome, and cystic fibrosis.

3. Ultrasound is the imaging modality of choice in cases of possible gallbladder disease. With the question of acalculous cholecystitis, nuclear medicine scan should be performed to evaluate gallbladder function. Magnetic resonance cholangiopancreatography is also useful to further evaluate gallbladder disease.

4. Obstruction and infection (cholecystitis, cholangitis, pancreatitis).

Reference

Siegel MJ, Coley BD: *Pediatric imaging*, Philadelphia, 2006, Lippincott Williams & Wilkins, pp 172–173.

Cross-Reference

Blickman JG, Parker BR, Barnes PD: *Pediatric radiology—the requisites*, ed 3, Philadelphia, 2009, Mosby, pp 107–108.

Comments

Gallstones are relatively rare in the pediatric population. Common causes include furosemide therapy, malabsorption, total parenteral nutrition, Crohn disease, cystic fibrosis, bowel resection, and hemolytic anemia such as sickle cell disease. Patients present with colicky right upper quadrant pain. Ultrasound is the imaging of choice and will demonstrate intraluminal echogenic shadowing structures within the gallbladder that may move with change in patient positioning. Differential diagnosis would also include gallbladder polyp and cholesterol granuloma. Complications of cholelithiasis include cholecystitis, choledocholithiasis, cholangitis, and pancreatitis. Gallbladder sludge may be a precursor to stone formation and is probably the result of stasis.

Causes: TPN
Malabs
CF
Crohns
Diuretic TX
Hemolytic Anemia

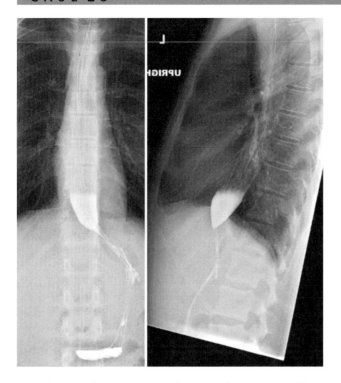

1. What are the imaging findings in this 12-year-old patient presenting with dysphagia? Frontal and lateral chest radiographs were obtained after the administration of oral contrast under fluoroscopy. What is the differential diagnosis?

2. What would the findings be on a chest radiograph?

3. What would be the typical findings on a dynamic esophagram?

4. What are the possible complications?

Diagnosis: Achalasia

1. Frontal and lateral views demonstrate dilated upper and midesophagus with nonobstructive tapered narrowing of the distal esophagus in the region of the lower esophageal sphincter. Differential diagnosis includes achalasia, esophageal stricture, gastroesophageal reflux, caustic ingestion, and epidermolysis bullosa.

2. On plain chest radiograph a dilated air-filled esophagus is classically seen in patients with achalasia.

3. A dilated proximal esophagus with distal beaking, failure of peristalsis to clear the esophagus in the recumbent position, antegrade and retrograde motion of barium in the esophagus, and pooling of barium in the esophagus that occurs late in the course of disease.

4. Esophagitis, increased risk for aspiration, and increased risk for esophageal carcinoma.

Reference

Schlesinger AE, Parker BR: Disorders of the esophago-gastric junction. In Kuhn JP, Slovis TL, Haller JO, editors: *Caffey's pediatric diagnostic imaging*, ed 10, Philadelphia, 2004, Mosby, pp 1575-1579.

Cross-Reference

Blickman JG, Parker BR, Barnes PD: *Pediatric radiology—the requisites*, ed 3, Philadelphia, 2009, Mosby, p 82.

Comments

Achalasia is an esophageal motility disorder with failure of the lower esophageal sphincter to relax, resulting in failure of the esophagus to advance food into the stomach. Often a deficiency of cells is found in Auerbach plexus. Although it is relatively rare in children, those children with achalasia present with dysphagia, chest pain, vomiting of undigested food, and severe bad breath. These children also may have prolonged coughing spells after meals. Weight loss is common. Definitive diagnosis is with manometry. On plain chest radiograph one may see a dilated air-filled esophagus. Classic findings on esophagram include dilated proximal esophagus with distal beaking; failure of peristalsis to clear the esophagus of barium with the patient in the recumbent position; antegrade and retrograde motion of barium in the esophagus secondary to uncoordinated, nonpropulsive, tertiary contractions; and pooling or stasis of barium in the esophagus that occurs late in the course of disease. Differential diagnosis includes esophageal stricture, gastroesophageal reflux, caustic ingestion, and epidermolysis bullosa. Treatment options include endoscopic balloon dilatation or surgical repair.

Complications include esophagitis as a result of stasis and the retention of foodstuff and upper gastrointestinal secretions in the esophagus, increased risk for aspiration, and increased risk for esophageal carcinoma, compared with the general population.

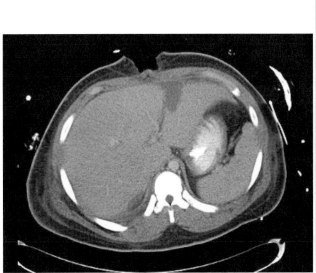
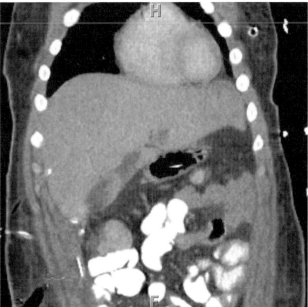

1. What are the imaging findings in this 4-year-old girl with injuries from a motor vehicle accident?

2. Would one expect to see associated injuries?

3. What is the differential diagnosis?

4. What is the cause?

Diagnosis: Liver Trauma

1. Subcutaneous tissue laceration is present in the anterior midabdomen. A focal intraparenchymal hypodensity extends from the left lobe of the liver continuing inferiorly along the inferior aspect of the right lobe of the liver, with subcapsular hypodense fluid collection in the left lobe representing a deep traumatic laceration and small subcapsular hematoma. No injury exists to the biliary tree, hepatic veins, or portal vein. In addition, a chest tube is noted in the left lower chest wall; however, the current image does not show the pneumothorax.

2. Forty-five percent of the cases have splenic injury, 33% have rib fractures, and some have duodenal hematoma or pancreatic injury.

3. In the correct clinical setting, this image is attributable to traumatic injury.

4. Blunt trauma is more common than penetrating injury.

Reference

Yoon W, Jeong YY, Kim JK, et al: CT in liver trauma, *Radiographics* 25(1):87–104, 2005.

Cross-Reference

Blickman JG, Parker BR, Barnes PD: *Pediatric radiology—the requisites*, ed 3, Philadelphia, 2009, Mosby, p 118.

Comment

Liver is the most commonly injured solid organ in abdominal trauma. The right lobe of the liver is more commonly affected than the left lobe. About two thirds of patients have accompanying hemoperitoneum. Blunt trauma is more frequent than penetrating trauma. Motor vehicle injuries are the leading cause, followed by fall and assault. Patients generally present with right upper quadrant pain and tenderness and hypotension. Male patients are more commonly affected than female patients.

Trauma to the liver may present as parenchymal laceration, subcapsular hematoma, parenchymal hematoma, active hemorrhage, infarction, periportal edema, or biliary injury. The most widely used grading system for blunt hepatic injury is the liver injury grading system established by the American Association of Surgery of Trauma (ASST). This system includes descriptions of injuries to abdominal organs that are based on the most accurate assessment at autopsy, laparotomy, or computed tomography (CT).

Grade 1: subcapsular hematoma (<10% surface area), laceration, less than 1 cm depth; grade 2: subcapsular hematoma 10% to 50% of surface area, parenchymal hematoma less than 10 cm in diameter or laceration 1 to 3 cm parenchymal depth; grade 3: subcapsular hematoma more than 50% surface area, intraparenchymal hematoma more than 10 cm or expanding, laceration more than 3 cm in depth; grade 4: parenchymal disruption involving 75% of hepatic lobe or more than three-segment involvement in a single lobe; grade 5: vascular hepatic avulsion.

Ultrasound imaging is very helpful to screen for abdominal injuries after trauma; however, contrast-enhanced CT is more widely used because it enables examination of the entire abdomen and pelvis in a very short time, including the skeleton.

Use of the ASST grading system is helpful when describing the injury, as well as when deciding on acute treatment options; however, the best predictor of the need for surgical intervention in patients with blunt liver trauma is hemodynamic instability, not the severity of injury as determined with CT. More than 90% of initially hemodynamically stable children with solid organ injuries can be successfully treated conservatively. Multiorgan involvement carries a higher risk of mortality. Complications include biloma, delayed hemorrhage, hemobilia, hepatic infarcts, and pseudoaneurysms.

Liver lac associated with:
- 45% splenic lac
- 33% Rib #
- duodenal hematoma
- pancreatic injury
- 66% hemoperitoneum
- MVC
- fall

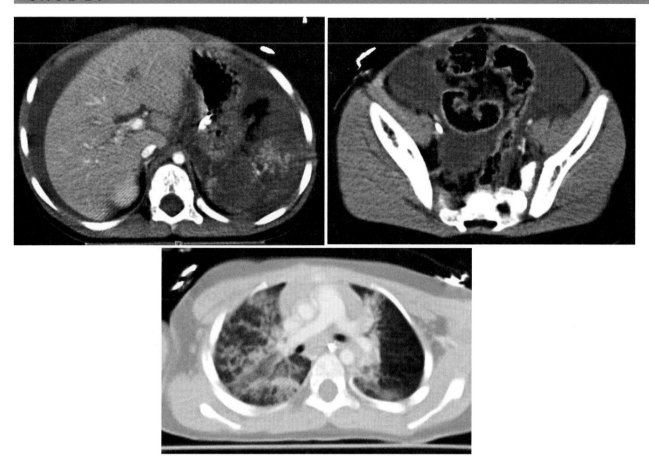

1. What are the imaging findings in this 11-year-old boy with injuries from a motor vehicle accident?

2. What is your diagnosis?

3. What is the classic radiographic triad in this entity?

4. What is the number one differential?

Diagnosis: Traumatic Splenic Injury: Grade 4-5

1. Hypodense nonenhancing spleen with small amount of enhancing parenchyma in the inferior and middle aspect of the organ. In addition, intraperitoneal fluid surrounds the liver and is seen in the cul de sac. The lungs show fluffy increased densities somewhat sparing the periphery representing lung contusion or, less likely, aspiration; relatively small caliber of the aorta and inferior vena cava compared with the portal vein suggest hypovolemic shock.

2. Traumatic splenic injury grade 4-5.

3. Elevated left hemidiaphragm, pleural effusion, left lower lobe atelectasis. In addition, rib fractures and findings of retroperitoneal hematoma, such as an obscured left kidney, psoas shadow, and medial displacement of the descending colon medially can be seen.

4. Too early arterial phase artifact that results from differences in enhancement of red and white pulp. The spleen appears heterogeneous and corrugated. Congenital cleft, splenic infarct, or abscess should also be considered in the differential.

References

Cloutier DR, Baird TB, Gormley P, et al: Pediatric splenic injuries with a contrast blush: successful nonoperative management without angiography and embolization, *Pediatr Surg* 39(6):969-971, 2004.

Upadhyaya P, Simpson JS: Splenic trauma in children, *Surg Gynecol Obstet* 126(4):781-790, 1968.

Cross-Reference

Blickman JG, Parker BR, Barnes PD: *Pediatric radiology—the requisites*, ed 3, Philadelphia, 2009, Mosby, pp 118-119.

Comment

The management of childhood solid organ injury has evolved from standard explorative laparotomy for suspected abdominal injury to routine nonoperative management. This approach has been validated as safe in hemodynamically stable children with splenic injury and has led to a decrease in childhood splenectomy. After a publication discussing the advantages of a conservative management of splenic injuries by Upadhyaya et al. in 1968, this strategy has been successfully applied to other solid organ injuries in children and also in the adult patient population.

Splenic trauma has been defined as the parenchymal injury to spleen with or without capsular disruption.

Blunt trauma is more frequently observed than penetrating trauma. Motor vehicle injuries are the leading cause followed by handlebar or bicycle injuries. Patients generally present with left upper quadrant pain and tenderness, hypotension, rib pain, and ecchymosis. Male patients are more commonly affected than female patients.

The American Association of Surgery of Trauma has established the most widely used grading system for splenic injury.

Grade 1: subcapsular hematoma (< 10% surface area), laceration, less than 1 cm depth; grade 2: subcapsular hematoma 10% to 50% of surface area, parenchymal hematoma less than 5 cm in diameter or laceration 1 to 3 cm parenchymal depth without involvement of trabecular vessels; grade 3: subcapsular hematoma more than 50% surface area, intraparenchymal hematoma more than 5 cm or expanding, laceration more than 3 cm in depth or involving the trabecular vessels; grade 4: laceration involving segmental or hilar vessels producing major devascularization, parenchymal disruption involving 25% of spleen; grade 5: completely shattered, hilar vascular injury that devascularizes spleen.

Ultrasound imaging is very helpful for initial screening after abdominal trauma; however, computed tomography is more widely used because it enables examination of the entire abdomen and pelvis in a very short time. Unlike in the adult patient population, the presence of arterial blush (active extravasation) does not dictate the need for embolization in all cases. Nonoperative management with monitoring of hemodynamic status is still the method of choice. In addition, unlike adults the grading system does not determine the outcome in children. Additional organ injuries should be actively searched for, such as pancreatic and renal injuries ipsilateral to the spleen, as well as rib fractures or bowel wall hematomas or perforations. Multiorgan involvement carries a higher risk of mortality. Prognosis is very good with early diagnosis and appropriate intervention.

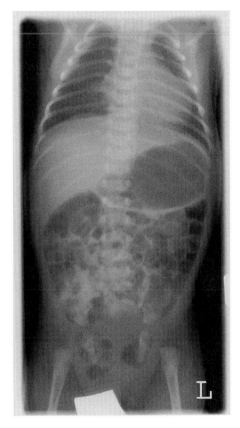

1. Why could this child be at risk for an intestinal incarceration?

2. Which anatomic structure is not closed?

3. Is there a sex predeliction?

4. Which imaging modality should be used for confirmation of the diagnosis?

Diagnosis: Bilateral Inguinal Hernias

1. Bilateral inguinal hernias.

2. Processus vaginalis.

3. Boys are more frequently affected than girls.

4. Ultrasound.

Reference

Siegel MJ, Coley BD: *Pediatric imaging*, Philadelphia, 2006, Lippincott Williams & Wilkins, pp 226-227.

Comment

Inguinal hernias can be seen as incidental findings on plain radiography of the abdomen. Most inguinal hernias are asymptomatic. Occasionally, herniated bowel loops may incarcerate with subsequent development of an acute abdomen. A less dramatic presentation may occur in so called sliding inguinal hernias. These children may present with intermittent episodes of mild intestinal obstruction. Most inguinal hernias in children are indirect (i.e., bowel loops herniate into the inguinal canal through a patent processus vaginalis). In boys the bowel loops may reach the scrotum; in girls they many reach the labia majora. Depending on the size of the processus vaginalis, a single bowel loop or multiple bowel loops may be herniated, as well as different amounts of omentum. Frequently a mild degree of free fluid is seen along the herniated bowel loops. Direct inguinal hernias in which the bowel loops herniate medially to the epigastric vessels, or femoral hernias in which the bowel loops herniated through the femoral sling, are uncommon in children.

Ultrasonography is the most sensitive imaging modality to identify the herniated bowel loops. Color Doppler sonography will also give valuable information about the bowel wall perfusion and will enhance differentiation between inguinal hernia and a hydrocele or varicocele.

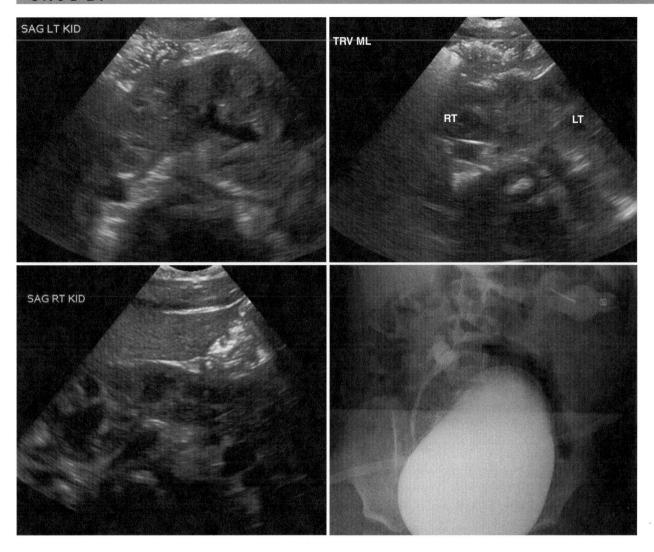

1. If not found by prenatal ultrasound, how might this lesion present in childhood (first, second, and third images)?

2. Which tumors have increased incidence?

3. Are the ureters long and redundant (fourth image)?

Diagnosis: Horseshoe Kidney

1. Urinary tract infection, urinary stone, trauma.

2. Wilms tumor in children; adenocarcinoma and transitional cell carcinoma in adults.

3. No, they are the appropriate length for their distance from the bladder.

Reference

Kuhn JP, Slovis TL, Haller JO: *Caffey's pediatric diagnostic imaging*, ed 10, Philadelphia, 2004, Mosby, pp 1764-1768.

Cross-Reference

Blickman JG, Parker BR, Barnes PD: *Pediatric radiology—the requisites*, ed 3, Philadelphia, 2009, Mosby, pp 125-129.

Discussion

This malformation represents fusion of primitive renal blastema resulting in lack of migration. It is quite frequent, found in 1 in 500 to 1000 autopsies. The kidneys are more medially oriented, with their fused lower poles anterior to the aorta and inferior vena cava. Often several renal arteries supply them from the aorta and a range of abnormality is seen—from a thin fibrous bridge to a single pelvic renal complex, from a symmetric V-shape to asymmetric fusion resembling crossed fused renal ectopia. The more distorted forms generally come more quickly to clinical attention. They are prone to ureteropelvic junction obstruction, vesicoureteral reflux, stones, and ureteral duplication. (However, they also frequently have an extrarenal pelvis, which should not be confused with hydronephrosis.) Their anterior position makes them more prone to traumatic injury. They have an association with trisomy 18, imperforate anus, Turner syndrome, and infants of diabetic mothers. When they are found clinically in the absence of those abnormalities, often an increased incidence of congenital cardiac anomalies is seen.

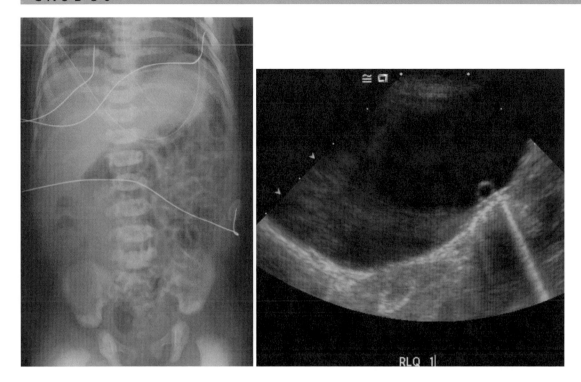

1. This newborn female had a palpable abdominal mass on physical examination. A plain film was obtained (first image). What do you see?

2. What is the differential diagnosis?

3. An ultrasound was ordered (second image). What are the findings?

4. What is the differential diagnosis now?

Diagnosis: Neonatal Ovarian Cyst with Second Follicle, Otherwise Uncomplicated

1. "Blank" area in the right lower quadrant with rounded margin, bowel loops displaced, no calcification.

2. Mesenteric cyst, ileal duplication cyst, ovarian cyst, meconium cyst, multicystic dysplastic kidney, unilateral hydronephrosis (e.g., ureteropelvic junction obstruction), choledochal cyst.

3. Clear fluid-filled single large cyst with second internal cyst.

4. Ovarian cyst, mesenteric cyst (other choices tend to contain more complex fluid or be multichambered).

Reference
Fotter R, editor: *Pediatric uroradiology*, Berlin-Heidelberg-New York, 2001, Springer, pp 345-347.

Cross-Reference
Blickman JG, Parker BR, Barnes PD: *Pediatric radiology—the requisites*, ed 3, Philadelphia, 2009, Mosby, pp 151-153.

Comment
Small follicular cysts can be seen on routine prenatal ultrasound after the twenty-sixth gestational week. Clinicians believe high levels of maternal or placental human chorionic gonadotropin cause large cysts. Additional maternal causes have been implicated (maternal diabetes, placental enlargement because of Rh sensitization), as well as adrenogenital syndrome in the fetus. The cysts can become very large and take up much of the abdomen. This increases the risk of ovarian torsion and amputation. The cyst fluid may show evidence of hemorrhage, with clot or resolving debris, depending on the timing of the event.

Most ovarian cysts will resolve as maternal hormones ebb in the newborn infant. However, large cysts that compromise bowel or respiratory function, have ruptured and caused ascites or are in danger of doing so, or cause pain suggesting ovarian torsion are either removed surgically (with ovarian salvage) or decompressed by needle aspiration.

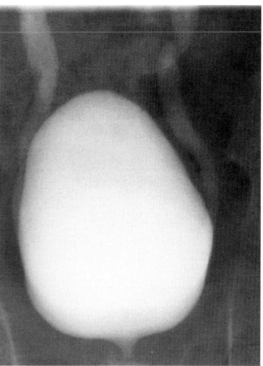

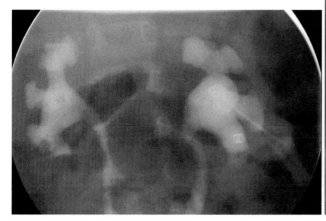

1. These figures show the upper and lower tract images from a voiding cystourethrogram (VCUG) in a 1-year-old male toddler who also has a gastrostomy tube. What is the grade of this vesicoureteral reflux (VUR)?

2. What factors make it more likely that reflux will resolve spontaneously?

3. This patient has an asymptomatic younger sister. Should she get tested?

4. What is the role of radionuclide cystography (RNC) in the evaluation of VUR?

Diagnosis: Vesicoureteral Reflux

1. Grade 3 on the right, grade 4 on the left

2. Young age at diagnosis, lack of associated renal anomalies (duplication, ureteropelvic junction obstruction), lack of associated ureteral anomalies (duplication, ectopic insertion, ureterocele)

3. Yes. The sibling has a 45% chance of having reflux.

4. RNC has a much lower radiation dose than fluoroscopic VCUG but less anatomic delineation. It is best suited for follow-up studies to track resolution of known VUR. Some centers use it for sibling screening studies.

Reference

Chow JS, Lebowitz RL: Vesicoureteral reflux. In Reid J, editor: *Pediatric radiology curriculum*, Cleveland, 2005, Cleveland Clinic Center for Online Medical Education and Training. Available from: https://www.cchs.net/pediatricradiology.

Cross-Reference

Blickman JG, Parker BR, Barnes PD: *Pediatric radiology— the requisites*, ed 3, Philadelphia, 2009, Mosby, pp 146–148.

Comment

VUR is more frequent in girls than in boys and less frequent in African-American children. Reflux of infected urine leads to scarring and stunted renal growth (reflux nephropathy), as well as pyelonephritis. Long-term sequelae include hypertension and renal failure. Normally, the ureters take an angled submucosal track through the muscular bladder wall to reach their orifices in the trigone, making a one-way valve that resists backflow of urine from the bladder. If this track is short, is distorted by a ureterocele or bladder diverticulum, or misses the trigone entirely, then reflux is more likely.

VCUG is the standard method for diagnosing reflux. The aim is to fill the bladder with contrast (retrograde, through a small-diameter urethral catheter) until the patient is able to void around the catheter, thereby exposing the ureterovesical junctions (UVJ) to maximum pressure. However, if the patient voids at a low volume (often the case with infants), maximum pressure may not be achieved. Additional filling through the same catheter usually results in greater volume on the second or third cycle. Oblique views isolate each UVJ in turn. Grading is on a 5-level scale, taking into account height of contrast ascent, configuration of the calyceal angles, and distension/ectasia of the ureter and collecting system:

Grade 1: contrast in ureter only

Grade 2: contrast in ureter and renal collecting system, with no distension

Grade 3: grade 2 + blunting of the calyceal angles

Grade 4: grade 2 + reversal of the calyceal angles + distension and mild ureteral ectasia

Grade 5: distended collecting system with bulbous calyces + distended, ectatic ureter

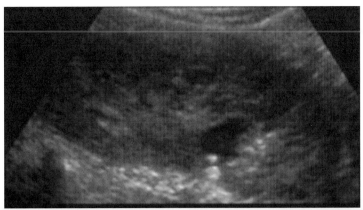

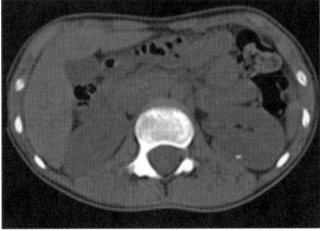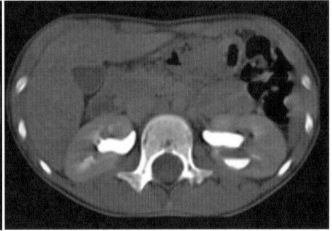

1. What are the findings in this teenage girl?

2. What is the diagnosis?

3. What are some complications of this malformation? Which is manifested in this patient?

4. How can this problem be treated?

Diagnosis: Calyceal Diverticulum

1. Ultrasound shows a cystic structure in the kidney with a small echogenic focus within it. Computed tomography (CT) shows the stone in the cystic space that, on delayed scan, contains dense contrast.

2. Calyceal diverticulum.

3. The diverticulum is the source of urinary stasis and may predispose to recurrent or refractory infection or, as in this case, stone formation.

4. A percutaneous approach was used in this patient with success. In some cases the diverticulum may need to be surgically removed.

Reference

Gearhart JP, Rink RC, Mouriquand PDE: *Pediatric urology*, Philadelphia, 2001, WB Saunders, p 134.

Comment

The calyceal diverticulum has also been called a congenital calyceal cyst. By ultrasound, the lesion appears cystic. In theory the location of the diverticulum may be more central within the kidney than the typical cortical cyst, which tends to be more peripheral. Their size is usually less than 1 cm, but they may be larger—especially if dilatation of the remainder of the collecting system exists for any reason. They usually freely connect to the collecting system and will fill with contrast on intravenous pyelogram or CT examination. It may be necessary to obtain delayed films or scans to observe the filling because the connection may be narrow. When the connection is actually stenotic, only faint contrast may be seen even on delayed imaging.

These lesions are usually asymptomatic, and no treatment is needed. In the example shown, the patient had recurrent urinary tract infection and flank pain.

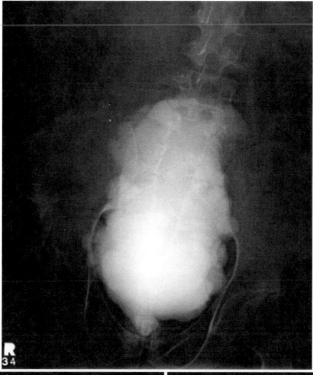

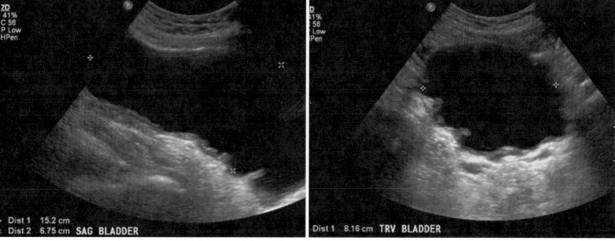

1. What are the findings in this teenage boy?

2. What is the likely cause?

3. What clinical test may be used to evaluate the patient?

4. What finding on the radiograph tells you the underlying cause of the bladder problem?

Diagnosis: Neurogenic Bladder

1. Cystogram showing elongated trabeculated bladder (Christmas tree shaped) with diverticulum formation and reflux into the prostatic ducts; sonographic evidence of thick-walled trabeculated bladder.

2. Neurogenic bladder.

3. Urodynamic study.

4. Absent posterior elements of the lower lumbar and sacral spine indicative of myelomeningocele (also note dislocated right hip).

Reference

Gearhart JP, Rink RC, Mouriquand PDE: *Pediatric urology*, Philadelphia, 2001, WB Saunders, pp 459–461.

Comment

Neurogenic bladder in children is most often associated with myelomeningocele and its variants, such as occult dysraphism and sacral agenesis. Trauma is a less likely cause; however, spinal cord, nerve root, or pelvic nerve injury can also result in neurogenic bladder. Spinal conditions such as neoplasm, infection, and transverse myelitis are the rarest causes of the condition.

Several types of neurogenic bladder exist, depending on the level of neurologic involvement (i.e., cerebral cortex, spinal cord, sacral micturition centers, or distal neural pathways). In myelomeningocele, a mixed type usually exists; the findings may change with time as the tethering of the cord may worsen and other factors, such as bowel function and urinary tract infection, come into play. Evaluation of the neurogenic bladder includes baseline and follow-up urodynamic studies, periodic ultrasound examinations, and baseline and follow-up voiding cystourethrograms as needed. The urodynamic study is done by the urologist and allows the measurement of the bladder capacities and detrusor pressures simultaneously with the electromyographic activity of the pelvic floor muscles indicative of sphincter function. Detrusor contractility may be normal, overactive, or underactive; the external sphincteric activity may be synergic (normal), dyssynergic (overactive), or inactive. The most common combination is overactive detrusor and dyssynergic sphincter activity, resulting in the elongated thick-walled bladder with trabeculations and diverticula (so-called spastic bladder) as in this example. Less commonly, normal detrusor and inactive sphincter activity results in the so-called flaccid bladder (one which empties continuously).

Treatment of the neurogenic bladder is dependent on the factors defined by the studies described previously. In most patients, clean intermittent catheterization (CIC) is the mainstay of management of the condition.

A child can accomplish CIC at a relatively young age if he or she has the mental and physical capacity to do so. The addition of pharmacologic agents and surgical procedures are reserved for special situations.

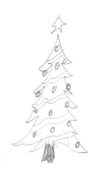

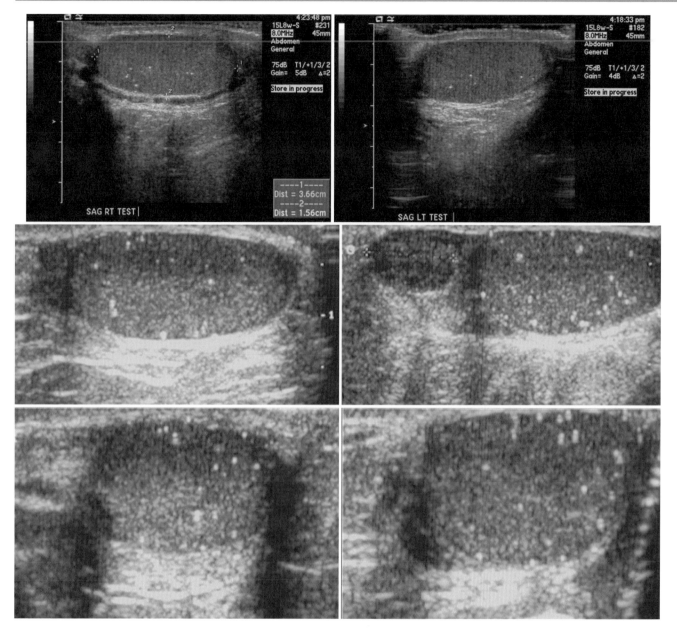

1. What is the diagnosis in this 9-year-old, previously healthy male who presented with scrotal pain and swelling?

2. What is the treatment?

3. What is the prognosis?

4. What are the predisposing or coexisting factors?

Diagnosis: Testicular Microlithiasis

1. Multiple tiny shadowing echogenic foci throughout both testes consistent with testicular microlithiasis.

2. Close follow-up is the only recommendation in cases of testicular microlithiasis.

3. The risk of testicular neoplasm, particularly germ cell tumors, increases 13 to 21 times in patients with testicular microlithiasis.

4. Coexistence of many benign and malignant pathologic conditions have been reported with testicular microlithiasis including cryptorchidism, Down syndrome, and infertility. The most important accompanying pathologic condition is testicular neoplasm, particularly germ cell tumors.

References

Cohen HL, Haller JO: Abnormalities of the male genital tract. In Kuhn JP, Slovis TL, Haller JO, editors: *Caffey's pediatric diagnostic imaging*, ed 10, Philadelphia, 2004, Mosby, p 1935.

Cast JEI, Nelson WM, Early AS, et al: Testicular microlithiasis: prevalence and tumor risk in a population referred for scrotal sonography, *AJR Am J Roentgenol* 175:1703-1706, 2000.

Comments

Testicular microlithiasis is the presence of calcifications within the lumina of the seminiferous tubules. It is an uncommon and usually incidental finding on testicular ultrasound. Studies report 13 to 21 times increased risk of testicular neoplasm, particularly germ cell tumors; therefore patients are monitored closely using ultrasound. However, imaging findings are nonspecific.

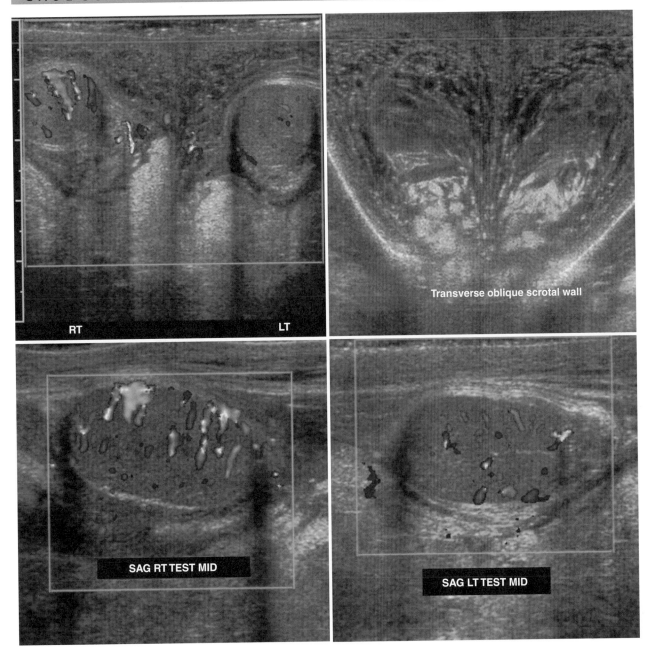

Transverse oblique scrotal wall

SAG RT TEST MID

SAG LT TEST MID

1. What are the imaging findings in this 6-year-old boy with acute scrotal swelling?

2. What is your diagnosis?

3. What is the clinical presentation?

4. What is the number one differential?

Diagnosis: Idiopathic Acute Scrotal Edema

1. Bilateral, diffuse severe edema of the scrotal wall, with normal testicles, no hydrocele; diffuse severe edema of scrotal wall is better depicted in transverse oblique images.

2. Acute scrotal edema.

3. An acute onset of scrotal swelling and erythema associated with scrotal discomfort.

4. It is most important to differentiate from entities that present with scrotal swelling that require immediate surgical attention (e.g., testicular torsion, incarcerated hernia, or other causes of acute scrotum that require immediate medical attention such as orchiepididymitis).

Reference

Lee A, Park SJ, Lee HK: Acute idiopathic scrotal edema: ultrasonographic findings at an emergency unit, *Eur Radiol* 19(8):2075-2080, 2009.

Cross-Reference

Blickman JG, Parker BR, Barnes PD: *Pediatric radiology—the requisites*, ed 3, Philadelphia, 2009, Mosby, pp 154-155.

Comment

Diffuse scrotal swelling in acute onset has a wide differential diagnosis including testicular torsion, orchiepididymitis, scrotal trauma, incarcerated inguinal hernia, testicular tumor with internal hemorrhage, and Fournier gangrene. The less commonly encountered entities are idiopathic scrotal swelling and scrotal swelling secondary to a systemic disease. The latter two entities are important to distinguish from the previously mentioned entities, because they can be treated medically and do not require surgical attention. These patients present with an acute onset of diffuse scrotal swelling without erythema or pain. In the idiopathic form, erythema always accompanies the swelling.

High-frequency ultrasonography performed with linear transducer with color Doppler analysis is the imaging modality of choice when evaluating scrotal disease. Diffuse edematous swelling in the subcutaneous fat in the scrotal wall, normal bilateral testicles with normal flow, and absence of hydrocele narrows the differentials to diffuse scrotal edema either idiopathic or secondary to a systemic disease. The idiopathic form can be unilateral or bilateral (often it is bilateral).

The presented case was known to have lupus nephritis and had laboratory evidence of nephrotic syndrome. Presence of diffuse edema in the scrotum may be explained by the inferior location of the scrotum and loose connective tissue thus enabling gravity to loculate edema. Treatment of underlying systemic disease will help to resolve scrotal edema. The idiopathic form is self-limiting and resolves spontaneously. Management includes reassurance, activity restriction, scrotal support, cooling of the scrotal wall, and close observation. Pain medication is advised as necessary. Use of medications such as steroidal and antihistaminic agents is controversial. Close follow-up with ultrasound is recommended to exclude late complications.

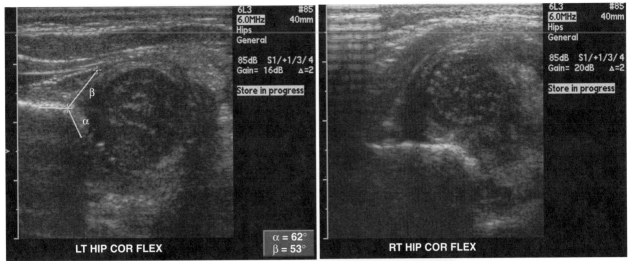

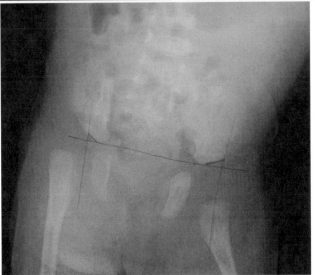

1. When is the best time to examine infants for this abnormality?

2. What clinical history raises or lowers your suspicion of a positive study?

3. What imaging procedures are used in evaluating this abnormality, and in what situations are they used?

Diagnosis: Developmental Dysplasia of the Hip

1. Because maternal hormones linger in the neonatal period and contribute to joint laxity, the first evaluation should be postponed until about 2 to 4 weeks of age.

2. Congenital developmental dysplasia of the hip (DDH) is seen more frequently in girls (8F:1M), multiple gestation, and breech presentation. Positive family history should also raise suspicion. Certain populations have higher frequency (some Asian and Native American tribal groups that swaddle infants with leg adduction and extension) and lower frequency (African-American infants).

3. Ultrasound in infants; plain film in older children; computed tomography (CT) for postoperative studies; magnetic resonance imaging (MRI) to detect complications.

Reference

Reid J: Developmental dysplasia of the hips. In Reid J, editor: *Pediatric radiology curriculum*, Cleveland, 2005, Cleveland Clinic Center for Online Medical Education and Training. Available from: https://www.cchs.net/pediatricradiology.

Cross-Reference

Blickman JG, Parker BR, Barnes PD: *Pediatric radiology—the requisites*, ed 3, Philadelphia, 2009, Mosby, pp 202–203.

Comment

The hips in infants are ideally evaluated with ultrasound, which allows both static and dynamic imaging. A linear, high-frequency transducer (7 to 10 MHz) is first oriented along the iliac bone with the femur in neutral position to obtain the coronal views. Acetabular angles are measured, using the horizontal line of the iliac bone for reference: the (alpha) angle of the iliac portion of the acetabulum should be close to 60 degrees and the (beta) angle of the cartilaginous labrum should be less than 70 degrees (first image). The femoral head should be covered at least 50% by the iliac portion of the acetabulum: this is illustrated by extending the horizontal iliac line though the femoral head (the center should lie at or below that line). The second image is a coronal view through a dysplastic, subluxed hip. Imaging the hip while rotating the femur with adduction and abduction should see the head remain stable in the joint. Transverse images through the posterior aspect of the acetabulum are obtained with the femur flexed. As the knee is pushed in a "piston" maneuver (Barlow test), the head should remain stable and not appear to rise over the acetabular margin.

Treatment initially consists of strategies to promote normal articulation, to mold the developing acetabulum and femoral head, through bracing the legs in flexion and abduction. Ultrasound can be used to follow hip development while the infant is in the brace. Pulvinar (a fibrofatty pad that normally cushions the hip joint) in abnormal position or amount can interfere with hip reduction. This is easily identified by ultrasound.

Progressive DDH can develop in older children who have spastic adduction of the lower limbs because of neurologic disease and do not go through the normal stages of motor development that lead to upright posture and walking. Anteroposterior plain film of the pelvis will reveal acetabular angles greater than 25 degrees, as demarcated by a horizontal line connecting the medial corners of the right and left triradiate cartilages (Hilgenreiner's line) and an angled line connecting the superior acetabular margin with Hilgenreiner's line on that side (third image).

Hip dysplasia develops gradually, and the accelerated pace of corrective bracing or operative reduction can lead to the treatment-related side effect of avascular necrosis of the femoral head. MRI scan may be necessary if this complication is suspected. Arthrography is usually used during open reduction to ensure anatomic placement. Low-dose CT scan of the hips is often performed to evaluate postoperative result when the child is in a spica cast.

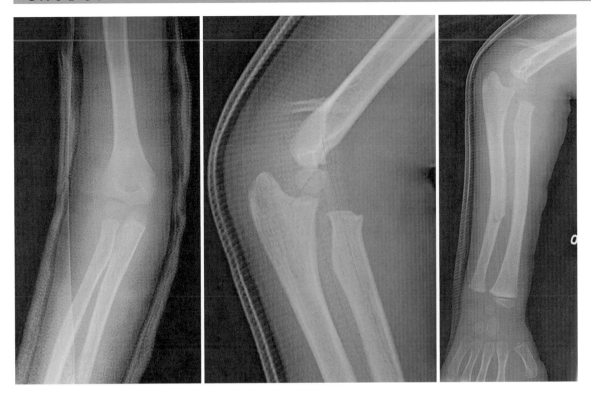

1. This 5-year-old boy fell on his outstretched arm and has pain in his elbow. He arrives in a splint and views of the elbow (first and second images) are given to you. What are the findings on the anteroposterior view of the elbow?

2. How does the lateral view of the elbow help you?

3. What do you ask for next? Why?

4. What eponym is associated with this injury?

Diagnosis: Monteggia Fracture

1. The elbow looks normal.

2. The anterior dislocation of the radial head is evident only on this view.

3. Ask for a view of the entire forearm (third image) because radial head dislocation is associated with ulna fracture.

4. Giovanni Battista Monteggia (Italian physician and surgeon, 1762 to 1815) described this fracture pattern in 1814.

Reference

Johnson KJ, Bache E: *Imaging in pediatric skeletal trauma*, Berlin-Heidelberg-New York, 2008, Springer, pp 270–272.

Cross-Reference

Blickman JG, Parker BR, Barnes PD: *Pediatric radiology— the requisites*, ed 3, Philadelphia, 2009, Mosby, pp 194–196.

Comment

These fractures occur most frequently in children between 5 and 7 years old. Seventy percent have this pattern, with anterior radial head dislocation and ulna fracture. Lateral dislocation and ulna fracture is the second-most common pattern, with posterior dislocation occurring rarely. It is also unusual to see fracture of *both* radius and ulna associated with anterior radial head dislocation. Because the forearm fracture is the more obvious injury, it can divert attention from the dislocation that, if untreated, can lead to loss of mobility.

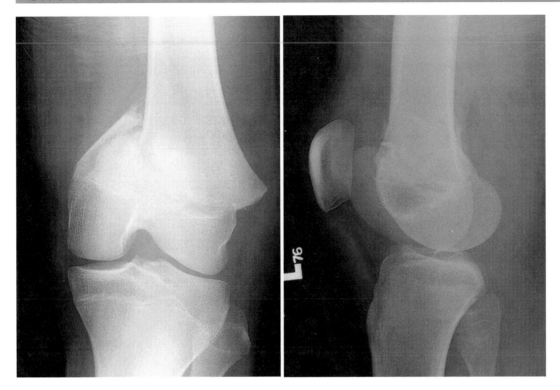

1. What kind of fracture is depicted in this teenage patient?

2. What are the other types of growth plate fractures?

3. What are the most significant complications of this type of fracture?

4. What imaging study is best in evaluating these complications?

Diagnosis: Salter-Harris Fracture

1. Salter-Harris II fracture.

2. These fractures all involve the physis but also include the metaphysis (as in this example), the epiphysis, or both.

3. Complications of this type of fracture are related to growth disturbance.

4. Plain films may be suggestive or diagnostic of premature growth plate fusion; magnetic resonance image (MRI) is more sensitive and informative.

Reference

Roger LF, Poznanski AK: Imaging of epiphyseal injuries, *Radiology* 191(2):297–308, 1994.

Cross-Reference

Blickman JG, Parker BR, Barnes PD: *Pediatric radiology—the requisites*, ed 3, Philadelphia, 2009, Mosby, pp 193–197.

Comments

Salter-Harris fractures include the following types:

Salter-Harris I: fracture completely across the physis with or without displacement

Salter-Harris II: fracture involving the physis and metaphysis

Salter-Harris III: fracture involving the physis and the epiphysis

Salter-Harris IV: fracture involving the physis, metaphysis, and the epiphysis

Salter-Harris V: axial load injury resulting in crush injury of the physis

The most common type is a Salter-Harris II fracture, representing about 75% of the injuries. These fractures are diagnosed with plain film radiography. Computed tomography is often useful to delineate multiplane complicated fractures, particularly in Salter-Harris III and IV types when the joint surface is involved.

Type II fractures infrequently result in growth disturbance. As the fractures become more severe, especially in the rare type V, growth interruption becomes more common. The prognosis is worse when the fracture involves the lower extremity, irrespective of the Salter-Harris classification. In general, the metaphysis and the epiphysis receive their arterial blood supply from separate sources so that a fracture through the physis does not result in arterial disruption. Two exceptions to this rule are the proximal femoral and distal radial epiphyseal centers, both of which receive arterial supply that crosses the physis and is disrupted in the fracture. The fracture outcome depends on the degree of arterial disruption. Early fusion of a portion or all of the growth plate is the outcome of arterial compromise. In partial fusion (i.e., involving only a portion of the growth plate), a tilted joint surface may result. In complete fusion, extremity length discrepancy is the result. Plain films are useful in monitoring healing, and growth abnormalities are often evident. Growth recovery lines not parallel to the epiphysis on follow-up films suggest a growth disturbance. MRI is the ideal imaging study to analyze the growth plate for this complication.

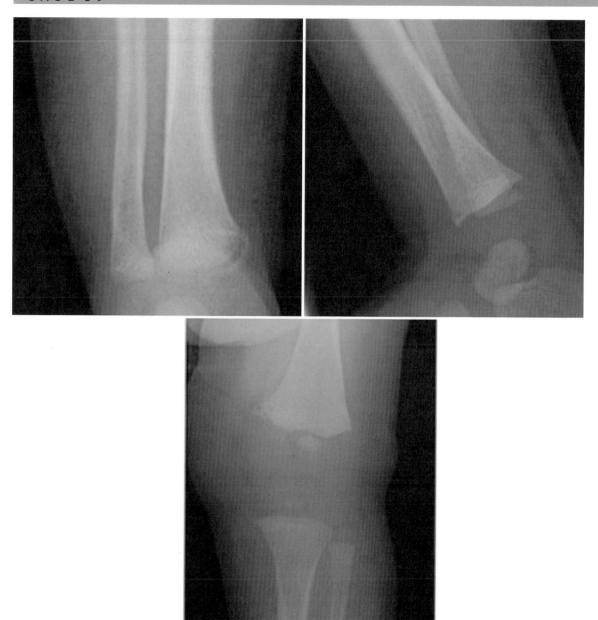

1. What do you see in the images of this 4-month-old infant?

2. In addition to these films, what other studies should be ordered on this patient?

3. Are the findings highly specific for any entity?

4. Will follow-up films be helpful?

Diagnosis: Child Abuse

1. Metaphyseal fractures.

2. Complete skeletal survey, head computed tomography and magnetic resonance imaging, ophthalmologic examination.

3. Nonaccidental trauma.

4. In situations that are highly suspicious clinically and/or in which few findings exist on the initial skeletal survey, a repeat study in 2 weeks may be useful.

Reference

Kleinman PK, Marks SC Jr: A regional approach to classic metaphyseal lesions in abused infants: the distal tibia, *AJR Am J Roentgenol* 166(5):1207-1212, 1996.

Cross-Reference

Blickman JG, Parker BR, Barnes PD: *Pediatric radiology—the requisites*, ed 3, Philadelphia, 2009, Mosby, pp 200-202.

Comments

The bucket handle fracture of the distal tibia was found first in this infant. The other fractures were clinically silent, which is usually the case in metaphyseal fractures. Any type of fracture may occur in child abuse; however, metaphyseal fractures, also referred to as classic metaphyseal lesions, are highly specific for this entity. These fractures are usually seen in the infant (younger than 12 months) and rarely seen in older children. They are frequently the result of shaking, which also may cause fatal or devastating neurologic injury. This mechanism helps to explain the often-symmetrical appearance of these fractures in the long bones. The fracture line extends for a variable distance in the primary spongiosa portion of the metaphysis of long bones and the metaphyseal equivalent elsewhere. The fracture may appear to involve the "corner" of the bone; in more extensive injury, a "bucket handle" fracture may be seen. These fractures may be more apparent in the healing phase, but dating of the injury is not usually possible because they do not heal with obvious callus formation. Over time, as the fractures heal, the metaphyseal fragments are incorporated into the adjacent bone and become less conspicuous; finally the bone becomes normal in appearance.

In addition to the metaphyseal fractures, fractures of the ribs posteriorly are also highly specific for child abuse. The mechanism for these posterior rib fractures is typically shaking with the chest gripped tightly during the assault. The fractures occur because squeezing of the thorax causes the posterior rib head to lever over the transverse process of the vertebra. This type of fracture is almost never seen in accidental trauma. Fractures can occur in other portion of the ribs as well, but these are less specific for abuse. Other mechanisms for fractures include direct blows or, in the extremities, twisting injuries.

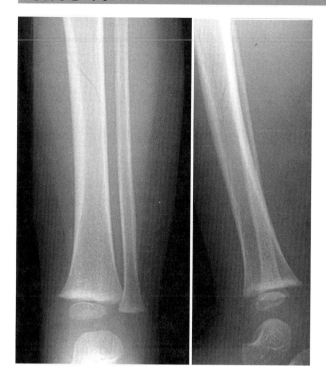

1. What is the imaging finding on the frontal and lateral views of the tibia and fibula in this 18-month-old child?

2. What is the most common presenting sign?

3. What is the mechanism of injury?

4. What other sites are common for this type of fracture?

Diagnosis: Toddler's Fracture

1. Nondisplaced spiral fracture of the midshaft tibia (i.e., toddler's fracture).

2. Refusal to bear weight or limping in a previously normally ambulating child.

3. Twist of the foot with the knee stable.

4. Midshaft, proximal or distal metaphysis of the tibia, cuboid (near calcaneal head), and calcaneus (near apophysis or along base).

Reference

Swischuk LE: *Imaging of the newborn, infant and young child*, ed 5, Philadelphia, 2004, Lippincott Williams & Wilkins, pp 775-779.

Cross-Reference

Blickman JG, Parker BR, Barnes PD: *Pediatric radiology—the requisites*, ed 3, Philadelphia, 2009, Mosby, p 197.

Comments

Toddler's fracture was originally described as a spiral fracture of the distal tibia resulting from torque or twisting of the lower leg. It has since been expanded to include other fractures that produce similar clinical findings, namely, refusal to bear weight or limp. Typically, there is a subtle, nondisplaced oblique fracture of the distal tibia in a child 9 months to 3 years of age. In addition, included are buckle fractures of the distal tibia and fibula. Fractures through the base of the first metatarsal, impaction cuboid fractures, and impaction fractures of the calcaneus are also considered toddler's fractures and typically result from direct compression. Toddler's fractures are often very difficult to identify on plain radiographs and may only be diagnosed on follow-up radiographs after 10 to 14 days with periosteal reaction and callus formation. They typically heal rapidly with no deformity. If seen in a nonambulating infant, nonaccidental trauma must be excluded.

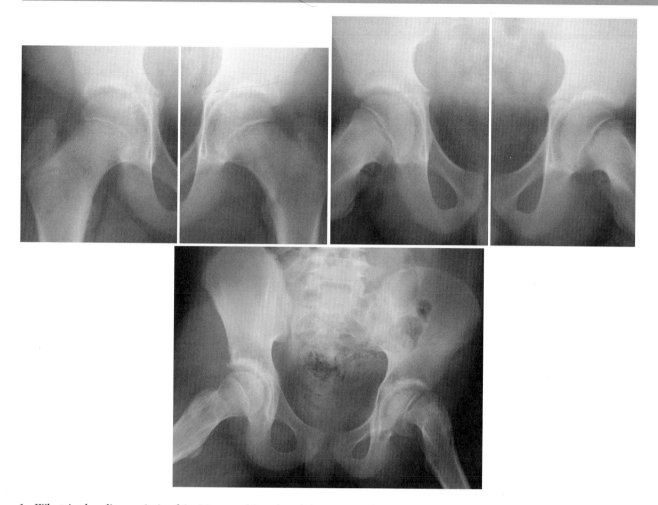

1. What is the diagnosis in this 12-year-old male adolescent? What type of Salter fracture is it?

2. How often is it bilateral?

3. Does a normal hip radiograph exclude the diagnosis?

4. What is the differential diagnosis?

Diagnosis: Slipped Capital Femoral Epiphysis

1. Slipped capital femoral epiphysis (SCFE), Salter-Harris I fracture caused by repetitive stress of weight bearing.

2. Up to 20% of SCFE injuries are bilateral at presentation.

3. No, normal hip radiograph does not exclude the diagnosis of SCFE.

4. Differential diagnosis includes Legg-Calvé-Perthes disease (younger) and inflammatory disease.

Reference

Harcke HT, Mandell GA, Maxfield BA: Trauma to the growing skeleton. In Kuhn JP, Slovis TL, Haller JO, editors: *Caffey's pediatric diagnostic imaging*, ed 10, Philadelphia, 2004, Mosby, pp 2277–2279.

Cross-Reference

Blickman JG, Parker BR, Barnes PD: *Pediatric radiology—the requisites*, ed 3, Philadelphia, 2009, Mosby, p 196.

Comments

SCFE is a Salter-Harris type I fracture of the capital femoral epiphysis, which slips posterior and medially relative to the metaphysis, toward or below Klein's line (a line drawn along the top of the femoral neck toward the acetabulum that usually transects a small portion of the capital femoral epiphysis). Findings are best seen on frog-leg views. SCFE most commonly presents with hip pain in boys (10 to 17 years old) more frequently than in girls (8 to 15 years old). African-Americans are at increased risk. Most patients are overweight. SCFE is the most common adolescent hip disorder. Radiographic findings include widening of the physis, medial and posterior displacement of the physis relative to the metaphysis, and irregularity of the metaphysis. Treatment is surgical and includes pinning to prevent further slippage and early closure of the physis. Complications include avascular necrosis.

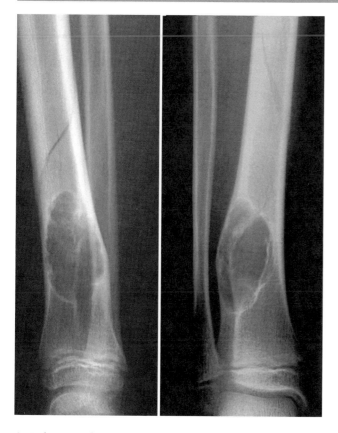

1. What are the imaging findings in this 12-year-old male patient with leg pain after trauma?

2. What is the diagnosis?

3. What is the typical prognosis?

4. What is Jaffe-Campanacci syndrome?

Diagnosis: Nonossifying Fibroma

1. Frontal and lateral views of the tibia and fibula demonstrate an eccentric oval radiolucency with a thin bulging cortex and multiple septations in the distal metaphysic of the tibia. A pathologic spiral fracture extends from the midshaft of the tibia through the lesion.

2. Nonossifying fibroma (NOF) with pathologic fracture.

3. Typically, NOFs undergo spontaneous resolution.

4. Multiple NOFs with extraskeletal congenital anomalies including café-au-lait spots, mental retardation, hypogonadism or cryptorchidism, ocular abnormality, and cardiovascular malformations is known as Jaffe-Campanacci syndrome.

Reference

Fletcher BD: Benign and malignant bone tumors. In Kuhn JP, Slovis TL, Haller JO, editors: *Caffey's pediatric diagnostic imaging*, ed 10, Philadelphia, 2004, Mosby, pp 2383-2385.

Cross-Reference

Blickman JG, Parker BR, Barnes PD: *Pediatric radiology—the requisites*, ed 3, Philadelphia, 2009, Mosby, p 189.

Comments

NOF, also known as fibroxanthoma, and fibrous cortical defect are nonaggressive developmental defects that typically occur within the metaphysis of growing long tubular bones in children, most commonly about the knee and close to the physis.

NOF typically occurs in children and adolescents; 70% occur in teenagers. The age range is reported to be 3 to 42 years.

On plain radiographs, NOF is usually an eccentric round or oval radiolucency measuring 1 to 3 cm with a thin bulging cortex. They are most commonly located within the posteromedial aspect of the distal femoral metaphysis. No associated soft tissue mass is present. These lesions are typically asymptomatic, but the increased risk of fracture, especially in larger lesions, leads to pain that is the most common presenting sign in those cases that are not diagnosed incidentally. Spontaneous resolution with associated ossification is the usual outcome of these lesions.

Differential diagnosis includes unicameral bone cyst, fibrous dysplasia, and chondromyxoid fibroma. The presence of extraskeletal congenital anomalies (e.g., café-au-lait spots, mental retardation, hypogonadism or cryptorchidism, ocular abnormality, cardiovascular malformations) in association with multiple NOFs constitutes the clinical and radiologic spectrum known as Jaffe-Campanacci syndrome.

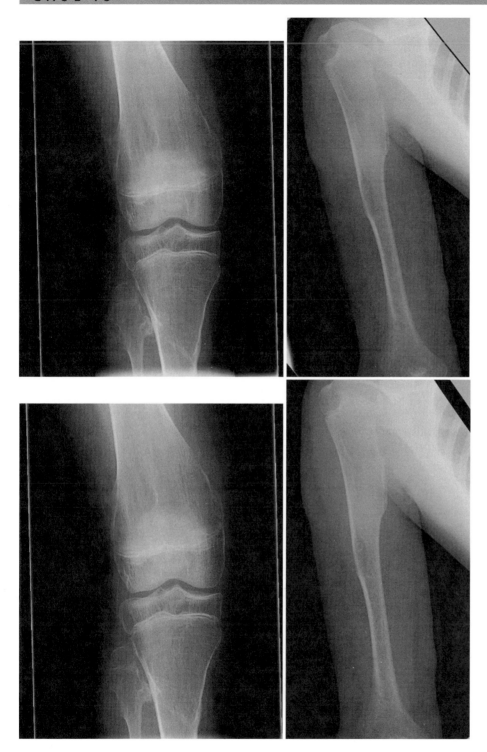

1. What is the diagnosis?

2. What are the complications of hereditary multiple exostosis (HME)?

3. Which bones are involved?

4. What is the cause of the condition?

Diagnosis: Hereditary Multiple Exostosis

1. HME, also known as *diaphyseal aclasia*

2. Complications of osteochondromas include fractures, bony deformities, neurologic and vascular injuries, bursa formation, and malignant transformation.

3. An osteochondroma can affect any bone preformed in cartilage—most frequently, the growing ends of long bones.

4. They may arise spontaneously or as a result of previous trauma.

Reference

Helms CA: Miscellaneous bone lesions. In Brant WE, Helms CA, editors: *Fundamentals of diagnostic radiology*, ed 3, Philadelphia, 2007, Lippincott Williams & Wilkins, pp 1186-1187.

Cross-Reference

Blickman JG, Parker BR, Barnes PD: *Pediatric radiology—the requisites*, ed 3, Philadelphia, 2009, Mosby, pp 168-169.

Comments

HME, also known as *diaphyseal aclasia*, is an inherited autosomal dominant disorder characterized by multiple osteochondromas or exostoses in a cartilage cap that arise from the metaphysis and point away from the adjacent joint. Osteochondromas are the most common bone tumors in children; they may be solitary or multiple and may arise spontaneously or as a result of previous trauma. When multiple, they can be associated with short stature and deformity as the result of asymmetric growth at the knees and ankles. The risk of malignant degeneration is between 1% and 20%.

In HME the osteochondromas are located close to the metaphyses and may be sessile or pedunculated. The cortex of the lesion is continuous with the cortex of the bone. Most are found at the rapidly growing ends of long bones, but they also commonly involve the medial borders of the scapulae, ribs, and iliac crests. Findings on plain radiographs are usually diagnostic; however, if a magnetic resonance image is taken, then visualization of a cartilaginous cap is typical.

Complications of osteochondromas include fractures, bony deformities, neurologic and vascular injuries, bursa formation, and malignant transformation. Axial lesions are more likely to undergo malignant transformation than peripheral lesions. HME affects both genders equally and usually appears in childhood between the ages of 2 and 10 years, with most cases discovered by the time the child is 4 years old.

HME should be differentiated from Ollier disease, which is a nonhereditary disorder characterized by multiple, usually unilateral, enchondromas that can be quite large and disfiguring. Enchondromas are benign cartilaginous neoplasms that are usually solitary lesions and arise in intramedullary bone. Plain radiographs demonstrate expansile lytic lesions containing chondroid calcifications. Solitary enchondromas have a predilection for the small bones of the hands and feet. In Ollier disease, most lesions occur in the long bones.

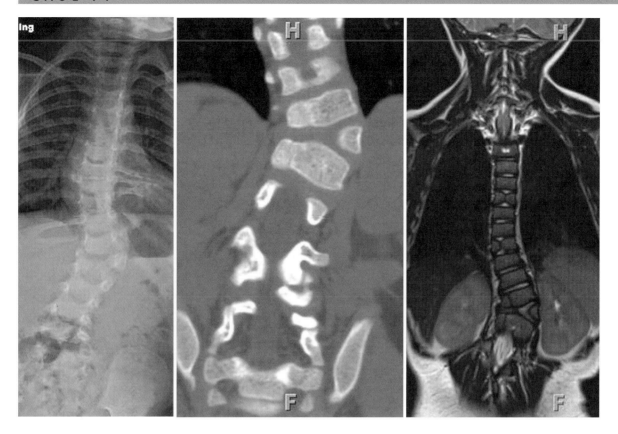

1. What are the imaging findings?

2. What is your diagnosis?

3. What is the classification system in approaching this anomaly?

4. How is the bone histology in this entity?

Diagnosis: Failure of Formation and Segmentation of the Vertebra

1. Plain anteroposterior view of the spine shows focal levoscoliosis centered in the proximal lumbar spine. The L1 is a left hemivertebrae (formation anomaly) resulting in levoscoliosis. Coronal reformat computed tomography (CT) of the lumbar spine depicts hemivertebra more clearly. Coronal T_2-weighted view shows the left L1 hemivertebra and lack of disk space between T12 and L2 on the right (segmentation anomaly). In addition, the magnetic resonance image (MRI) shows butterfly vertebrae at T6 and T9, which were not as clearly visualized on the plain radiography.

2. Segmented hemivertebrae and fused hemivertebra.

3. Formation failure can be partial or complete, and segmentation anomaly can be fully segmented, partially segmented, or unsegmented depending on the relative development of the intervertebral disk.

4. The bone histology is completely normal unless a concurrent metabolic abnormality is present.

Reference

Grimme JD, Castillo M: Congenital anomalies of the spine, *Neuroimaging Clin N Am* 17(1):1-16, 2007.

Comment

Failure of the formation and segmentation of the vertebrae are generally studied under the same title as segmentation anomalies; however, they refer to failure of different embryologic processes. Vertebral formation occurs in three steps: (1) membrane development, (2) chondrification, and (3) ossification. Failure of vertebral formation can be partial (wedge vertebrae) or complete (vertebral aplasia, hemivertebra). Abnormal vertebrae can be supranumerary or replace the normal vertebral body. Imaging findings of vertebral body formation failure is determined by deficient vertebral body failure: lateral formation failure (common) results in classic hemivertebrae; anterior formation failure (common) results in sharply angulated kyphosis; and posterior formation failure (rare) results in hyperlordotic curve. Segmentation and fusion anomalies result from aberrant vertebral column formation.

The thoracolumbar region is the most common site. Asymmetric height with relative hypoplasia of one of the chondrification centers results in a wedge vertebrae (*hemivertebrae* is the term used when one half of the vertebrae fails to form). The process may involve single or multiple levels, which may result in congenital scoliosis, kyphosis, and rotational abnormalities. Hemivertebra can be fully segmented, partially segmented, or unsegmented depending on the relative amounts of intervertebral disk space and fusion present at the levels above and below it. Most cases are asymptomatic or detected during scoliosis evaluation.

Congenital scoliosis is often associated with abnormalities of other organ systems, such as those seen in VACTERL (vertebral anomalies, anorectal atresia, cardiac defects, tracheoesophageal fistula, renal anomalies, and limb defects) syndrome. Spinal dysraphism may be associated with congenital scoliosis. Abnormal formation and segmentation of the spine can be associated with genitourinary malformations such as cloacal exstrophy. In addition, they can be encountered in various spinal cord malformations such as diastematomyelia.

Plain radiography is often used to classify the scoliotic deformity and to monitor its progression over time. CT of the spine with two-dimensional coronal and sagittal reformats allows for detailed evaluation of the anatomy. MRI provides benefits similar to CT, but it has the advantage of a lack of ionizing radiation. In addition, it provides detailed information about the spinal cord and the nerve roots. Spinal cord tethering is a contraindication to implantation of fixation devices.

Differential diagnosis would include inherited spinal dysplasias, such as mucopolysaccharidosis, and achondroplasia or vertebral fractures (pathologic or traumatic). Knowing the pedicle count per vertebral level is helpful in differential diagnosis; in a case of dysplasia or fracture, the count would be normal.

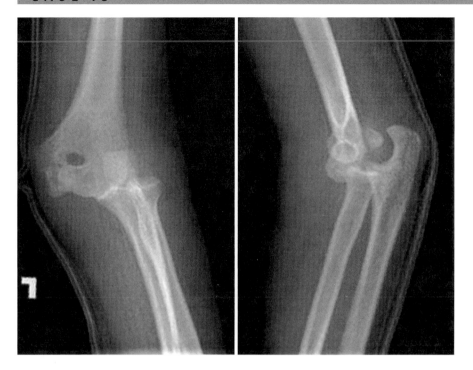

1. What are the imaging findings?

2. What is your diagnosis?

3. Does treatment require surgery?

4. Are computed tomography and magnetic resonance imaging (MRI) part of the diagnosis?

Diagnosis: Medial Elbow Dislocation and Avulsion Fracture of the Medial Epicondyle

1. Medial dislocation of the elbow with posteroinferior dislocation of the medial epicondyle, representing an avulsion fracture of the medial epicondyle.

2. Posteromedial elbow dislocation with avulsion fracture of the medial epicondyle.

3. Most cases can be reduced without surgery unless other associated fractures exist that may require surgical intervention.

4. In a great majority of the cases, plain radiographs are sufficient to evaluate the elbow before and after reduction. MRI is only necessary in cases that present with instability of the joint status postreduction to document the integrity of the ligaments and repair the ones that show impairment.

Reference

Kuhn MA, Ross G: Acute elbow dislocations, *Orthop Clin North Am* 39(2):155-161, 2008.

Cross-Reference

Blickman JG, Parker BR, Barnes PD: *Pediatric radiology—the requisites*, ed 3, Philadelphia, 2009, Mosby, pp 194-196.

Comment

The elbow is the most commonly dislocated major joint in the pediatric population, with a peak between 5 and 10 years old. The elbow joint is highly stable, relying more on the bony anatomy for stability rather than the ligaments, which explains the relatively higher incidence in the developing bony skeleton. Elbow dislocations make up 10% to 25% of all elbow injuries, and a male predominance (M:F/2:1) is seen. Sports injuries make up 40% of the cases. The mechanism of injury is believed to be a hyperextension moment. A fall on the outstretched hand is a common event.

Elbow dislocations have been traditionally described by the resulting location of the involved radius and ulna in relation to the distal humerus. This classification divides elbow dislocations into posterior, anterior, and divergent. Posterior elbow dislocations make up over 90% of all elbow injuries. Associated injuries with elbow dislocation are common in children and seen in 50% of the cases. With open physes, a medial epicondyle avulsion is the most common associated injury. Incarceration of the fragment into the elbow joint can occur. Although prereduction and postreduction radiographs reveal periarticular fractures in 12% to 60% of dislocations, operative findings have revealed unrecognized osteochondral injuries in nearly 100% of acute elbow dislocations. Anterior dislocations are usually the result of a direct posterior force to a flexed elbow. Associated fractures of the olecranon are commonly seen with anterior dislocation. Before any reduction maneuvers, assessment of neurovascular status is mandatory. Neurovascular injuries are rare but can be potentially devastating. Multiple case reports exist of brachial artery injuries with posterior dislocation.

Plain films are the modality of choice, performed in two orthogonal planes. Postreduction radiographs should be obtained, and the affected limb's neurovascular status should be documented before and after reduction. Recreation of a normal radiocapitellar line should be evident on all radiographic views.

Immediate atraumatic reduction is the goal before muscle spasm and swelling begins. Otherwise, conscious sedation or general anesthesia may be needed for muscle relaxation. If the patient complains of persisting pain and limited elbow mobility, magnetic resonance arthrography of the elbow should be considered. In the appropriate setting (and with a dedicated musculoskeletal sonographer) high-resolution ultrasound can be helpful to exclude effusion and/or osteochondral lesions.

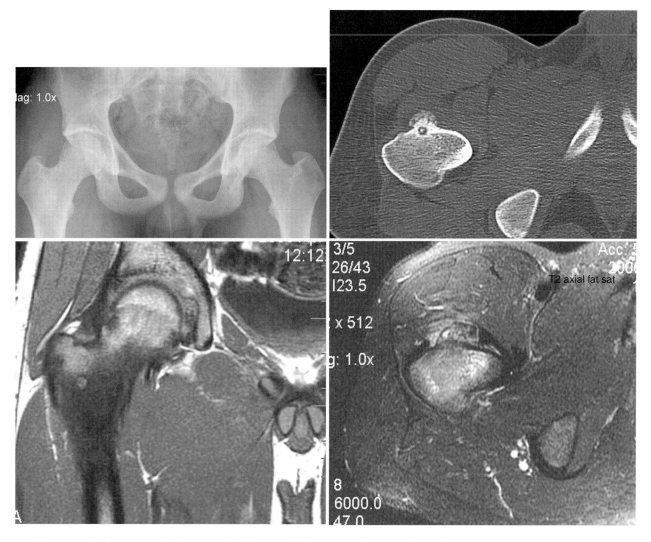

1. What are the imaging findings in this 13-year-old boy complaining of pain?

2. What is your diagnosis?

3. What is the differential diagnosis?

4. What is the commonly accepted upper limit of lesion diameter?

Diagnosis: Osteoid Osteoma

1. Plain radiography shows a radiolucent cortical lesion less than 1.5 cm in size surrounded by a sclerotic rim. Computed tomography (CT) shows the nidus more clearly. On T_1-weighted magnetic resonance image (MRI), the nidus is seen as a hyperdense focus. A T_2-weighted image shows edema in the surrounding bone marrow.

2. Osteoid osteoma.

3. Brodie abscess, stress fracture, osteoblastoma, osteoma.

4. The commonly accepted upper limit of lesion diameter is 1.5 to 2 cm. This measurement helps distinguish these lesions from osteoblastomas.

Reference

Gangi A, Alizadeh H, Wong L, et al: Osteoid osteoma: percutaneous laser ablation and follow-up in 114 patients, *Radiology* 242(1):293–301, 2007.

Cross-Reference

Blickman JG, Parker BR, Barnes PD: *Pediatric radiology—the requisites*, ed 3, Philadelphia, 2009, Mosby, p 189.

Comment

Osteoid osteomas are benign bone-forming tumors affecting the cortical bone that commonly present between 10 and 20 years of age. Most patients display classical symptoms of bone pain that flares nocturnally but is promptly relieved with salicylate agents. Osteoid osteoma has a male predominance and a male-to-female ratio of at least 2:1. The most common location of osteoid osteoma is the long bones of the lower extremities; the proximal femur is the most commonly affected, followed by the tibia. However, virtually any bone can be affected. Metaphysis and diaphysis are commonly affected sites. Sometimes the tumor can be intraarticular, where it presents with joint pain and effusion.

A plain radiograph is the initial modality of choice. CT and MRI are found to work equally well in establishing an accurate radiologic diagnosis. MRI is performed with contrast enhancement that shows peak enhancement in the early arterial phase followed by washout. Edema can be seen surrounding the nidus and may obscure visualization of the nidus. 99mTc-methylene diphosphonate (99mTc-MDP) bone scintigraphy shows increased uptake and can be used to localize the lesion.

Osteoid osteomas do not reveal progressive growth or malignant transformation. They may regress spontaneously. Therapy changes from conservative treatment using analgesic agents to surgical excision of the nidus.

A successful alternative to open surgical excision is image-guided thermal, radiofrequency, or laser ablation, which is more commonly performed because of a decreased risk of complications such as fractures.

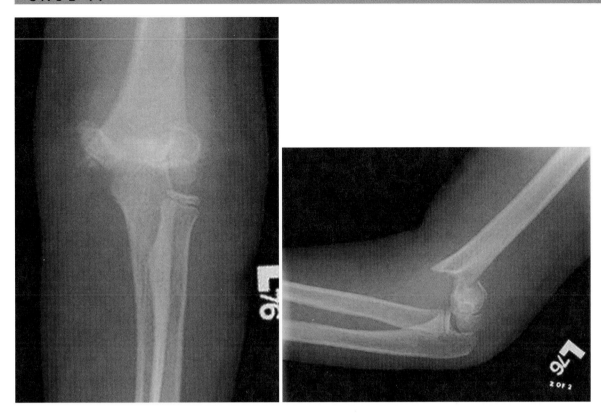

1. What is the most common stress that results in this type of fracture?

2. Name the commonly affected bones in elbow fractures in the decreasing order of frequency.

3. Describe the classification system for elbow fractures.

4. What does CRITOE stand for?

Diagnosis: Supracondylar Elbow Fracture

1. Hyperextension-rotation injuries with valgus or varus stress are the most common cause of supracondylar elbow fracture in children.

2. Supracondylar humerus (80%), lateral epicondyle of the humerus, medial epicondyle of the humerus, radius, and ulna.

3. The classification system is used for extension type injuries, which are classified according to both the direction and the degree of displacement. Gartland type I fracture, minimally displaced; Gartland type II fracture, displaced with intact posterior cortex; Gartland type III fracture, displaced with no cortical contact.

4. Ossification centers of the elbow: capitellum, radius, internal (medial) epicondyle, trochlea, olecranon, and external lateral epicondyle. Knowing the age of appearance is important for appropriate diagnosis: Capitellum, 1 year; Radial head, 5 years; Internal epicondyle (medial epicondyle), 7 years; Trochlea, 10 years; Olecranon, 10 years; External epicondyle (lateral epicondyle), 11 years. Girls tend to have an earlier appearance of ossification centers by 1 to 2 years (compared with boys).

Reference

Omid R, Choi PD, Skaggs DL: Supracondylar humeral fractures in children, *J Bone Joint Surg Am* 90 (5):1121–1132, 2008.

Cross-Reference

Blickman JG, Parker BR, Barnes PD: *Pediatric radiology—the requisites*, ed 3, Philadelphia, 2009, Mosby, pp 194–196.

Comment

Supracondylar humerus fractures are the most common elbow fractures in children, accounting for 60% to 80% of pediatric elbow fractures. These injuries are usually seen in skeletally immature patients in the first decade of life and are associated with a high rate of complications, with rates of nerve injury reported between 6% to 16%, and a high incidence of malunion leading to cubitus varus/valgus. The majority of the fractures are of the extension type, resulting in posterior displacement of the distal fracture fragment, as presented in this case. Flexion injuries are less common, result from a direct blow to the posterior aspect of a flexed elbow, and are often unstable.

Elbow radiographs are performed in two standard planes: (1) the anteroposterior view with the elbow fully extended and the forearm in supination, and (2) the lateral view, with the elbow in 90-degree flexion and the forearm in neutral position.

Many radiologic landmarks and lines are defined to help describe and diagnose elbow fractures. The anterior humeral line is defined in the lateral view as a longitudinal line drawn along the anterior cortex of the humerus and should traverse the middle third of the capitulum. The radiocapitellar line is defined in the lateral view as a line along the center of the radius and should intersect the capitulum. The articular surfaces of the elbow are contained within the joint capsule. Three fat pads lie over the capsule: (1) the anterior over the coronoid fossa, (2) the posterior over the olecranon fossa, and (3) the third over the supinator as it wraps around the radius. Fracture, hematoma, and effusion into an intact capsule may cause capsular distension, improving the visibility of the fat pads and identifying the occult fractures. In the setting of acute trauma, a visible posterior fat pad should be regarded as abnormal, particularly to the radial head or to a nondisplaced supracondylar fracture. The anterior fat pad can be seen in normal conditions; if the pad displaced anteriorly, then it is regarded as abnormal.

It is important to distinguish between flexion and extension fractures because flexion injuries often require surgical stabilization and open reduction.

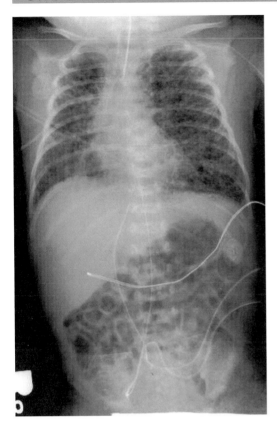

1. Is the umbilical arterial catheter (UAC) line properly placed?

2. Is the umbilical venous catheter (UVC) line properly placed?

3. Would you recommend advancement of the peripherally inserted central catheter (PICC) line?

4. Does neck extension move the endotracheal (ET) tube cranially or caudally?

Diagnosis: Supporting Devices in a Neonate

1. The UAC line is seen to the left of UVC line, making a curve at the insertion site at the site of umbilicus, downward to the iliac artery and then looping up and into the aorta. It terminates at T9, above the expected major branches of abdominal aorta, in a good location for high UAC line placement.

2. The UVC line is to the right of UAC line, terminating close to the right atrium base, in a good location.

3. No. The left-sided PICC line terminates in the mid/distal superior vena cava, central location. In addition to the placement of the catheters, the lungs are hyperinflated in this premature infant. The interstitial markings are coarse, and focal round lucencies extending from the hilum to the periphery of the lungs indicate developing interstitial emphysema.

4. Neck flexion moves the ET tube caudally, and extension moves the ET tube cranially. When evaluating proper positioning of the ET tube, attention should be paid to the location of the chin. If the chin goes down, the ET tube goes down.

Reference

Lobo L: The neonatal chest, *Eur J Radiol* 60(2): 152–158, 2006.

Comment

Vascular catheters, ET tubes, and enteric tubes are of crucial importance in a sick neonate to support the lungs, the circulatory system, and the gastrointestinal system. Plain films are essential in ensuring proper placement of these devices.

UVCs are commonly used in the first week of life. They are introduced through the umbilical stump, follow the umbilical vein, left portal vein, ductus venosus, middle or left hepatic vein, inferior vena cava, and right atrium. UVCs provide general venous access, commonly used for premature infants. They can be used for total parenteral nutrition, exchange transfusions, and central venous pressure monitoring. Ideally, the distal tip should be just above the hemidiaphragm, which generally correlates with level of T8 through T9.

UACs are used for frequent blood sampling, continuous monitoring of arterial blood pressure, and administration of medications. Ideally, for high approach UAC line placement the distal tip should be between T6 and T10 to avoid major aortic branches; for low UAC placement the distal tip should be below L3. The UAC is introduced from the umbilical stump, follows the umbilical artery, common iliac artery, and aorta. The downward looping is characteristic.

Complications of UAC and UVC include malpositioning, thrombus, thrombus along the tip of the catheter or portal venous thrombosis, pseudoaneurysm (usually arterial), and abscess formation. High positioning of the UVC in the right atrium can cause fibrillations. Plain radiographs are very helpful in determining the appropriate positioning. Ultrasound imaging with Doppler is very helpful in evaluation of thrombus or abscess formation.

ETs are used to provide respiratory support and surfactant administration in neonates. The ET tube is introduced via the upper airways, and the distal tip should reach no lower than midtrachea. This can be determined based on the visualization of the air-filled lucent trachea and carina. In cases in which the airway cannot be clearly visualized as a radiolucent column, placement of the distal tip in relation to the thoracic vertebra becomes helpful. The carina is generally at the T4 and T5 disk spaces, and the distal tip should be above the carina. Complications include migration of the ET tube to mainstem bronchi, resulting in atelectasis of the contralateral site and hyperinflation of the ipsilateral site. Misplacement of the ET tube in the esophagus may result in perforation of the esophagus or stomach.

Enteric tubes can be aimed for the stomach or duodenum as the distal locations, via nasal or oral approach. Misplacement in airways may result in pneumothorax and bronchopleural fistula, as well as hypoventilation asphyxia and accidental infusion of fluids into the lungs.

Fair Game

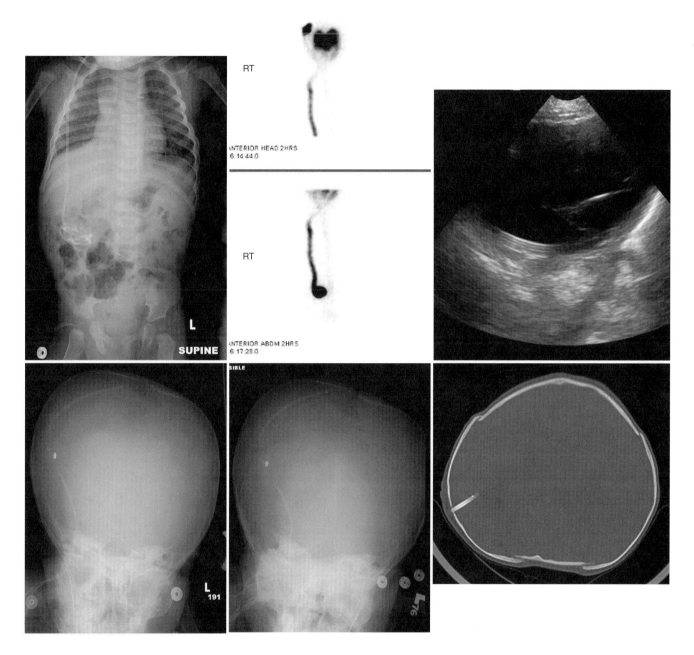

1. Patient A: This 2-year-old boy with posthemorrhagic hydrocephalus and treated with ventriculoperitoneal (VP) shunt presented with vomiting. What does the abdomen and chest view from the shunt survey show (first image)? What study is shown in the second image, and what are the findings?

2. Patient B: This 2-year-old boy with VP shunt also has gastroesophageal reflux and has been hospitalized on previous occasions with feeding intolerance. The fourth figure is a skull view from a shunt survey from one of those previous occasions. He now presents with vomiting again, and the fifth image is taken. What has changed? What is seen in the third image?

3. Patient C: This female infant was shunted soon after birth for Dandy-Walker malformation. At 5 months, a head computed tomographic (CT) scan showed what findings the last image? What complication can result from this?

Diagnosis: Ventriculoperitoneal Shunt Complications

1. The first image shows the VP shunt coiled tightly in the right upper quadrant, where before it had been free in the peritoneum. The second image is an indium 111 diethylenetriamine pentaacetic acid (In 111 DTPA) scan in which the isotope was injected in the shunt bulb. Imaging after 30 minutes shows collection of the cerebrospinal fluid (CSF) around the catheter tip, with no free drainage to the peritoneum.

2. In the month between the fourth and fifth images, the sutures have expanded. Ultrasound (third image) found an abdominal fluid collection around the tip of the shunt *(arrow)*.

3. Findings include overshunting, resulting in overlapping sutures. To prevent the complication of craniosynostosis, drainage pressure was adjusted to reexpand the brain slightly.

Cross-References

Kuhn JP, Slovis TL, Haller JO: *Caffey's pediatric diagnostic imaging*, ed 10, Philadelphia, 2004, Mosby, pp 633-636.

Aldana PR, James HE, Postlethwait RA: Ventriculogallbladder shunts in pediatric patients, *J Neurosurg Pediatr* 1(4):284-287, 2008.

Comment

As better medical care ensures greater survival of premature infants with posthemorrhagic hydrocephalus, children with closed-head trauma, and children with brain tumors, the population of children with shunted central nervous system ventricles is growing. About 40% of shunts will eventually fail, either because of infection or mechanical dysfunction. Shunting in an individual patient generally begins with the VP approach. In a tiny, premature infant, a temporizing reservoir might be installed that drains to the subgaleal space; peritoneal drainage can be established when the infant gains sufficient size and cutaneous thickness. As the child grows, infection and fibrotic reactions can render the peritoneal space unusable. The neurosurgeon can attempt to establish drainage sites in the pleural spaces, the right atrium and superior vena cava, and even in the gallbladder.

Complications of overshunting include subdural hemorrhage (occurring when the shrinking brain disrupts bridging vessels) and craniosynostosis, necessitating later surgical cranial expansion.

When the child with a shunt has a medical problem, it is axiomatic that the shunt is responsible until proven otherwise. Therefore the child generally receives a head CT scan to assess the ventricular size and position of the intracranial catheter. Next, plain films are taken that cover the pathway of the extracalvarial shunt tubing. It is essential to have comparison studies, both for the head CT scan and for the plain-film survey. Large ventricles on head CT scan may be the normal, balanced state for that patient, just as small ventricles may represent overshunting. Disconnection of the distal shunt tubing can be difficult to see when the valve is radiolucent: increasing space across the connection may be the only clue. Breakage most often occurs at the base of the neck—the point of maximum flexion stress. The tip should move around in the abdomen between studies. If it stays in one place, then it may be surrounded by fibrotic tissue and a high-pressure fluid collection might form. One exception to this is the recently perfected practice of inserting the shunt tip into the gallbladder; the tubing will remain closely coiled in the right upper quadrant, so clinical information is important to distinguish this from shunt fixation. The child can outgrow the shunt: as the torso lengthens, distal tubing is retracted from the peritoneum into the subcutaneous tunnel and can become obstructed. The chest and abdomen should also be assessed for signs of pneumonia, enteritis, or other medical problems that could cause the child's symptoms.

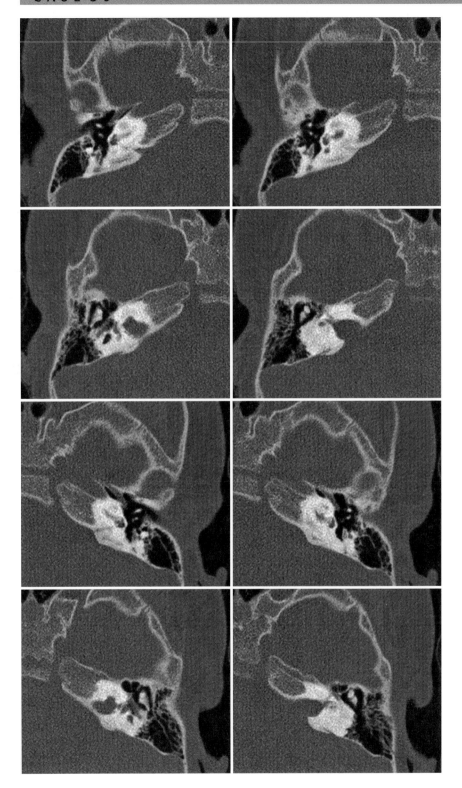

1. What are the computed tomographic (CT) findings in this 9-month-old girl?

2. Which structures are involved?

3. What is your diagnosis?

4. What is the most likely cause?

Diagnosis: Labyrinthitis Ossificans

1. Increased density of the cochlea, vestibulum, and semicircular canals.

2. Membranous labyrinth.

3. Labyrinthitis ossificans and bony obliteration of membranous labyrinth.

4. Secondary ossification after acute meningitis with *Streptococcus pneumoniae* or *Haemophilus influenzae*.

Reference

Aferzon M, Reams CL: Labyrinthitis ossificans, *Ear Nose Throat J* 80:700–701, 2001.

Comment

Membranous labyrinthitis with secondary ossification of the membranous labyrinth is the most common cause of acquired, bilateral sensorineural hearing loss (SNHL) in children. Ossification of the membranous labyrinth usually results from an infectious or traumatic insult. In children, typically SNHL occurs 2 to 18 months after an acute meningitis episode. The most frequent agents include *S. pneumoniae* and *H. influenzae*. The ossification occurs within the lumen of the otic capsule in response to the destructive, inflammatory process. The most common involved inner ear structure is the scala tympani of the basal turn. Clinically, a near complete deafness and vestibular malfunction may develop. Clinicians believe that extension of bacterial meningitis into the inner ear structures evolves along the cochlear aqueduct or internal auditory canal. Deafness after bacterial meningitis is observed in 5% to 20% of cases. Unfortunately, profound labyrinthine ossification is associated with a very poor prognosis.

Diagnosis is likely based on the combination of findings on high-resolution petrous bone CT and a matching positive, previous history of bacterial meningitis. CT may reveal an increased density of the cochlea and vestibulum. In early cases or in mild forms, the fibrosis and osteoid deposition may go undetected by CT. Magnetic resonance imaging (MRI) is especially helpful to rule out other reasons for acute deafness. In rare cases, during the acute phase, contrast-enhanced MRI may show an increased enhancement of the labyrinthine membrane. Prognosis has significantly improved because of the advent of cochlear implants.

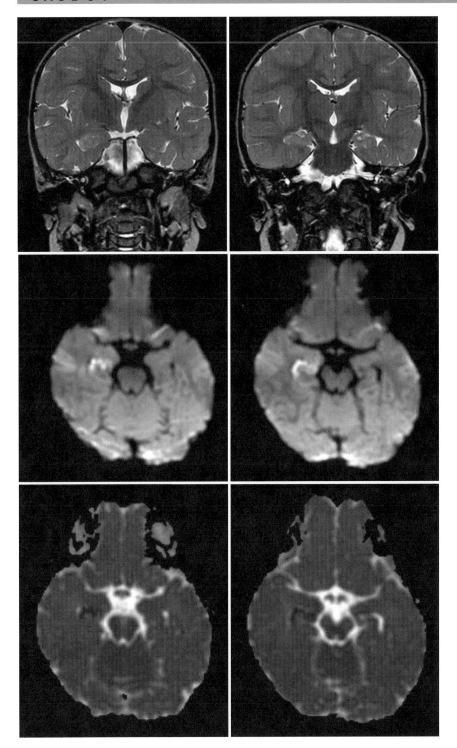

1. What are the imaging findings on the T$_2$-magnetic resonance image (MRI) in this 16-month-old girl with respiratory infection and a prolonged febrile seizure?

2. Which additional functional information is seen on diffusion-weighted imaging?

3. What is the most likely diagnosis?

4. What condition is this child at risk to develop on follow-up?

Diagnosis: Acute Hippocampal Injury after Febrile Seizure

1. T_2-hyperintense swelling of the right amygdaloid body and hippocampus.

2. Restricted diffusion and cytotoxic edema within the right hippocampus.

3. Ischemic injury of the right hippocampus because of prolonged febrile seizure.

4. Mesial temporal sclerosis with intractable seizures.

Reference

Provenzale JM, Barboriak DP, VanLandingham K, et al: Hippocampal MRI signal hyperintensity after febrile status epilepticus is predictive of subsequent mesial temporal sclerosis, *AJR Am J Roentgenol* 190:976–983, 2008.

Comment

Prolonged or complex febrile seizures in early childhood may result in ischemic injury of the hippocampus with subsequent development of mesial temporal sclerosis. Mesial temporal sclerosis is associated with temporal lobe seizures. Febrile status epilepticus is defined as a seizure that lasts at least 30 minutes or a series of seizures lasting more than 30 minutes without interictal recovery in the setting of a febrile disease. Experimental animal studies showed that seizure-related injury is especially pronounced in the pyriform cortex and amygdale; however, the hippocampus is also involved. Acute MRI showed that the T_2 hyperintensity of the hippocampal structures is preceded by a reduction of the apparent diffusion coefficient indicating cytotoxic edema. Histologically, the edema is rapidly followed by neuronal necrosis and tissue fragmentation. Provenzale and colleagues showed a strong correlation between the degree of hippocampal signal abnormality on acute imaging and subsequent hippocampal damage (respectively, development of mesial temporal sclerosis). Provenzale and colleagues also concluded that the identification of a marked signal abnormality after a prolonged febrile seizure might warrant the use of neuroprotective agents in the future.

Differential diagnosis may include a low-grade ganglioneuroma, astrocytoma, or a dysembryoplastic neuroepithelial tumor. High-resolution imaging of the temporal lobe usually allows the clinician to differentiate between acute postictal hippocampal swelling and a neoplasm or malformation.

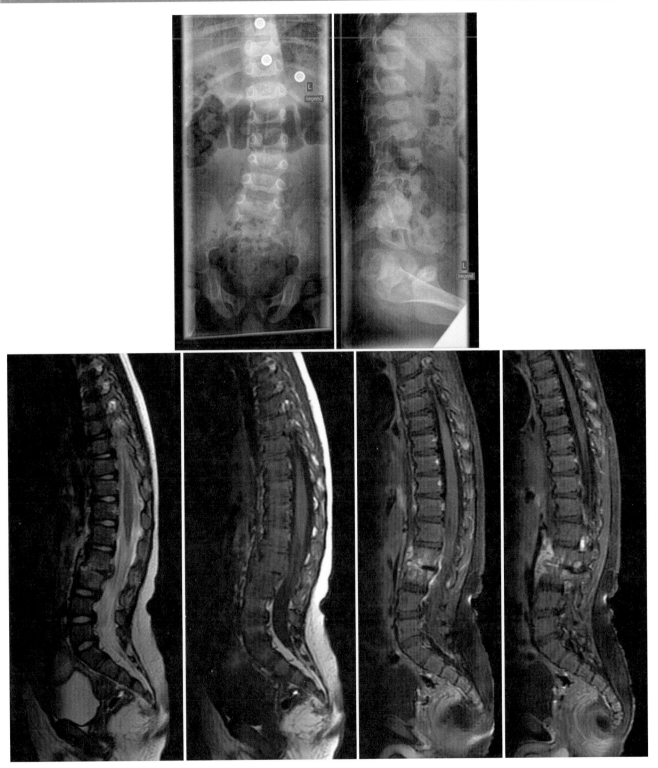

1. What are the imaging findings in this 14-month-old boy with left hip pain?

2. What is seen on contrast-enhanced magnetic resonance imaging (MRI)?

3. What is the final diagnosis?

4. What is the most frequent causative agent?

Diagnosis: Spondylodiscitis

1. Levoscoliosis, narrowed disk space between L2 and L3, and irregular endplates L2 and L3.

2. Narrowed disks L2 and L3, adjacent bone marrow edema and contrast enhancement, and mild epidural enhancement.

3. Spondylodiscitis.

4. *Staphylococcus aureus.*

Reference

Kayser R, Mahlfeld K, Greulich M, et al: Spondylodiscitis in childhood: results of a long-term study, *Spine* 30:318–323, 2005.

Cross-Reference

Blickman JG, Parker BR, Barnes PD: *Pediatric radiology—the requisites*, ed 3, Philadelphia, 2009, Mosby, pp 290–291.

Comment

Childhood spondylodiscitis is a rare disease; the exact incidence is unclear. In spondylodiscitis, both the disk and the adjacent vertebral bodies are infected. In adults, rarely an isolated diskitis is seen. In children, because of the differences of the blood supply of the developing spine, an isolated diskitis may be observed more frequently. The clinical presentation is frequently non-specific and may include refusal to walk or sit, back pain, inability to flex the lumbar spine, spinal scoliosis, and a loss of the normal lumbar lordosis. In addition, children may present with hip pain. Laboratory tests usually show nonspecific signs of infection, with a slight to moderately increased white blood cell count. Blood cultures are frequently negative. Initial radiographic studies frequently include an ultrasound of the hip as a first step, combined with radiography of the pelvis and spine. The radiography of the spine is frequently negative in the acute phase, because the typical radiographic findings usually do not appear until 2 to 3 weeks after onset of symptoms. Consequently, the diagnosis of a spondylodiscitis is usually delayed. Imaging findings on radiography include narrowing of the intervertebral disk, irregularity of the vertebral endplates, scoliosis, and possibly a widened paraspinal soft tissue line or an obscured psoas contour. Gas inclusions indicate abscess formation. MRI is the imaging modality of choice. The disk is usually narrowed and may show a strong contrast enhancement. In addition, T_2-hyperintense bone marrow edema is seen in the adjacent vertebral bodies. The adjacent soft tissue may enhance, and an extension into the spinal canal with a possible epidural abscess should be excluded. In addition, a typical complication is an abscess formation in the adjacent paravertebral soft tissues, including a psoas abscess.

The cause of childhood spondylodiscitis remains unclear. Most frequently a generalized infection with sepsis is considered. Trauma, injections, or punctures may also be considered. *S. aureus* is the most frequently found organism in nontuberculous spondylodiscitis. Pneumococci, salmonella, and *Escherichia coli* infection are less common. Tuberculous spondylodiscitis is again on the rise and should always be considered. The therapeutic consequences are considerable. In nontuberculous spondylodiscitis, antibiotic agents and immobilization are usually recommended. If an epidural or paravertebral abscess develops, then abscess drainage is recommended. After the acute infection has resolved, frequently local fibrosis or bony ankylosis develops in the affected spinal segment.

Back pain may also result from spondylolysis; spondylolisthesis; traumatic injuries; disk degeneration and herniation; Scheuermann disease; tumors (primary, secondary, and hematogenous); and miscellaneous conditions (e.g., metabolic disorders, sickle cell disease, osteoporosis).

Refusal to walk, nocturnal waking with crying, and back pain in general in a child should always alert the clinician to the possibility of a spondylodiscitis.

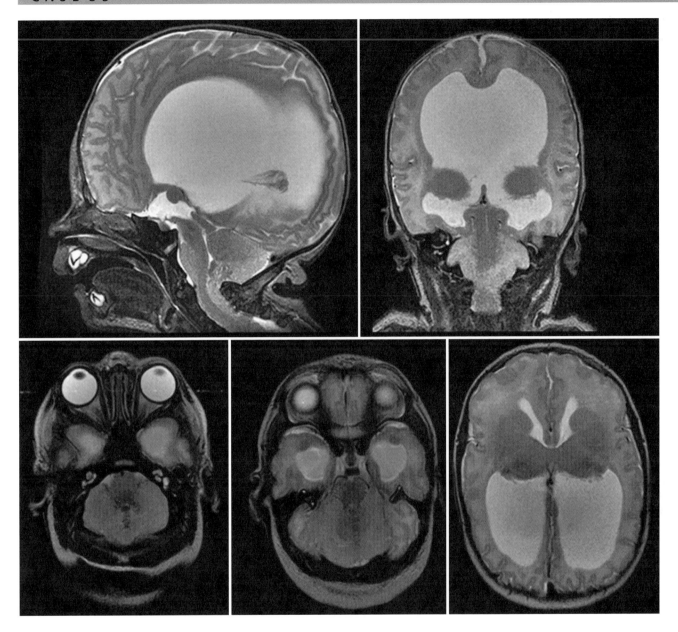

1. Summarize all visible imaging findings.

2. What is the diagnosis?

3. This condition is usually associated with what problem?

4. Which fruits are used to describe the findings on prenatal ultrasound?

Diagnosis: Arnold-Chiari II Malformation

1. Small posterior fossa, embracement of the brainstem, tectal beaking, tonsillar herniation, kinking of the cervical cord, compressed brainstem, colpocephaly, hypoplastic falx cerebelli, corpus callosum dysgenesis or agenesis, large massa intermedia, and occipital stenogyria.

2. Arnold-Chiari II malformation.

3. Open (nonskin covered) myelomeningocele.

4. Lemon-shaped calvarium and banana-shaped cerebellum.

Reference

Barkovich AJ: *Pediatric neuroradiology, diagnostic imaging*, Salt Lake City, 2007, Amirsys Inc, pp III 16–III 19.

Cross-Reference

Blickman JG, Parker BR, Barnes PD: *Pediatric radiology— the requisites*, ed 3, Philadelphia, 2009, Mosby, pp 272–274.

Comment

The Arnold-Chiari II malformation is named after Dr. Julius Arnold and Dr. Hans Chiari. This is a complex malformation that primarily involves the posterior fossa, which is too small. An extensive, complex combination of supra- and infratentorial malformations (and therefore findings) result from this condition. Arnold-Chiari II malformation is present in all patients with an open, nonskin-covered myelomeningocele. Clinicians believe that Arnold-Chiari II malformation results, at least in part, from leakage of cerebrospinal fluid from the open neural tube, which may prevent an adequate expansion of the rhombencephalic vesicle (believed to produce the small posterior fossa). Most patients are diagnosed prenatally. Functional outcome depends on the degree of hydrocephalus and the extent of the cerebral- and cerebellar-associated malformations. Magnetic resonance imaging is the best imaging modality to summarize all findings. Imaging findings include the small posterior fossa, a squeezed cerebellum and brainstem (resulting in a compression of the brainstem against the clivus), herniation of the cerebellar tonsils into the upper cervical spinal canal with kinking of the spinal cord, embracement of the brainstem by the cerebellar hemispheres, deformity (beaking) of the tectal plate, ascending herniation of the superior cerebellum through the tentorium cerebelli, supratentorial hydrocephalus with colpocephaly, thinning and/or dysgenesis of the corpus callosum, large massa intermedia, and a fenestrated hypoplastic falx cerebri with interdigitation of the mesial gyri.

The occipital cortex may mimic polymicrogyria, which Barkovich has described as stenogyria.

Arnold-Chiari II malformation may be associated with syringohydromyelia in 50% to 70% of children. An increased incidence of diastematomyelia also exists.

Diagnosis is frequently made during the prenatal screening. Increased α-fetoprotein is highly suggestive of an open myelomeningocele. On prenatal ultrasound the downward displacement of the flattened and elongated cerebellum mimics a banana, whereas the inward depression of the frontal bones mimics a lemon.

Most children require a ventriculoperitoneal shunt to treat the hydrocephalus. Prognosis is variable and depends on the degree of hydrocephalus and associated malformations.

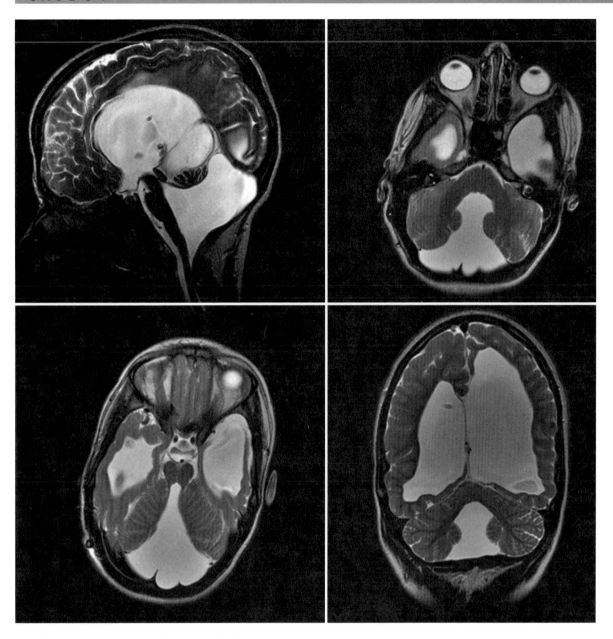

1. What are the presented imaging findings?

2. What is your diagnosis?

3. What are the differential diagnoses of cystic posterior fossa lesions?

4. What additional lesions may occur with the presented syndrome?

Diagnosis: Dandy-Walker Malformation

1. Cystic dilation of the fourth ventricle, hypoplastic elevated and rotated upper vermis, enlarged posterior fossa, hydrocephalus, and keyhole appearance of the fourth ventricle.

2. Dandy-Walker malformation (DWM).

3. Blake pouch, retrocerebellar arachnoid cyst, and mega cisterna magna.

4. Hydrocephalus, corpus callosum dysgenesis, migrational abnormalities (gray matter heterotopias, polymicrogyria, schizencephaly), occipital encephaloceles, and hydromyelia of the cervical cord.

Reference

Patel S, Barkovich AJ: Analysis and classification of cerebellar malformations, *AJNR Am J Neuroradiol* 23:1074–1087, 2002.

Cross-Reference

Blickman JG, Parker BR, Barnes PD: *Pediatric radiology— the requisites*, ed 3, Philadelphia, 2009, Mosby, pp 212–214.

Comment

DWM is named after the neurosurgeon Walter E. Dandy and the neurologist Arthur E. Walker. A DWM is characterized by a cystic dilation of the fourth ventricle because of defective development of the anterior and posterior velum medullare. The vermis is hypoplastic or may be completely absent. A spectrum of DWM is known, and depending on the degree of malformation, different names are used. The more extensive anomalies are known as classic DWM or DW-variant; the less severe forms are known as *Blake pouch cyst* or mega cisterna magna. It should be kept in mind that not every cystic lesion within the posterior fossa is a DWM. Differential diagnosis includes a retrocerebellar cyst. In addition, DWM should be differentiated from a cerebellar hypoplasia or brainstem malformation, as well as from an infarcted cerebellum. The classic DWM is characterized by a cystic dilation of the fourth ventricle, usually with an absent choroid plexus, an upward rotated hypoplastic vermis, a large posterior fossa with elevation of the torcular herophili, and elevated straight sinus. The tentorium cerebelli may be hypoplastic. Frequently a supratentorial hydrocephalus occurs. Hydrocephalus does not have to be present at birth. In 60% of patients, associated findings are seen that include hydrocephalus, corpus callosum dysgenesis, migrational abnormalities (gray matter heterotopias, polymicrogyria, schizencephaly), occipital encephaloceles, and hydromyelia of the cervical cord. The neurocognitive development depends on the associated malformations; a majority of children will have a mental retardation. In addition, DWM is reported to be associated with cardiac anomalies and polydactyly. Magnetic resonance imaging (MRI) easily makes the diagnosis. A multiplanar MRI depicts all previously described findings. Differential diagnosis from a Blake pouch cyst and a mega cisterna magna may be challenging. A key feature is the identification of an intact vermis. In addition, DWM should be differentiated from acquired injuries of the cerebellum and vermis. Prognosis may differ significantly. Frequently, a DWM is diagnosed intrauterine by prenatal ultrasound examination. The fourth ventricle may have a typical keyhole appearance.

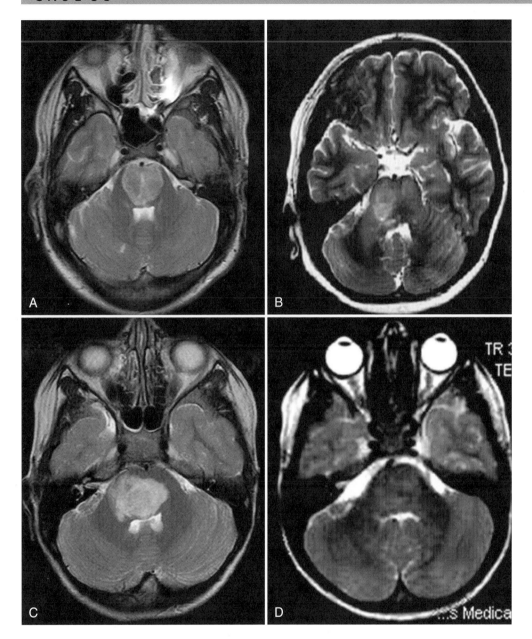

1. What are the four categories of the pathologic condition shown in these four different children?

2. What are the four diagnoses?

3. Place these children in order according to their prognosis, from good to poor.

4. Which child or children will most likely display additional lesions in the brain?

C A S E 5 5

Diagnosis: Various Brainstem Lesions

1. Ischemia, infection, tumor, and phakomatose.

2. Acute brainstem ischemia, acute disseminated encephalomyelitis (ADEM), diffuse infiltrative brainstem glioma, and unidentified bright objects (UBOs) in neurofibromatosis.

3. D, B, C, and A.

4. The children in categories B (basal ganglia and thalami) and D (related to the neurofibromatosis).

Cross-Reference

Blickman JG, Parker BR, Barnes PD: *Pediatric radiology—the requisites*, ed 3, Philadelphia, 2009, Mosby, pp 264–265.

Comment

In children, many lesions may mimic primary brain tumors. A diffuse infiltrative brainstem glioma may have a long, benign course with only minimal clinical symptoms, significantly delaying diagnosis. In addition, symptoms may be attributed to various other causes. Diffuse infiltrative brainstem gliomas have a very slow growth and respect functional neurological center for a long time. Hydrocephalus occurs usually late during the course of the disease. Acute brainstem infarction is rare in children and presents with an acute onset of severe neurologic deficits, including various cranial nerve palsies and frequently dysregulation of respiration, hypoventilation, and dysregulation of temperature control. Prognosis is poor; most children die in the acute phase or may progress into a *locked in* syndrome. Acute brainstem infarction shows restricted diffusion on diffusion-weighted imaging and is usually symmetric in distribution. A thrombus within the basilary artery should be excluded. A mild mass effect may be observed because of the reactive edema. ADEM is an autoimmune reactive inflammation in response to a previous infection—frequently an upper respiratory tract infection. Lesions are frequently multifocal and involve the brainstem, basal ganglia, and thalami. Symptoms may be acute and diffuse. On imaging, lesions are T_2 hyperintense, ill defined, and show a mild mass effect. On diffusion-weighted imaging, lesions usually show an increased diffusion compatible with vasogenic edema. If treated early, symptoms and lesions may resolve completely. UBOs are seen in neurofibromatosis and are not yet completely understood. These lesions are benign and usually without any clinical symptoms related to their location, extent, and size. Lesions are ill defined and T_2 hyperintense, may show mild mass effect, and infrequently show a contrast enhancement. Lesions may change over time or disappear completely. Diagnosis is made in the setting of a neurofibromatosis. Multiple additional lesions may be seen throughout the brain.

It is essential to correlate imaging findings with the clinical findings to identify or rule out additional lesions and to use all current imaging modalities and functional sequences available to differentiate and characterize tumors from the various tumorlike lesions.

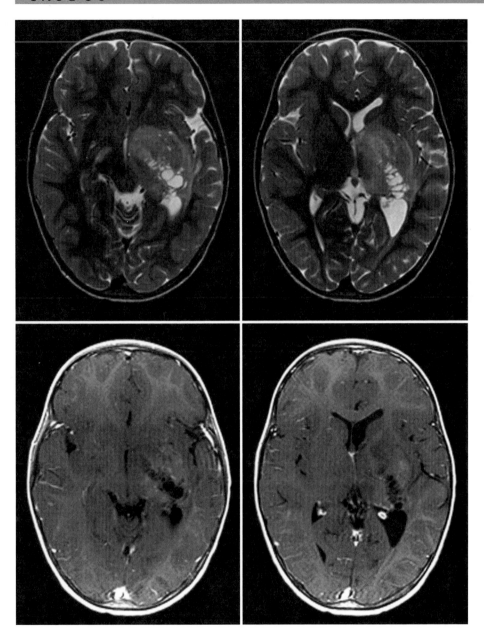

1. What are the imaging findings in this 12-year-old girl with dystonia?

2. What is the diagnosis?

3. What are the most likely histologic diagnosis and grade?

4. What are the most likely findings on proton magnetic resonance spectography (^{1}H-MRS) measured within the lesion?

CASE 56

Diagnosis: Cerebral Astrocytoma

1. Ill defined, T_2-hyperintense mass lesion within the left thalamus, internal capsule and basal ganglia, minimal contrast enhancement, multiple small cysts, minimal edema, mild obstruction of left lateral ventricle.

2. Cerebral astrocytoma.

3. A low-grade fibrillary astrocytoma.

4. Increased cholin and reduced N-acetylaspartate (NAA) concentration.

Cross-Reference

Blickman JG, Parker BR, Barnes PD: *Pediatric radiology— the requisites*, ed 3, Philadelphia, 2009, Mosby, p 252.

Comment

Cerebral astrocytomas are the most frequent supratentorial neoplasms in childhood. They represent more than 30% of all childhood supratentorial tumors. The majority of cerebral astrocytomas are fibrillary astrocytomas and may be of various degrees of malignancy; most of them are, however, low grade. Pilocytic astrocytomas are, with exception of a location within the hypothalamic-chiasmatic region, rare in a supratentorial location. The tumor may be solid, solid with necrosis, or solid with multiple cysts. Tumors are frequently in a deep location involving the thalamus or basal ganglia and may extend into the mesencephalon. On magnetic resonance image, low-grade variants are typically T_2 hyperintense and show minimal or no contrast enhancement. Because the lesion diffusely infiltrates the adjacent brain, tumor borders are usually ill defined. The mass effect can be minimal or significant and complicated by obstructive hydrocephalus because of a compression of the adjacent ventricles. Higher-grade malignancies, especially a grade IV astrocytoma or glioblastoma multiforme, typically show a more extensive degree of contrast enhancement with big tumor cysts and extensive vasogenic edema. These lesions may be mistaken for abscesses. Diffusion-weighed imaging (DWI) is especially helpful in differentiating abscesses from tumor necrosis, because an abscess will be characterized by a restricted diffusion, whereas a necrotic tumor cyst will show an increased diffusion rate. Symptoms depend on the location of the tumor and may include seizures, focal neurologic deficits, or symptoms related to increased intracranial pressure, either by the tumor or by a complicating obstructive hydrocephalus. Currently, functional imaging, including DWI, diffusion tensor imaging, perfusion-weighted imaging, and ^{1}H-MRS may help to characterize and determine the grade of malignancy of the tumor; however, a final histologic diagnosis is not yet possible. Tumor biopsy remains the gold standard for diagnosis. Therapy is determined by the location, age, and clinical symptoms. A deep, central location usually prevents surgical resection; a hemispheric location is more accessible for a surgical resection or at least tumor debulking followed by either chemotherapy and/or radiotherapy.

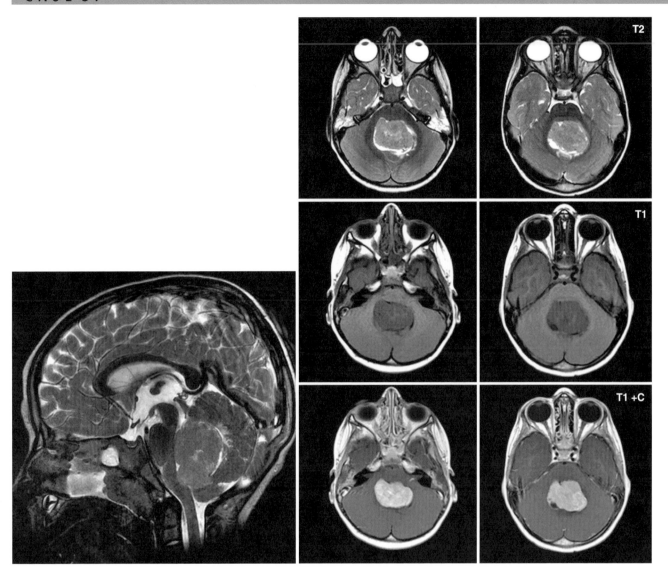

1. What are the imaging findings in this 15-month-old boy?

2. What is the most likely diagnosis?

3. What are the four most frequent tumors in the posterior fossa in children?

4. What is one of the most significant prognostic factors for long-term survival?

Diagnosis: Medulloblastoma

1. A large, solid, and contrast-enhancing tumor dorsal to the fourth ventricle; an ill-defined dorsal tumor border with some edema within the vermis; and T_2 hypointense with high cellularity.

2. Medulloblastoma dorsal to the fourth ventricle originating in the vermis.

3. Pilocytic astrocytoma, medulloblastoma, brainstem glioma, and ependymoma.

4. Residual tumor volume after neurosurgical resection.

Cross-Reference
Blickman JG, Parker BR, Barnes PD: *Pediatric radiology—the requisites*, ed 3, Philadelphia, 2009, Mosby, p 243.

Comment
Medulloblastoma is, depending on the age and gender of the patient, one of the most frequent primary neoplasms of the posterior fossa. Medulloblastoma is especially frequent in boys in their first decade of life. Overall, medulloblastoma (25%) is second to pilocytic astrocytoma (35%). Brainstem gliomas (25%) and ependymomas (12%) are the third and fourth most frequent tumors of the posterior fossa in children. In total, these four variants represent 97% of all posterior fossa tumors. Medulloblastomas most frequently arise dorsal to the fourth ventricle either in the midline (vermis, 75% to 90%) or in a somewhat more lateral position (10% to 15%; also known as lateral medulloblastoma). Consequently, the fourth ventricle is pushed anteriorly and serves as an anterior tumor border. The compression of the fourth ventricle may result in an obstructive hydrocephalus. Clinical symptoms are either related to the obstructive hydrocephalus or to local tumor infiltration and may include ataxia, gait disturbance, nausea, vomiting, and headaches. Medulloblastomas have a high cellularity and are consequently dense on computed tomography. On magnetic resonance imaging the lesions can be differentiated from ependymomas, which are typically located within the fourth ventricle (in contrast to the medulloblastomas, which are primarily located dorsal to the fourth ventricle). Medulloblastomas usually display an ill-defined dorsal border because of infiltration of the adjacent vermis or cerebellar hemispheres; they are T_1 hypointense to isointense and T_2 isointense or hyperintense. Contrast enhancement may be strong but is occasionally absent. Cerebrospinal fluid (CSF) metastases may occur when the tumor has invaded the fourth ventricle. Tumor metastases may be seen within the third ventricle and lateral ventricles or along the spinal cord. A preoperative work-up should include the entire spinal axis. Prognosis depends on the residual tumor bulk after neurosurgical resection. The smaller the residual component, the better the prognosis. The residual tumor component is even of higher prognostic significance than the initial tumor size. In addition, the histology, immunohistochemistry, and neurogenetic results will also help to determine prognosis. Adjuvant treatment is decided by the combined information collected by imaging, immunohistochemistry, neurogenetic analysis, and residual tumor bulk after neurosurgery. Prognosis significantly improved in the last decade, with good long-term prognosis in most cases.

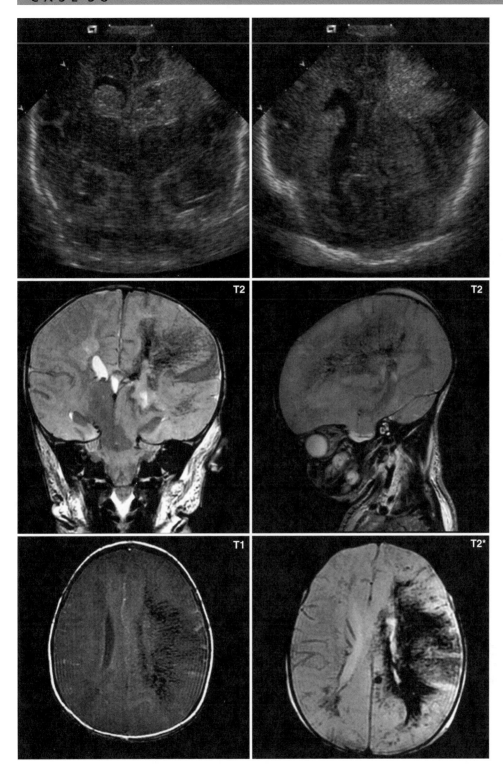

1. What are the findings on head ultrasonography for this preterm neonate?

2. What is the diagnosis and grading?

3. What are the findings on magnetic resonance imaging (MRI)?

4. What is the anatomic correlation to the T_2 and T_2 hypointense lines and lesions?

Diagnosis: Germinal Matrix Hemorrhage with Venous Infarction

1. Bilateral germinal matrix hemorrhage, mild hydrocephalus, and focal fan-shaped hyperechoic signal of the left periventricular white matter.

2. Bilateral germinal matrix hemorrhage (GMH). Grading is: right, grade III; left, grade IV.

3. Extensive T_2 and T_2 hypointense lesions with confluent areas within the left hemispheric white matter and mild diffuse brain edema.

4. Thrombosed intramedullary veins because of obstructed, subependymal veins.

Cross-Reference

Blickman JG, Parker BR, Barnes PD: *Pediatric radiology— the requisites*, ed 3, Philadelphia, 2009, Mosby, p 235.

Comment

The germinal matrix is a highly perfused cell layer located along the ventricles from which the neurons originate that migrate toward the cerebral cortex. The germinal matrix is characterized by a high metabolic activity and is vulnerable for focal hemorrhages, especially in the preterm child. During ongoing development and maturation, the germinal matrix will progressively involute and finally disappear completely. Consequently, the risk for developing a GMH decreases with progressive gestational age.

GMHs are classified into four grades. Grade I is defined as a focal hemorrhage confined to the germinal matrix. In grade II the hemorrhage will rupture into the ventricles that are not widened, whereas in grade III GMH the ventricles will be widened. This hydrocephalus is believed to result from focal adhesions along the ventricles, especially at the sylvian aqueduct and the outlets of the fourth ventricle, as well as by obliteration of the pachionic granulations. GMH grade IV has previously been defined as a GMH with extension into the adjacent hemispheric white matter (grade IV GMH is believed to represent a venous ischemia of the periventricular white matter because of compression and/or thrombosis of the deep, subependymal venous system by the hemorrhage). Secondary hemorrhagic conversion may complicate the hemorrhage. Clinically, grades I and II GMH may go undetected or may result in a focal seizure. Grade III is evident because of an increasing head circumference and neurologic instability. The development of a hydrocephalus is the major complication of GMH. Obstructive hydrocephalus may require frequent cerebrospinal fluid (CSF) punctures or even placement of a ventriculoperitoneal shunt. Diagnosis is usually made by transfontanellar ultrasound. GMH grade I is characterized by a focal, hyperechoic subependymal lesion along the ventricles (most frequently at the caudothalamic groove). Grade II hemorrhage is seen as a larger GMH in which blood products may cover the choroid plexus, resulting in a CSF-blood sedimentation level in the dependent parts of the ventricles or by a hyperechoic lining of the ventricles. Grade III is easily recognized by the enlarging ventricles. In grade IV hemorrhage, a hyperechoic signal is seen within the periventricular white matter (frequently in a fan-shaped pattern that follows the distribution of the venous drainage of the white matter into the deep venous system). A focal hemorrhage is seen as a focal hyperechoic mass lesion within the ischemic white matter. MRI is helpful for a better delineation and estimation of the degree of injury to the white matter. Functional sequences may give important information about functional outcome and prognosis. Follow-up examinations of GMH are usually done by serial bedside head ultrasound examinations. Color-coded duplex sonography with spectral analysis of the arterial flow profile with estimation of the resistive index may give important, indirect information about the intracranial pressure and the amount of brain edema. Serial, routine head ultrasound examinations are especially useful in children who are sedated and relaxed because of, for example, extracorporeal membrane oxygenation in heart failure.

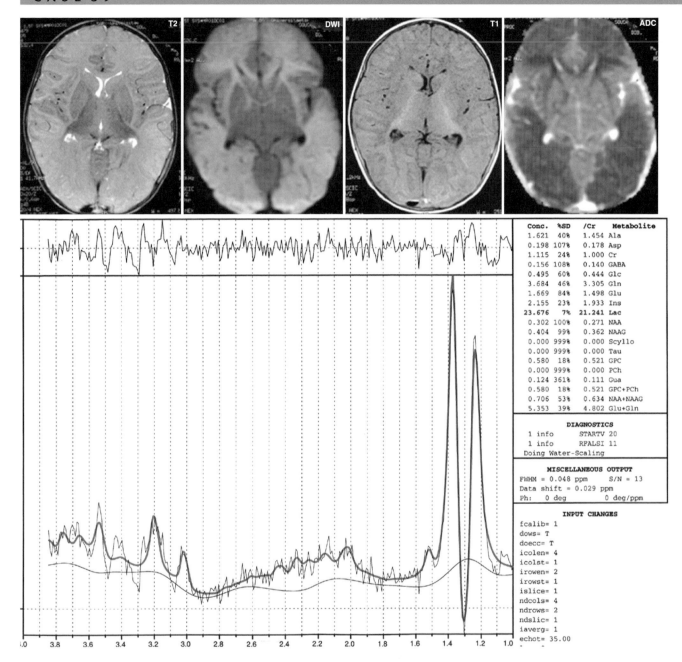

1. What are the imaging findings in this 3-year-old child?

2. What is the diagnosis and what could be the cause?

3. What is the added value of diffusion-weighted imaging (DWI)?

4. What is the prognosis?

Diagnosis: Hypoxic-Ischemic Injury

1. T_2-hyperintense swelling of the cerebral cortex; extensive white matter edema with corresponding cytotoxic edema on DWI and apparent diffusion coefficient; basal ganglia, thalami, and insular cortex preserved.

2. Hypoxic-ischemic injury (HIE) of the brain, after drowning or cardiac arrest.

3. DWI allows for differentiation between cytotoxic and vasogenic edema; cytotoxic edema linked to irreversible cell injury.

4. Poor because of extensive, probably irreversible injury of the cerebral cortex and white matter.

Cross-Reference

Blickman JG, Parker BR, Barnes PD: *Pediatric radiology— the requisites*, ed 3, Philadelphia, 2009, Mosby, pp 233-234.

Comment

HIE is a very unfortunate combination of hypoxic injury to the brain because of hypoventilation and simultaneous ischemic injury to the brain (because of hypoperfusion resulting from, for example, cardiac arrest). HIE is a devastating injury that can occur intrauterine, perinatally during birth, or postnatally. HIE may also occur in near sudden infant death syndrome, after drowning, and in children with congenital heart diseases complicated by a sudden cardiac arrest. Depending on the age of the child (preterm versus term), the degree of hypoxia-ischemia, and the duration of hypoxia-ischemia, the distribution and severity of brain injury will vary. Preterm children with perinatal HIE will have injury to the periventricular white matter, which can evolve into periventricular leucomalacia (PVL), whereas term babies typically infarct their basal ganglia and thalami. Depending on the severity and duration of hypoxia-ischemia, various overlapping combinations of injury may be encountered. In addition, complicating germinal matrix hemorrhages may be seen in preterm neonates. Transfontanellar ultrasound is believed to be limited in the early detection of HIE. High-end ultrasound examination with combined color-coded duplex sonography and spectral analysis may, however, identify brain edema by measuring the resistive index. In addition, ultrasound may exclude other causes for the observed neurology. Neonates with severe HIE may be floppy, lethargic, have a low Apgar score, or may present with seizures. In older children with HIE, decreased consciousness, hypoventilation, hypothermia, or focal neurologic deficits may be observed. Magnetic resonance imaging (MRI), including DWI and quantitative proton magnetic resonance spectography (^{1}H-MRS), give important functional data about the degree of injury. DWI can reveal ischemic injury to the brain before conventional MRI (T_1- and T_2-weighted imaging) shows pathologic condition. ^{1}H-MRS may show increased concentrations of lactate within the brain, indicating anaerobic metabolism, while a decreased concentration of N-acetylaspartate (NAA) and creatine indicates neuronal cell injury and energy failure. On conventional MRI a reduced corticomedullary differentiation with swelling and increased T_2 hyperintensity of the white matter are the most striking findings. Depending on the mechanism of injury, the basal ganglia and/or thalami may also be swollen. In neonates the T_1-hyperintense and T_2-hypointense signal of the myelinated white matter tracts in the posterior limb of the internal capsule (PLIC) have proven to be of prognostic value for outcome. If the PLIC signal is lacking, prognosis is poorer. In addition, intracortical T_1-hyperintense foci within the central region indicate HIE with intracortical petechial hemorrhages. The intramedullary veins may also be prominent because of increased venous pressure or thrombosis. Functional MRI is especially helpful in examining children with HIE because it gives valuable, early information before conventional MRI shows the pathologic condition. Consequently, neuroprotective treatments can be started earlier and more selectively.

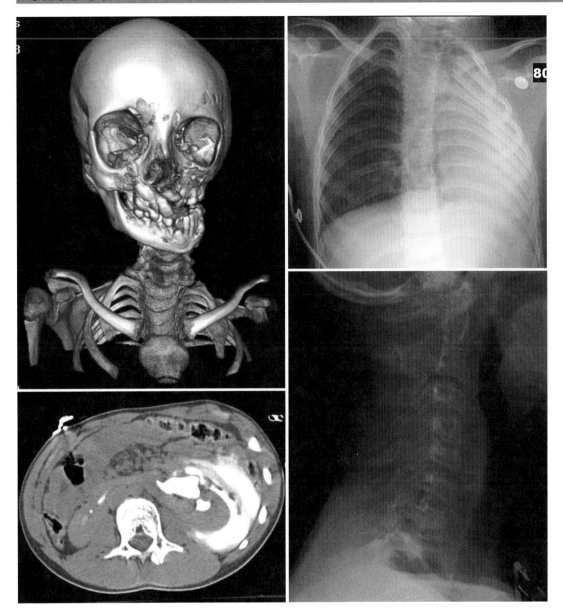

1. Patients A and B illustrate different aspects of the same condition. What are the findings in patient A (first and second images)?

2. Patient B was involved in a motor vehicle accident and complained of abdominal and neck pain. Abdominal computed tomography (CT) and cervical spine plain films were obtained (third and fourth images). What are the condition-related findings that made the patient uniquely vulnerable to injury?

3. What other systems can be involved with this condition?

4. What is one embryologic explanation of some of the findings?

Diagnosis: Goldenhar Syndrome (Goldenhar-Gorlin Syndrome, Facioauriculovertebral Sequence)

1. Left hemifacial microsomia (left auditory canal also aplastic), and left pulmonary aplasia with fusion of left ribs 1 and 2.

2. Horseshoe kidney (a low, transverse position that makes it more likely to be crushed against the lumbar spine); laceration and extravasation of contrast seen here; the fusion of C4 and C5 (the cervical spine is less flexible and more prone to injury at the levels above and below the fusion).

3. Cardiovascular, central nervous system (CNS), or limbs.

4. Unilateral insult at the time of formation of the first and second branchial arch derivatives.

Reference

Taybi H, Lachman RS: *Radiology of syndromes, metabolic disorders and skeletal dysplasias*, ed 4, Baltimore, 1996, Mosby, pp 356–358.

Cross-Reference

Blickman JG, Parker BR, Barnes PD: *Pediatric radiology— the requisites*, ed 3, Philadelphia, 2009, Mosby, p 305.

Comment

The striking facial, ocular, and auricular anomalies in this syndrome are what usually bring it to clinical attention and obtain a diagnosis for the child. However, the associated anomalies in other systems may be subtler and can be missed without rigorous search. These abnormalities are highly varied and have no particular pattern; screening echocardiogram, frontal radiograph of the chest, renal ultrasound, head CT and magnetic resonance imaging, and physical examination will provide a complete picture for the individual patient.

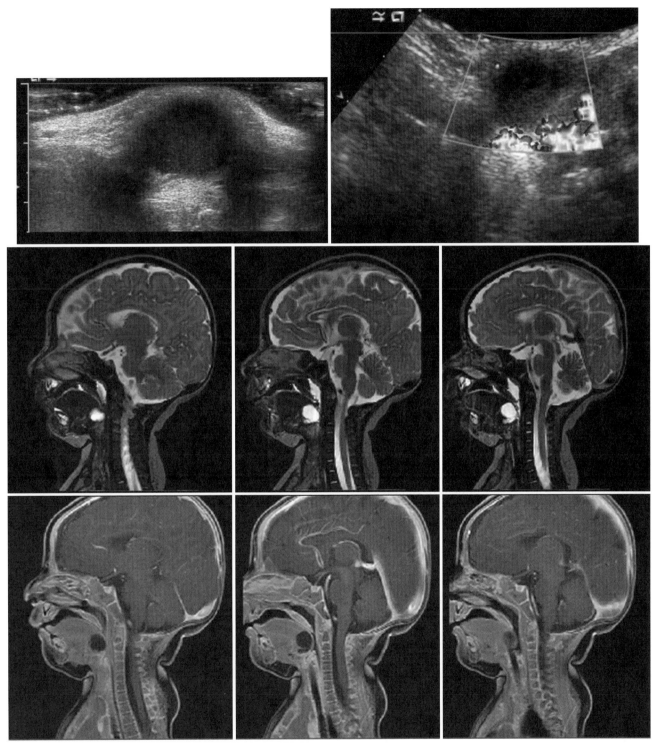

1. A 9-year-old girl has a lump on her anterior neck in the midline that has recently enlarged. The first and second images are taken from an ultrasound study. What does it show?

2. The plastic surgeon wants to remove it. What should be done *before* surgery?

3. The third and fourth images are from the magnetic resonance imaging (MRI) scan of a 1-month-old girl with feeding difficulty. What are the findings?

4. What is the final diagnosis?

Diagnosis: Thyroglossal Duct Cyst

1. Spheric cystic and solid subcutaneous mass about 1 cm in diameter, with no vascular flow; dermoid cyst, thyroglossal duct cyst (especially if it has been previously infected), thyroid rest, branchial arch remnant cyst.

2. A thyroid ultrasound to make sure the child has a normal thyroid.

3. Cystic mass in base of the tongue, cordlike structure extending from the cyst to the level of thyroid.

4. Persistent thyroglossal duct with a cyst inside the tongue, just below site of the foramen cecum.

References

Moore KM: *The developing human*, ed 2, Philadelphia, 1977, Saunders, pp 160-180.

Barkovich AJ, Moore KR, Jones BV, et al, editors: *Diagnostic imaging: neuroradiology,* Salt Lake City, 2007, Amirsys, II 4:18-21.

Cross-Reference

Blickman JG, Parker BR, Barnes PD: *Pediatric radiology— the requisites*, ed 3, Philadelphia, 2009, Mosby, pp 309-311.

Comment

The thyroid begins to form in the fourth week of fetal life as a pit in the base of the tongue, at the junction of the proximal one third (derived from the third branchial arch) and the distal two thirds (derived from the first branchial arch). As the fetus enlarges, the pit deepens, forming a duct in the midline—the thyroglossal duct—with the developing thyroid at its distal tip. Ultimately this duct passes inferiorly through the base of the tongue; then it passes anteriorly to the surface of the neck, passing superior and anterior to the hyoid bone and anterior to the thyroid and cricoid cartilages. The rapidly enlarging bilobed thyroid reaches its place in the lower neck by the end of the seventh week; usually by that time the duct above it has disappeared, persisting only as the vestigial pit in the tongue—the foramen cecum—and occasionally as the pyramidal lobe of the thyroid, projecting upward from the isthmus. However, remnants of the duct can persist as cysts anywhere along its pathway. Similarly, remnants of thyroid can be left behind as solid masses.

The complexity of the duct's path complicates its imaging workup. Cysts in the anterior neck are easily studied using ultrasound. However, cysts or masses in the base of the tongue may not be accessible, and computed tomography or MRI might be necessary. In some cases the thyroid is completely arrested in its descent, and the mass may actually represent the patient's entire complement of thyroid tissue. Therefore ultrasound of the thyroid to establish its normal configuration is mandatory before surgery is contemplated. If thyroid tissue is not in its normal place, then nuclear medicine thyroid scan must be done to determine its presence and location.

Because the path of the thyroglossal duct crosses the territories of the second, third, and fourth branchial arches, the differential diagnosis of a mass in the base of the tongue or anterior neck must also include cystic remnants of these structures. Generally these structures are off-midline and more lateral.

can exist positioned along at any part of the path of the thyroglossal duct

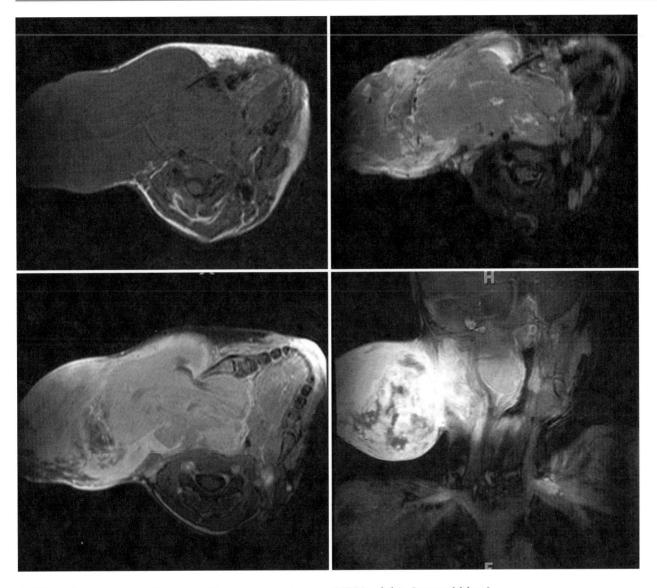

1. What do you see on the magnetic resonance images (MRIs) of this 8-year-old boy?

2. What is the differential diagnosis?

3. What are the different cell types of rhabdomyosarcoma?

4. What is the prognosis?

Diagnosis: Rhabdomyosarcoma

1. A large exophytic mass in the right neck and a lymphadenopathy in the left neck.

2. A primary tumor such as rhabdomyosarcoma, Ewing sarcoma, peripheral neuroectodermal tumor, or other rare sarcomas (less likely lymphoma).

3. Embryonal, botryoid (embryonal variant), alveolar, and undifferentiated.

4. The prognosis in rhabdomyosarcoma varies widely based on the location, cell type, and stage. Those with localized disease have a 5-year survival rate of 85% with combined treatment including chemotherapy, surgery, and radiotherapy.

Reference

Arndt CAS, Crist WM: Common musculoskeletal tumor of childhood and adolescence, *N Engl J Med* 341:342–352, 1999.

Cross-Reference

Blickman JG, Parker BR, Barnes PD: *Pediatric radiology— the requisites*, ed 3, Philadelphia, 2009, Moby, pp 325–338.

Comment

Rhabdomyosarcoma is the most common soft tissue sarcoma in childhood. The name comes from the Greek words *rhabdo,* meaning rod shaped, and *myo,* meaning muscle. The tumor arises from primitive muscle cells; tumor cells are usually positive for desmin, vimentin, myoglobin, actin, transcription factor myoD, and elements of differentiated muscle cells. The incidence is four to seven per 1 million children younger than 15 years old in the United States (or about 250 cases annually). Two thirds of the patients are younger than 10 years old. The boy-to-girl ratio is 1.2:1.4 to 1. Most cases occur sporadically and the cause is unknown. However, a pattern of familiar cancer exists, including osteosarcoma and rhabdomyosarcoma in the Li-Fraumeni syndrome, which is seen in children with first-degree relatives with adrenocortical carcinoma, breast cancer, or other tumors that occur before the age of 45 years. Tumor-suppressor gene p53 mutations are associated with this syndrome.

Rhabdomyosarcoma can occur anywhere in the body but does not arise primarily in bone. The most common sites are the head and neck (28%), extremities (24%), and genitourinary (GU) tract (18%). Other sites include the trunk (11%), orbit (7%), retroperitoneum (6%), and other sites in less than 3% of patients. The botryoid variant of embryonal rhabdomyosarcoma arises in mucosal cavities, such as the bladder, vagina, nasopharynx, and middle ear. Lesions in the extremities are most likely to have an alveolar type of histology. Metastases are found predominantly in the lungs, bone marrow, bones, lymph nodes, breasts, and brain.

The images shown in this case are of an unfortunate boy who was noted to have an egg-sized mass 3 months before this MRI was obtained. Initial treatment with antibiotic agents had had no effect on the mass, and biopsy 1 month later showed embryonal rhabdomyosarcoma. The mass grew rapidly. The family sought several medical opinions, and he was first treated with herbal supplements. He never received conventional therapy and died at home 8 months after the MRI examination.

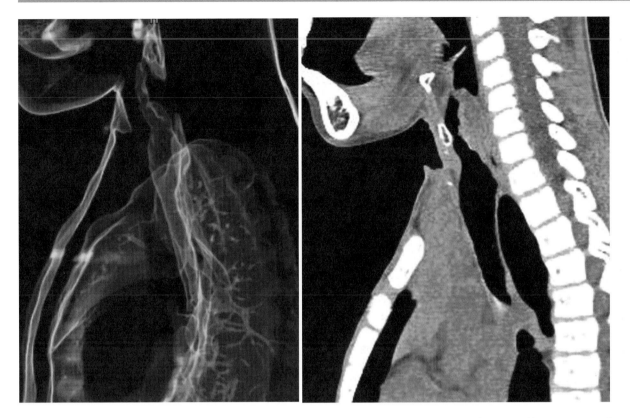

1. What are the imaging findings in this 11-year-old boy with stridor and a previous history of long-term tracheostomy?

2. What is the diagnosis?

3. Why is airway obstruction more detrimental in children compared with adults?

4. What are the most common laryngeal anomalies?

Diagnosis: Subglottic Stenosis

1. Three-dimensional (3D) virtual bronchoscopy image reconstructed from axial thin-slice noncontrast computed tomography (CT) scan shows narrowing of the subglottic airway with irregular contours. Two-dimensional (2D) sagittal reformat at the same level shows increased soft tissue density, likely from granulation, causing stenosis of the subglottic trachea.

2. The diagnosis is subglottic stenosis.

3. In children the larynx and trachea are significantly smaller than in adults. This discrepancy is because of the increased relative size of the child's adenoids and lingual and palatine tonsils, leaving little margin for obstruction. One millimeter of glottic edema leads to 35% obstruction of the airway. In the subglottis, 1 mm of edema leads to a 44% narrowing. In addition, the resistance to airflow is inversely proportional to the fourth power of the radius of the airway. Therefore 1 mm of concentric edema in a newborn trachea (radius approximately 2 mm) increases resistance 16 times, resulting in significant airway compromise.

4. Laryngomalacia, vocal fold paralysis, and congenital subglottic stenosis are the most common anomalies.

Reference

Tekes A, Flax-Goldenberg R: Diagnostic imaging of the pediatric airway. Operative techniques in otolaryngology, *Head Neck Surg* 18(2):115–120, 2007.

Cross-Reference

Blickman JG, Parker BR, Barnes PD: *Pediatric radiology— the requisites*, ed 3, Philadelphia, 2009, Mosby, pp 13–15.

Comment

Subglottic stenosis is one of the most common causes of airway obstruction in infants and children. It is the second most common cause of stridor in infants and the most common laryngotracheal anomaly requiring tracheostomy in children younger than 1 year old. It is the most common serious long-term complication of endotracheal (ET) intubation in neonates. Subglottic stenosis may be categorized as congenital or acquired. The diameter of the normal subglottic lumen is 4.5 to 5.5 mm in a full-term neonate and approximately 3.5 mm in a preterm baby. A subglottic airway diameter of 4 mm or less in a full-term infant or 3 mm or less in a premature infant is considered narrow and consistent with a diagnosis of subglottic stenosis. Subglottic stenosis is considered congenital when no other apparent cause of the stenosis exists. Congenital subglottic stenosis implies that a child is born with a small laryngeal lumen and that trauma of intubation or another cause did not contribute to the stenosis. After intubation, it is difficult to distinguish congenital from acquired stenosis. A congenitally malformed larynx leads to respiratory distress that may require intubation. Inflammation and scarring may occur even though an age-appropriate size of ET tube was used. Therefore the true incidence of congenital subglottic stenosis is difficult to determine. The majority of cases of subglottic stenosis are acquired and most commonly associated with ET tube intubation and many other factors, including laryngopharyngeal reflux, infection, and the associated inflammatory response. ET tubes may cause pressure injury to the glottis, whereas tracheotomy tubes may cause severe stomal stenosis in the trachea or infraglottic region.

Plain films may be the first modality of choice; however, thin-slice CT images provide better anatomic detail and allow for 3D reconstructions of the larynx and airways. Short scan time allows for scanning of the child without intubation or sedation, making it more preferable than magnetic resonance imaging.

Acquired subglottic stenosis may present years after ET intubation. Surgical correction of subglottic stenosis aims to provide an adequately enlarged lumen while preserving vocal quality and airway protection. Treatment success is predicted on a thorough preoperative evaluation and tailoring the repair to address the severity and location of the individual lesion.

Differential diagnosis is broad and includes—but is not limited to—tracheomalacia, laryngomalacia, laryngeal cleft, vascular compression, teratoma, vascular anomalies (e.g., hemangiomas, lymphatic malformation), and recurrent respiratory papillomatosis.

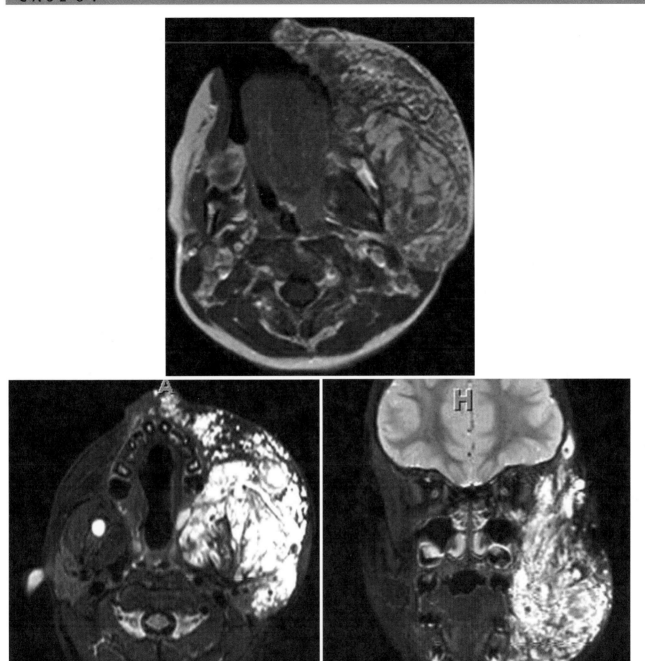

1. What are the imaging findings?

2. What is the diagnosis?

3. In 1982, Mulliken and Glowacki introduced a classification system of vascular anomalies. When did the International Society for the Study of Vascular Anomalies (ISSVA) accept this system?

4. What are the differential diagnoses?

Diagnosis: Venous Malformation

1. A large serpiginous, tubular, T_2-bright, enhancing left facial soft tissue mass exists, involving the subcutaneous fat extending into the masticator space and within the fossa for the left temporomandibular joint.

2. Venous malformation.

3. Eleventh meeting of ISSVA in 1996 (Rome, Italy).

4. Hemangiomas and lymphatic malformations. Hemangiomas are soft tissue mass lesions that show arterial flow within their parenchyma; venous malformations do not have any arterial flow. Venous malformations typically present with tubular serpiginous T_2-bright avidly enhancing mass lesions, whereas lymphatic malformations are generally cystic lesions that are again T_2 bright but do not enhance except for the wall of the cysts or septations.

Reference

Mulliken JB, Fishman SJ, Burrows PE: Vascular anomalies, *Curr Probl Surg* 37(8):517-584, 2000.

Cross-Reference

Blickman JG, Parker BR, Barnes PD: *Pediatric radiology—the requisites*, ed 3, Philadelphia, 2009, Mosby, pp 314-315.

Comment

Venous malformations represent a subcategory of vascular malformations that are congenital malformations of vessels that are *not* true neoplasms.

In 1982, Mulliken and Glowacki published a landmark article proposing characterization of vascular anomalies based on biologic and pathologic differences. This classification system clarified the misconceptions and misnomers that had been developing within the group of vascular anomalies during the past 200 years. Vascular anomalies are divided in two major groups: (1) hemangiomas (true vascular tumors) and (2) vascular malformations (including venous malformations, lymphatic malformations, capillary malformations, mixed type of venolymphatic malformations, arteriovenous malformations, and arteriovenous fistulas).

Venous malformations represent dysplasia of small and large venous channels. They generally present as painful soft tissue masses, sometimes with a bluish hue. They may bleed and result in cosmetic problems. Venous malformations are commonly diagnosed at birth but may become apparent at any age. They may suddenly enlarge secondary to hemorrhage or hormonal influences.

Radiographs may show a soft tissue mass. Computed tomography is typically not used in the diagnostic workup. Ultrasound can show mixed echogenicities within tangles of hypoechoic tubular structures. Color Doppler sonography does not show any arterial flow. Venous malformations reveal increased T_2 signal and appear as channel-like serpiginous areas. They show avid contrast enhancement and can have calcifications that appear as signal voids (phlebolith). Venous malformations are infiltrative lesions crossing multiple soft tissue planes involving subcutaneous fat, bone, neurovascular bundles, or even viscera. Magnetic resonance imaging is preferred for monitoring the disease, whereas ultrasound is commonly used to rule out deep venous thrombosis after treatment.

Differential diagnosis includes hemangiomas and lymphatic malformations. Hemangiomas are soft tissue mass lesions that show arterial flow within their parenchyma; venous malformations do not have any arterial flow. Venous malformations typically present with tubular serpiginous T_2-bright, avidly enhancing mass lesions, whereas lymphatic malformations are generally cystic lesions that are again T_2 bright but do not enhance except for the wall of the cysts or septations.

Aspirin may be used to avoid thrombosis. Elastic compression garments are recommended. The primary modality of treatment is percutaneous sclerosis, such as direct injection with ethanol or other sclerotic agents under fluoroscopy or ultrasound guidance (performed under general anesthesia). Potential complications of percutaneous treatment of vascular malformations include skin necrosis, nerve damage, extremity swelling, muscle atrophy, and deep vein thrombosis. Often this is a life-long problem, with treatment aimed at reducing symptoms rather than eliminating disease. A multidisciplinary approach facilitates appropriate diagnosis, management, and treatment of these cases.

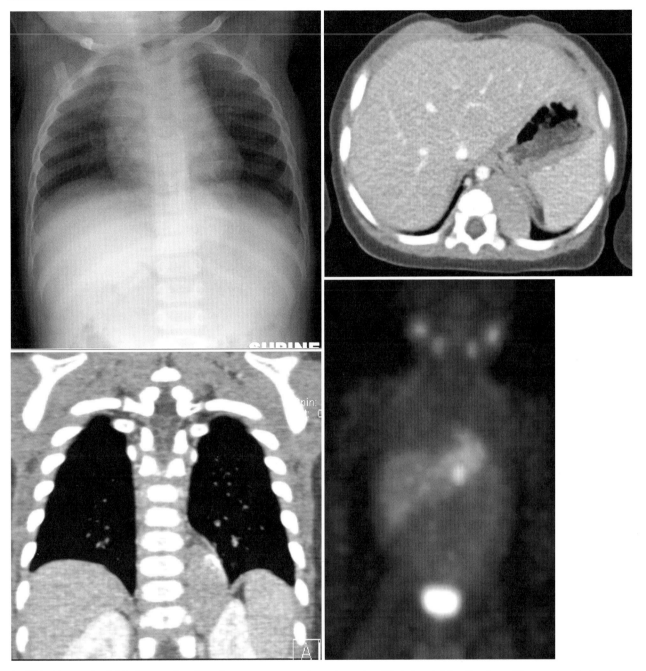

1. This 7-month-old infant arrived at the emergency department with intractable diarrhea. He received chest and abdomen films. What do you see on the chest film (first image)?

2. What are the differential diagnoses for this age group?

3. What are the findings on the computed tomography scan (second and third images)?

4. What does the metaiodobenzylguanidine (MIBG) scan show (fourth image)?

Diagnosis: Paraspinal, Posterior Mediastinal Neuroblastoma

1. The left paraspinous line is elevated away from the spine.

2. Infection; neuroenteric cyst; meningocele; pulmonary sequestration; tumor originating in neural elements (neurofibroma, neuroblastoma, ganglioneuroma) or in the left adrenal gland (adenoma, neuroblastoma). (Diarrhea can be caused by high circulating catecholamines, making neuroblastoma more likely in this patient.)

3. The mass is solid, paraspinal, contains calcium, lies above the diaphragm, and does not involve the adrenal gland.

4. High uptake in the left paraspinal area, where no physiologic uptake is expected.

Reference

Kuhn JP, Slovis TL, Haller JO: *Caffey's pediatric diagnostic imaging*, ed 10, Philadelphia, 2004, Mosby, pp 1210-1215.

Cross-Reference

Blickman JG, Parker BR, Barnes PD: *Pediatric radiology—the requisites*, ed 3, Philadelphia, 2009, Mosby, pp 43-45, 143-144.

Comment

Neuroblastomas can form anywhere along the parasympathetic neuronal chain. Sixteen percent of neuroblastomas are found in the chest (almost all in the posterior mediastinum). Forty percent show calcification. Up to 20% have extradural extension, even in the absence of symptoms. The tumor may also extend along the spine superiorly and inferiorly, as well as through the retrocrural space. However, because thoracic neuroblastoma tends to present at an earlier age and at an earlier stage than abdominal neuroblastoma, the prognosis is better.

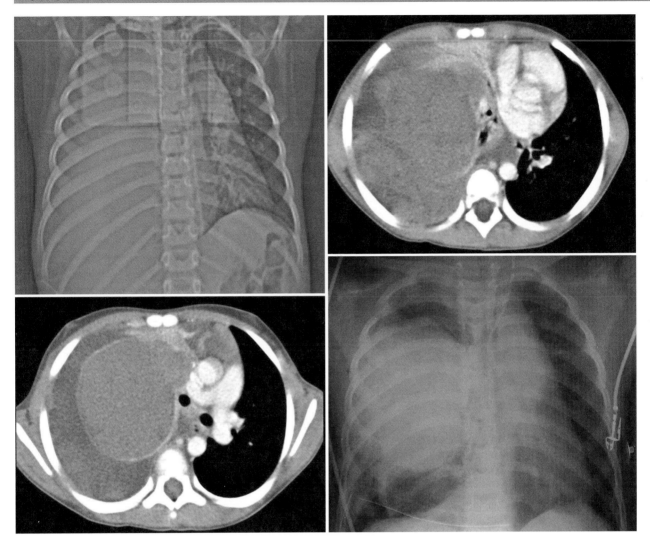

1. This 3½-year-old girl had a 1-week history of dyspnea on exertion. What are the findings in the first, second, and third images?

2. After a chest tube was placed, the fourth image was obtained. What is seen now?

3. What are the differential diagnoses?

Diagnosis: Pleuropulmonary Blastoma

1. A cystic and solid tumor displacing and compressing the normal right lung medially.

2. Evacuation of pleural effusion; a large round tumor mass extending from the right lung.

3. Cystic adenomatoid malformation, lung abcess, hamartoma, malignant mesenchymal tumor, and intraparenchymal bronchogenic cyst.

References

Kuhn JP, Slovis TL, Haller JO: *Caffey's pediatric diagnostic imaging*, ed 10, Philadelphia, 2004, Mosby, pp 1134-1137.

Priest JR, McDermott MB, Bhatia S, et al: Pleuropulmonary blastoma: a clinicopathologic study of 50 cases, *Cancer* 80(1):147-161, 1997.

Cross-Reference

Blickman JG, Parker BR, Barnes PD: *Pediatric radiology— the requisites*, ed 3, Philadelphia, 2009, Mosby, p 38.

Comment

The pluripotent mesodermal layer in the developing embryo gives rise to cartilage, skeletal and smooth muscle, and fibrous tissue. Its persistence in the mature infant, however, makes it a source of malignant growths. These tumors are named for the predominant tissue found on histology, but their radiographic features are similar. Foci of mesenchyme can be found in developmental cystic lesions that are otherwise thought to be benign (e.g., bronchogenic cyst, cystic adenomatoid malformation, congenital pulmonary cyst, cystic hamartoma); clinicians theorize that these foci account for the malignant transformation seen in some lesions. Pleuropulmonary blastoma is the most frequently found representative of this group of tumors. Unlike the adult tumor of the same name, the epithelial elements in the pediatric tumor are benign; the malignant elements have sarcomatous and blastematous features.

Three subtypes are described. Type I is purely cystic and found in young infants. Type II (cystic and solid) and type III (purely solid) occur later, but this tumor is found almost exclusively in children younger than 5 years old. Type I has a slightly better prognosis.

This tumor can be regarded as a dysontogenetic analog to Wilms tumor, neuroblastoma, and hepatoblastoma.

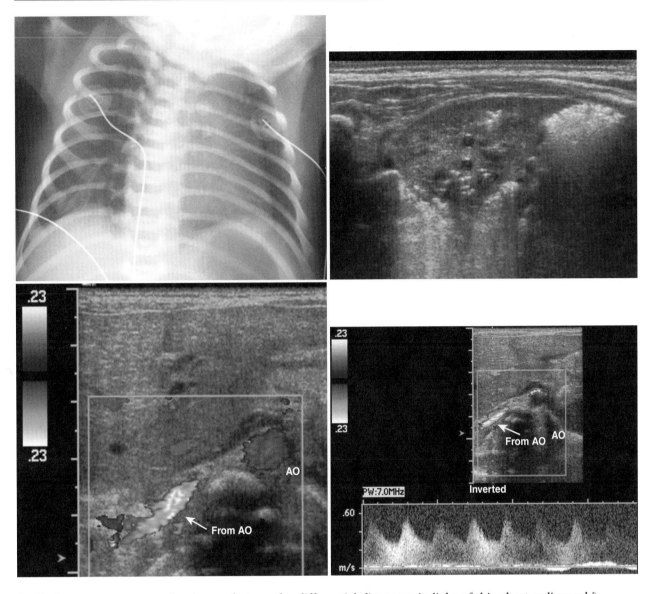

1. If a lung mass was seen in utero, what are the differential diagnoses in light of this chest radiograph?

2. Does the location of the abnormality help in the differential diagnoses?

3. Name the two major types of this entity.

4. The venous drainage was likely to the inferior vena cava. Which type is this example?

Diagnosis: Pulmonary Sequestration

1. Sequestration, congenital cystic adenomatoid malformation (CCAM), or bronchogenic cyst.

2. Yes, sequestration usually occurs in the lower lobes.

3. Intralobar and extralobar.

4. Extralobar; the small cysts seen in the lesion by ultrasound suggest a possible component of CCAM.

Reference

Patterson A: Imaging evaluation of congenital lung abnormalities in infants and children, *Radiol Clin North Am* 43(2):303–323, 2005.

Cross-Reference

Blickman JG, Parker BR, Barnes PD: *Pediatric radiology—the requisites*, ed 3, Philadelphia, 2009, Mosby, pp 25–26.

Comment

Pulmonary sequestration usually presents as an asymptomatic mass seen in an imaging study or is found before birth by fetal ultrasound (as in this example). These masses are usually located in the lower portion of the lung (more commonly on the left than on the right). When located beneath the diaphragm in unusual cases, it is called extrapulmonary sequestration. The mass is usually solid in appearance and does not contain air-filled alveoli. No bronchial connection exists.

Diagnosis can usually be made by a combination of chest radiograph, sonography, and computed tomography or magnetic resonance imaging. The key to diagnosis is the identification of the blood supply.

Sequestration is characterized by its blood supply and pleural investment. A large systemic artery (often from the aorta) leads to the mass, and its venous drainage is either to the pulmonary venous system (intralobar type, which accounts for 75% of all sequestrations) or the systemic venous system (extralobar type, which accounts for 25% of the total). Some variability exists in the venous drainage. The extralobar type has a separate pleural investment. This type is more likely to be associated with other congenital abnormalities such as diaphragmatic hernia, heart disease, and CCAM. The intralobar sequestration is considered more likely to become infected, because some connections may exist to the adjacent lung via the pores of Kohn, adjacent bronchi, or foregut communication. One could make an argument for observation in some cases; however, in the United States most sequestrations are resected because of the risk (or prior occurrence) of infection.

The mass in this patient was electively resected; it had elements of CCAM, as well as the anomalous arterial and venous blood supply. It is not unusual to see a combination of lesions as in this case.

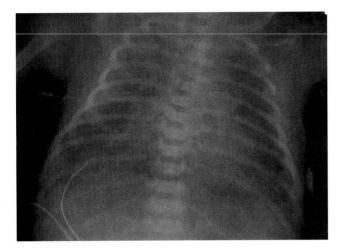

1. What are the differential diagnoses of this neonatal chest image?

2. Is this patient likely to have surfactant deficiency? Why or why not?

3. What pathophysiologic result can you report regarding the initial findings in this disease?

4. What is the outcome of this condition?

CASE 69

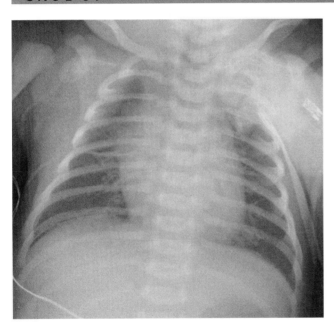

1. What are the findings in this term newborn with respiratory distress?

2. What are the differential diagnoses?

3. If a chest radiograph taken on day 2 of life is normal, what is the most likely diagnosis?

4. What is the natural history of this condition?

Diagnosis: Meconium Aspiration Syndrome

1. Meconium aspiration syndrome and, less likely, group B streptococcal pneumonia.

2. Yes; not for the same reason as in premature infants but because of the depletion effect of meconium on the surfactant normally present in term or postterm infants.

3. Partial and/or complete obstruction of the airways with the particulate matter (meconium).

4. Most patients do not have serious sequelae; however, a higher incidence of reactive airway disease occurs later in childhood when compared with controls.

Reference

Taussig LM, Landau LI: *Pediatric respiratory medicine*, ed 2, Philadelphia, 2008, Mosby.

Cross-Reference

Blickman JG, Parker BR, Barnes PD: *Pediatric radiology—the requisites*, ed 3, Philadelphia, 2009, Mosby, pp 30-31.

Comment

Meconium aspiration syndrome is the most common cause of respiratory distress in the term or postterm neonate. It is caused by the aspiration of meconium before, during, or immediately after delivery. The diagnosis may be obvious to the neonatologist, but the radiologist must consider other causes when the clinical information is incomplete. The aspiration of meconium results initially in the paradoxic combination of atelectasis and hyperinflation, both manifestations of varying degrees of bronchial and bronchiolar obstruction. Surfactant is depleted by components of meconium, especially the free fatty acids, which also results in atelectasis. This leads to the classic radiographic appearance of large lungs with diffuse patchy opacities (atelectasis). Later the radiographic findings reflect more of a chemical pneumonitis or persistent pulmonary hypertension. Air leaks into the mediastinum, pleural space, or pericardium may occur as a result of barotrauma and the inherent obstructive nature of the initial aspiration of particulate meconium. General respiratory support and surfactant administration is the usual treatment. Antibiotic agents are not routinely recommended but may be needed if secondary bacterial pneumonia develops. Extracorporeal membrane oxygenation is sometimes necessary in the most severely affected patients.

Diagnosis: Transient Tachypnea of the Newborn

1. Mild hyperinflation, interstitial prominence, fluid in the fissures, and possibly a small amount of right pleural fluid.

2. Transient tachypnea of the newborn (TTN), mild meconium aspiration, or neonatal pneumonia.

3. TTN.

4. The infant may require some supplemental oxygen but will generally normalize within 1 to 2 days.

Reference

Kuhn JP, Slovis TL, Haller JO: *Caffey's pediatric diagnostic imaging*, ed 10, Philadelphia, 2004, Mosby, pp 72-73.

Cross-Reference

Blickman JG, Parker BR, Barnes PD: *Pediatric radiology—the requisites*, ed 3, Philadelphia, 2009, Mosby, p 30.

Comment

TTN is caused by the retention of fetal lung fluid in the lungs after birth. It is also known as the wet lung syndrome, and its clinical presentation is tachypnea with minimal or no oxygen requirement. Often a history exists of prolonged maternal labor, caesarian section (25%), maternal asthma, or diabetes. Lung fluid is normally removed by capillary resorption, lymphatic resorption, and retrograde flow out of the trachea. The reason for delayed resorption is obvious in some (but not all) cases. A genetic predisposition may exist to diminished β-adrenergic responsiveness in the infant and mother. An increased incidence of asthma and atopy is noted at 4- to 5-year follow-up of children who had TTN.

Radiographic findings include mild hyperinflation, as well as fluid in the alveolar space, in the interstitial space, and/or in the pleural space.

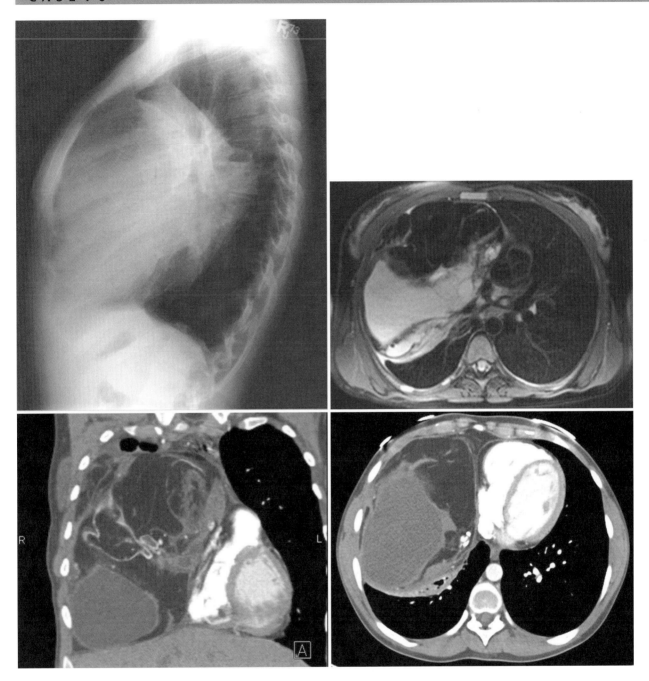

1. What is seen in this teenage patient?

2. What are the differential diagnoses?

3. Is this type of tumor ever malignant?

4. What is the treatment?

Diagnosis: Mediastinal Teratoma

1. Computed tomography and magnetic resonance imaging show a large anterior mediastinal mass with calcification and fatty and cystic components.

2. The components of this mass make teratoma, a type of germ cell tumor, the only diagnosis. Other anterior mediastinal masses include lymphoma, thymoma, and ectopic thyroid gland.

3. Yes.

4. Resection alone, if benign.

Reference

Sellke FW, editor: *Sabiston and Spencer surgery of the chest*, Philadelphia, 2005, Saunders.

Cross-Reference

Blickman JG, Parker BR, Barnes PD: *Pediatric radiology—the requisites*, ed 3, Philadelphia, 2009, Mosby, p 40.

Comment

Knowing the site from which the tumor arises can help the clinician to narrow down the differential diagnosis of masses in the mediastinum. The mediastinum is divided into three parts: (1) anterior, (2) middle, and (3) posterior. In the anterior mediastinum, masses are most likely the result of teratoma, other germ cell tumors, lymphoma, thymoma, and substernal thyroid. The mediastinum is the most common site of extragonadal germ cell tumor. Germ cell tumors may be benign or malignant. Benign tumors are called teratomas if they have tissue from at least two out of three primitive germ cell layers. Theories for their development include derivation from the cells in the region of the third brachial cleft or pouch, origination from totipotent cells, and initiation from germinal nests of cells located along the urogenital ridge that failed to migrate to the gonads in embryologic development.

Teratomas in the mediastinum can become extremely large; in older children and adults they may produce no symptoms. In younger patients, symptoms because of mass effect (particularly on the trachea and bronchial tree) are more common.

There are three types of teratomas: (1) mature, (2) immature, and (3) teratoma with malignant components. The mature type is benign, accounts for 85% of these tumors, and is the diagnosis in this case. The immature type contains mature epithelial and connective tissue components, as well as immature elements with neuroectodermal and mesenchymal elements. This type may be cystic and contain calcification, as well as hair and sebaceous material. Clinicians classify teratomas with malignant components by the type of malignant tissue seen histologically; these are nonseminomatous germ cell types, adenocarcinoma or squamous carcinomas, mesenchymal or sarcomatous types (or a combination).

No imaging can absolutely distinguish between the three types of teratoma. The malignant types are likely to be poorly marginated and to invade adjacent structures. Serum markers, such as α-fetoprotein, β-human chorionic gonadotropin, and lactate dehydrogenase, may be elevated. Surveillance of these markers can be used to monitor tumor response to therapy. In the latter two types of teratoma, therapy is often a combination of surgery, chemotherapy, and radiation therapy.

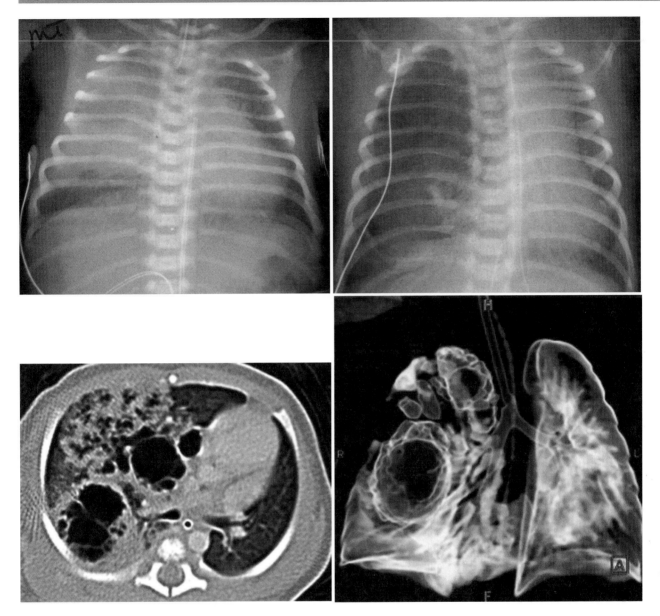

1. What are the imaging findings in this neonate? What is the most likely diagnosis?

2. How is this different than a pulmonary sequestration?

3. Which type is associated with other congenital anomalies?

4. Should intravenous (IV) contrast agents be used for computed tomography (CT)? Why or why not?

Diagnosis: Congenital Cystic Adenomatoid Malformation

1. Frontal chest radiograph demonstrates large cystic and solid mass in the right upper and midlung. Axial and coronal reformatted CT scans further delineate the multiple small and large cysts within the lesion.

2. Congenital cystic adenomatoid malformation (CCAM) typically has no connection with systemic arterial circulation, no lobar predominance, and contains air. Pulmonary sequestration has a connection with the arterial circulation, has a predilection for the left upper lobe, and typically does not contain air.

3. Type II CCAM is associated with other congenital anomalies in 50% of patients (skeletal, intestinal, renal, and cardiac).

4. Yes. When CT is performed with the possible diagnosis of CCAM, IV contrast agents must be used to prove that no systemic arterial supply exists (to rule out pulmonary sequestration).

Reference

Swischuk LE: *Imaging of the newborn, infant and young child*, ed 5, Philadelphia, 2004, Lippincott Williams & Wilkins, pp 86-88.

Cross-Reference

Blickman JG, Parker BR, Barnes PD: *Pediatric radiology—the requisites*, ed 3, Philadelphia, 2009, Mosby, pp 24-25.

Comment

CCAM is a relatively rare congenital lung abnormality that is often identified on prenatal ultrasound. Some cases regress before birth. Imaging findings depend on the size of cysts and the absence or presence of fluid within the cysts. Classically, the cysts communicate with the bronchial tree and are air filled early on; most lesions are solitary. CCAM is usually unilateral with no lobar predilection. Fifty percent of cases are classified as type I and contain one or more large (2 to 10 cm) cysts. Forty percent are type II, which contain numerous small cysts that are uniform in size. This type is associated with other congenital anomalies in 50% of the cases, including renal, skeletal, cardiac, and intestinal anomalies. Type III is the most rare (< 10% of cases) and appears solid but contains microcysts. Ultrasound and CT are used to better delineate the size of cysts. A risk of infection exists, and surgical removal is recommended in these symptomatic cases. In addition, a small risk of malignant degeneration (rhabdomyosarcoma) exists; therefore many clinicians advocate surgical removal even if the CCAM is asymptomatic. Differential diagnosis includes pulmonary sequestration (systemic arterial supply, usually left lower lobe), congenital diaphragmatic hernia, and necrotizing pneumonia.

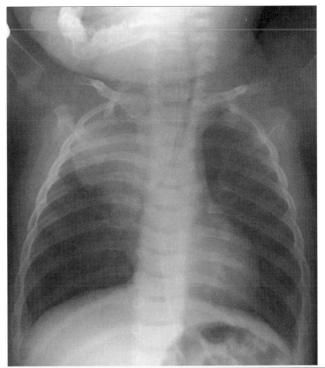

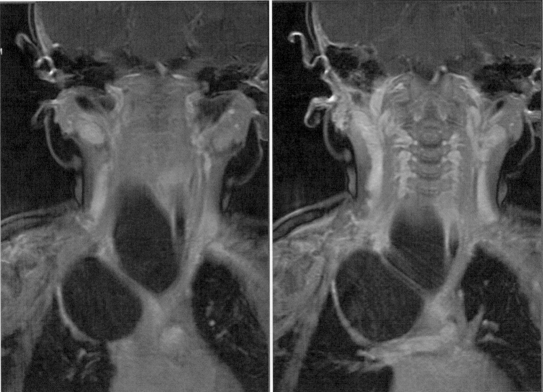

1. What are the imaging findings on the frontal chest radiograph and the contrast enhanced T_1-weighted coronal magnetic resonance image (MRI) in this child with respiratory distress? What is the most likely diagnosis?

2. What are the different types of foregut duplication cysts?

3. What are the differential diagnoses of a well-defined soft tissue density mass with smooth borders seen on chest radiograph?

4. What are some of the complications of bronchogenic cysts that can be seen on a chest radiograph?

Diagnosis: Bronchogenic Cyst

1. The frontal radiograph of the chest demonstrates a well-defined soft tissue mass with smooth borders overlying the right upper lung zone. The contrast enhanced T_1-weighted MRI images demonstrate a well-defined, thin-walled cystic structure in the right paratracheal region, consistent with a bronchogenic cyst.

2. Bronchogenic cyst, enteric cyst, and neurenteric cyst.

3. Fluid-filled bronchogenic cyst, round pneumonia, congenital cystic adenomatoid malformation (CCAM), and neurogenic tumor.

4. Mass effect and airway compression.

Reference

Effmann EL: Anomalies of the lung. In Kuhn JP, Slovis TL, Haller JO, editors: *Caffey's pediatric diagnostic imaging*, ed 10, Philadelphia, 2004, Mosby, pp 904-905.

Cross-Reference

Blickman JG, Parker BR, Barnes PD: *Pediatric radiology—the requisites*, ed 3, Philadelphia, 2009, Mosby, pp 23-24.

Comment

A bronchogenic cyst is a type of foregut duplication cyst and is a developmental lesion probably resulting from abnormal airway branching. These cysts are most commonly mediastinal (85%) but may be intrapulmonary or even found in the neck or pericardium. Occasionally, prenatal diagnosis of an intrapulmonary bronchogenic cyst is made. They often communicate with the bronchial tree, and about two thirds are aerated. Radiographically, mediastinal bronchogenic cysts present as a well-defined mass in the paratracheal or subcarinal region. Intrapulmonary bronchogenic cysts are usually in the medial third of the lung and more frequently in the lower lobes. Infants present with respiratory distress or feeding difficulties; the condition may cause airway or esophageal compression. Differential diagnosis of fluid-filled cysts includes round pneumonia, neoplasm (neurogenic tumor), lymphadenopathy, and loculated effusion. Differential diagnosis of air-filled cysts includes CCAM, pneumatocele, abscess, and cavitating nodule.

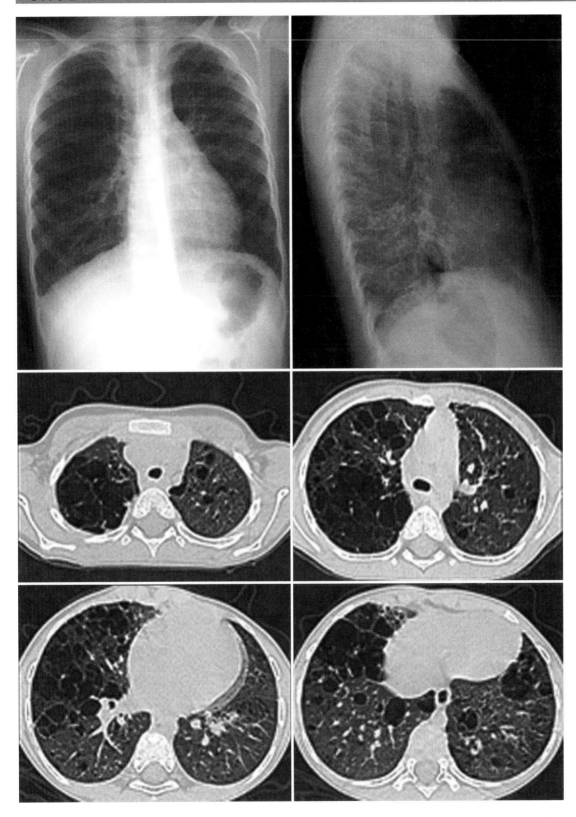

1. What is the diagnosis?

2. What is the most common site of involvement in this disease?

3. What are the most common extraosseous sites of involvement?

4. What are the most common findings in the lungs?

Diagnosis: Langerhans Cell Histiocytosis

1. Langerhans cell histiocytosis (LCH).

2. The skeletal system.

3. The skin, central nervous system (CNS), liver, spleen, lungs, lymph nodes, soft tissue, and bone marrow.

4. Initially diffuse interstitial disease with progression to honeycomb pattern and large cysts.

Reference

Schmidt S, Eich G, Geoffray A, et al: Extraosseous Langerhans cell histiocytosis in children, *Radiographics* 28:707–726, 2008.

Cross-Reference

Blickman JG, Parker BR, Barnes PD: *Pediatric radiology— the requisites*, ed 3, Philadelphia, 2009, Mosby, pp 39–40.

Comment

The most common manifestations of LCH are bone lesions, with extraosseous involvement less frequently seen. Extraosseous sites of involvement include skin (55%), CNS (35%), hepatobiliary system and spleen (32%), lungs (26%), lymph nodes (26%), soft tissues (26%), bone marrow (19%), salivary glands (6%), and digestive tract (6%). Approximately 10% of patients with LCH present with lung manifestations that are typically 1 to 10 mm nodules, usually cavitated, with a slight predominance of upper lobe involvement. Spontaneous pneumothorax occurs in approximately 10% of cases and may be the presenting feature. Lung lesions may remain static or progress rapidly.

Initial chest radiographs may show diffuse, bilateral, symmetric interstitial disease with a characteristic reticulonodular pattern resulting from the summation of nodules and thin cystic walls. As the disease progresses, the radiographic features gradually evolve into a honeycomb-like pattern.

Thin-section computed tomography is valuable for the diagnosis and follow-up of pulmonary LCH. Multiple bilateral small nodules with early signs of cavitation or cysts with varied wall thickness (preferentially in the upper and middle lobes with sparing of the costophrenic angles) are highly suggestive of LCH.

The peak age at initial diagnosis is from 1 to 3 years, but the disease may manifest at any age. Boys are more often affected than girls.

With CNS disease, the pituitary stalk is typically involved; patients present with diabetes insipidus. Mastoid air cells may also be involved, with patients presenting with hearing loss.

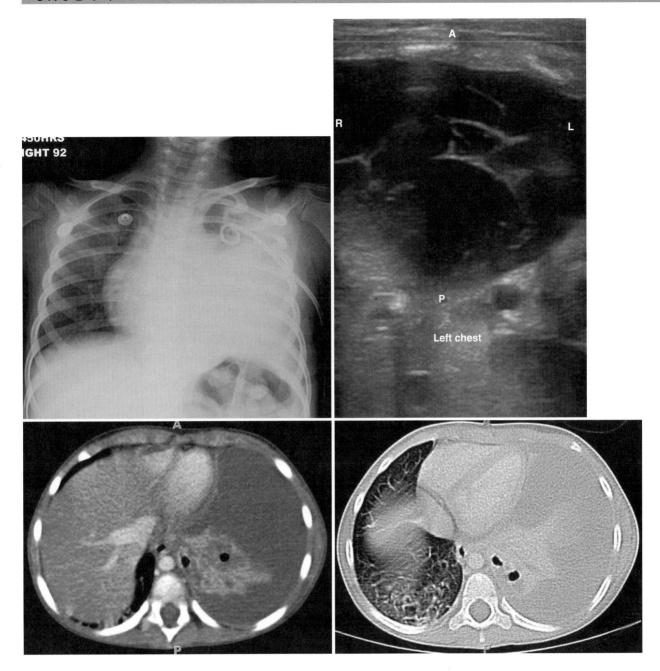

1. What are the imaging findings in this 8-year-old girl?

2. What is the diagnosis?

3. Ultrasound is superior to computed tomography (CT) in characterizing the nature of fluid collection in the pleural space. True or false?

4. Describe the three stages of this entity.

Diagnosis: Empyema as a Complication of Pneumonia

1. Radiographic findings reveal a near complete opacification of the left hemithorax with mediastinal shift to the right and a right lateral displacement of the trachea. (These findings confirm that the opacification is from a process that results in increased volume.) The ultrasound reveals a loculated septated fluid collection in the left pleural space. The CT scan shows that pneumatoceles may be noted in opacified left lower lobe with enhancement of the left pleura.

2. Pneumonic infiltrate in the left lower lobe with pneumatoceles and adjacent pleural fluid is the diagnosis. (In the presence of the infiltrate with pneumatoceles, the pleural fluid is considered to represent empyema.)

3. True.

4. Stages are (1) exudative stage in which protein-rich pleural fluid remains free flowing; (2) fibrinolytic stage in which viscosity of the pleural fluid increases; and (3) organizing stage in which loculations form.

Reference

Eastham KM, Freeman R, Kearns AM: Clinical features, etiology and outcome of empyema in children in the north east of England, *Thorax* 59:522–525, 2004.

Cross-Reference

Blickman JG, Parker BR, Barnes PD: *Pediatric radiology— the requisites*, ed 3, Philadelphia, 2009, Mosby, pp 32–35.

Comment

Pleural empyema is defined as pus in the pleural cavity and has significant clinical morbidity. Empyema is an exudative effusion with pH less than 7.2, and lactate dehydrogenase greater than 1000 mg/dl. Most empyema in childhood follows acute bacterial pneumonia (most commonly streptococcus pneumonia). In rare instances it can be associated with viral infections or tuberculosis. More unusual causes of empyema include spread from other sites of sepsis, such as from septic emboli, lung abscess, subphrenic abscess, osteomyelitis of a rib, or as a result of a missed inhaled foreign body. The most common clinical presentation is persistent fever and sepsis, respiratory distress, and persistent elevated C-reactive protein despite antibiotic treatment for pneumonia. Radiologic workup starts with a plain radiograph of the chest. The imaging findings on the plain radiograph can range from presence of pneumonic infiltrate along with pleural effusion (as evidenced by blunting of the ipsilateral costophrenic sinus) to complete opacification of the entire hemithorax, depending on the severity of the disease. Mediastinal shift can be observed if the volume of the fluid is high. Ultrasound imaging is very helpful to differentiate exudative from transudative effusion. Transudate appears as anechoic fluid, whereas transudate contains echogenic debris, septations, and loculations. In addition, ultrasound is helpful for image-guided drainage. CT is helpful in cases with progressive and persisting illness, despite adequate antibiotic treatment and pleural drainage. The CT examination should be performed with intravenous contrast agents where additional findings such as lung abscess, cavitary necrosis of pneumonic infiltrate, and pericarditis can be visualized. CT should not be used to differentiate free fluid from loculated fluid or transudative effusion from exudative effusion. Typically the pleura will enhance, and calcification may occur. Plain radiographs obtained in anteroposterior and decubitus positions and ultrasound are sufficient to make that differentiation.

Management of pleural empyema depends on the size of the effusion and symptoms; generally, conservative treatment with antibiotic agents is the first line of choice. In severe cases, drainage with thrombolytic therapy to the pleural space, video-assisted thoracscopic surgery, or thoracotomy may be necessary. Pleural empyema is more frequently seen in immune-compromised children (e.g., human immunodeficiency virus, posttransplant status, and severe combined immunodeficiency).

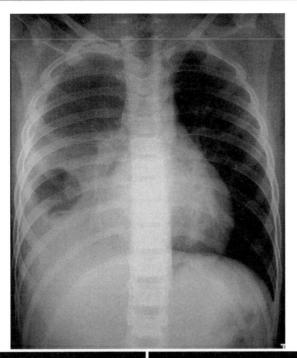

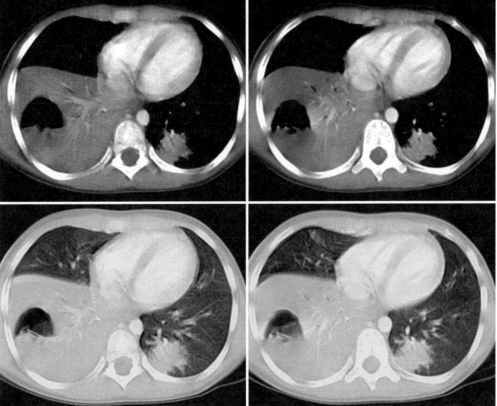

1. What are the findings on the chest radiography?

2. What are the imaging findings on the computed tomography (CT)?

3. What is the most likely diagnosis?

4. What is the anatomic correlation for the structure within the cyst?

Diagnosis: Pulmonary Hydatid Cyst

1. A right-sided, air-filled intrapulmonary cystic lesion with a *floating membrane* in the base and an adjacent pneumonic infiltrate and pleural effusion.

2. An air-filled intrapulmonary lesion with a *serpent* or *whirl* sign.

3. Hydatid cyst of the lung.

4. A collapsed parasitic membrane after bronchial rupture.

Reference

Ramos G, Orduña A, García-Yuste M: Hydatid cyst of the lung: diagnosis and treatment, *World J Surg* 25:46–57, 2001.

Comment

Hydatid disease is a primary or secondary infestation of the lung caused by *Echinococcus granulosus*. Hydatid disease is an anthropozoonosis, which is endemic in several regions of the world and is considered to be a major health problem affecting both humans and animals. Humans are intermediary hosts, becoming infested by eating food that is contaminated with the feces of a primary host (e.g., dog) containing *Taenia* spp. eggs. The ingested eggs reach the liver via the portocaval system and the lungs or other organs via the general circulation. The *Taenia* spp. eggs may also directly reach the lungs via inhalation and/or lymphatic distribution. The development of the parasitic larval stage in the host's organs manifests in the form of a cyst (hydatid). The liver is most frequently affected (50% to 60%), followed by the lung (10% to 30%). Hematogenous spread may result in hydatid cysts in almost every part of the body.

The hydatid cyst can develop anywhere in the lung; however, it is more frequently noted in the lower lobes. The intact hydatid cyst is liquid and may have remnants of hooklets and scolices in the base of the cyst. The cysts range from a few centimeters to large cysts that fill out an entire hemithorax. On plain radiography a well-defined, rounded, soft tissue lesion may be seen. If the cyst ruptures into the bronchial system, the fluid within the cyst will be replaced by air. Frequently, the scolices and collapsed parasitic membrane are visible within the dependant part of the cyst floating on residual fluid within the cyst. On CT the collapsed parasitic membrane results in the serpent or snake sign and the spin or whirl sign. The cyst may be surrounded by an allergic or inflammatory pulmonary infiltration or atelectatic lung. Rarely the cyst may rupture into the pleural cavity. In the majority of cases only one cyst is encountered; multiple cysts are much more rare but may be unilateral and/or bilateral. Either ultrasound or CT should be used to exclude additional lesions within the liver.

Next to imaging studies, serologic assays using immunoglobulin G enzyme-linked immunosorbent assay and immunoelectrophoresis are helpful in confirming diagnosis.

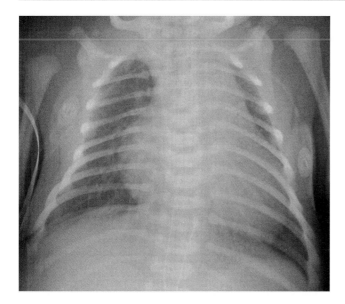

1. This term newborn was discharged and then returned at 3 days of age in cardiopulmonary collapse, when this chest radiograph was obtained. What happened physiologically that led to readmission? What are the findings?

2. What are the ultimate goals of repair?

3. At what age are the surgeries performed?

4. What is the only other alternative therapy at this time?

Diagnosis: Hypoplastic Left Heart Syndrome

1. Pulmonary vascular resistance fell on schedule toward the normal range, allowing the ductus arteriosus to close. Unfortunately, the ductus was supplying all systemic flow because this patient has a tiny aorta, atretic aortic valve, and diminutive left ventricle and atrium. On the image, cardiomegaly (reflecting dilated right ventricle and atrium) and pulmonary arterial and venous overload are seen.

2. To allow the right ventricle to be the systemic ventricle, pumping through a neoaorta; supply the pulmonary arteries with low-pressure blood; stop the mixing of oxygenated and deoxygenated blood in the heart.

3. At presentation, between 3 and 6 months, and between 18 months and 4 years.

4. Cardiac transplantation.

Reference

Sena L: Coarctation of the aorta and hypoplastic left heart, 2005: In Reid J, editor: *Pediatric radiology curriculum*, Cleveland, 2005, Cleveland Clinic Center for Online Medical Education and Training. Available from: https://www.cchs.net/pediatricradiology.

Cross-Reference

Blickman JG, Parker BR, Barnes PD: *Pediatric radiology—the requisites*, ed 3, Philadelphia, 2009, Mosby, pp 56-57.

Comment

This cardiac defect is entirely compatible with fetal life, because it relies on the high pulmonary vascular resistance, patent foramen ovale, and wide-open ductus that are naturally present to bypass the inadequate systemic cardiac chambers and outflow tract. The coronary arteries connect to the tiny aorta and are perfused by retrograde flow. Most of the time this defect is diagnosed on prenatal ultrasound. At birth, prostaglandin infusion is begun to prevent ductus closure, and the atrial septum is assessed for adequacy of communication to allow oxygenated left atrial contents to flow into the right atrium. Balloon septostomy and even extracorporeal membrane oxygenation (ECMO) may be needed for stabilization. Chest radiograph findings reflect right heart dilatation and small left ventricle. The pulmonary arteries can be large if the atrial left-to-right shunt is unrestricted. If the defect is small, then the pulmonary veins obstruct and venous edema occurs.

Stage 1 repair takes place as soon as the patient is stable. The main pulmonary artery is separated from its bifurcation and main branches. The right pulmonary artery and right subclavian artery are connected side to side (modified Blalock-Taussig shunt). Alternatively, the right ventricle is connected directly to the right pulmonary artery (Sano connection). The main pulmonary artery and tiny ascending aorta (with its coronaries) are incorporated, augmented with graft material, and connected to the descending aorta. The ductus arteriosus is tied off, and the atrial septum is excised to maximize mixing of left atrial inflow. Thus the first of the three goals (mentioned in question two) is satisfied but the other two are not.

Stage 2 repair seeks to accomplish the second goal, because prolonged exposure to systemic blood pressure leads to irreversible changes in the pulmonary arteries. However, it can only take place when the patient's pulmonary vascular resistance finally falls below systemic venous pressure. The surgeon replaces the Blalock-Taussig shunt with a Glenn shunt, which connects the superior vena cava to the right pulmonary artery. It is termed a bidirectional Glenn because blood flows to both the right and left pulmonary arteries. However, systemic venous blood still reaches the right atrium through the inferior vena cava (IVC), allowing admixed blood to flow out through the neoaorta.

Stage 3 is performed when the patient's growth outstrips the supply of available oxygenated blood and cyanosis deepens. The surgeon connects the IVC to the right pulmonary artery. A baffle in the right atrium directs blood through the connection.

Chest radiograph appearance after repair may reflect some asymmetry in pulmonary blood flow (R > L), but the difference should not be great unless an obstruction exists. Aneurysmal dilation or leakage of the grafted neoaorta can occur.

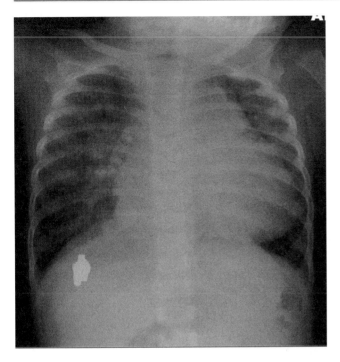

1. What are the imaging findings in this tachypneic, acyanotic 2-month-old child?

2. What other anatomic regions should be closely inspected for signs of associated abnormality?

3. What cardiac defect is most likely to be uncovered on a teenage girl's camp physical?

Diagnosis: Left-to-Right Shunt (This Patient: Trisomy 21 with Complete Atrioventricular Canal)

1. Cardiomegaly, *wormlike* hilar shadows, pulmonary arterial congestion, and mild pulmonary edema.

2. Ribs, shoulders, vertebrae, and sternum.

3. Atrial septal defect (ASD).

Reference

Pennington DJ: Acyanotic congenital heart disease, 2005: In Reid J, editor: *Pediatric radiology curriculum*, Cleveland, 2005, Cleveland Clinic Center for Online Medical Education and Training. Available from: https://www.cchs.net/pediatricradiology.

Cross-Reference

Blickman JG, Parker BR, Barnes PD: *Pediatric radiology—the requisites*, ed 3, Philadelphia, 2009, Mosby, pp 47-51.

Comment

In fetal life the heart begins as a single tube that divides both transversely (into atria, ventricles, and inflow-out-flow tracts) and longitudinally (separating pulmonary from systemic circulation). Abnormal connections between the systemic and pulmonary circuits can persist that, because of the lower resistance on the pulmonary side, result in blood shunting across from the systemic side. Because the shunted blood is already oxygenated, the patient is not cyanotic. Clinical and plain film findings relate to the size and position of the shunt and associated intra- and extracardiac malformations.

Plain film findings relate to volume overload: blood recirculates on the pulmonary side, effectively increasing blood volume. Both atria and the right ventricle dilate and dilatation of pulmonary arteries occurs, eventually leading to leakage and interstitial edema. These shunts can occur as part of various syndromes that can be suspected from chest imaging signs such as vertebral anomaly (vertebrae, anus, cardiovascular tree, trachea, esophagus, renal system, and limb buds syndrome), right-sided aortic arch (tetralogy of Fallot, mirror image branching), omphalocele (general association), Sprengel deformity (Holt-Oram Syndrome), asplenia (general association), heterotaxy (general association), 11 or 13 pairs of ribs ± hypersegmented sternum (trisomy 21 [Down syndrome]), and hypoplastic or missing ribs (trisomy 13 and 18).

Patent ductus arteriosus (PDA): The ductus arteriosus is a normal fetal structure that connects the descending aorta to the main pulmonary artery, allowing blood to bypass the high-resistance pulmonary bed. After birth, intrinsic muscles should close the ductus. As breathing opens the alveoli and resistance falls, flow can reverse in a ductus that is still patent, overloading the pulmonary circuit.

Ventriculoseptal defect (VSD): Incomplete division of the ventricles may leave small defects that close on their own or large ones that need surgical patching. The most common location is in the membranous septum (70% to 80%), but spontaneous closure is more common in muscular VSDs. They have equal incidence in males and females. Presentation can be insidious, with feeding fatigue and increased respiratory infections.

ASD: This is the most frequent shunt lesion of all and predominates in female patients (2:1). It is also the lesion most frequently found in teenagers. The atrial septum forms first from the septum primum that, in its late development, forms a defect—the ostium secundum. If the septum secundum that forms later fails to cover this hole, the most frequent type (75%) of defect is formed—the ostium secundum ASD. These also most frequently close spontaneously. Ostium primum ASDs and sinus venosus ASDs form earlier in fetal cardiac development and usually need surgical repair.

Atrioventricular (AV) canal: Also known as endocardial cushion defect, these fetal structures form the core of the heart, their malformation resulting in various combinations of mitral and tricuspid valve leaflet deformities, ostium primum ASD, and membranous VSD. About 40% of patients with AV canal will have trisomy 21.

Aorticopulmonary window: This is a persistent defect in the spiral septum that divides the ascending aorta from the main pulmonary artery. It is a rare anomaly and may be associated with ASD, PDA, and aortic coarctation.

Systemic shunts: Shunt vascularity and cardiomegaly with negative echo raises the possibility of shunts outside the heart such as vein of Galen malformation, soft tissue hemangioma, and hepatic hemangioendothelioma. Ultrasound and magnetic resonance imaging (MRI) are appropriate diagnostic examinations for these entities.

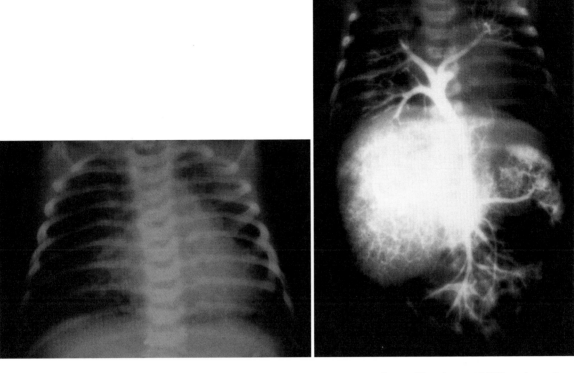

1. What are the chest radiograph findings in this cyanotic term newborn (first image)? What does the angiogram (second image, postmortem) show?

2. What helps differentiate this entity on plain film from other entities causing cyanosis?

3. What intracardiac connection is necessary for survival?

4. Why is such a patient more hypoxemic with feeding?

Diagnosis: Total Anomalous Pulmonary Venous Connection

1. The chest shows hazy pulmonary edema in the classic venous pattern and a normal heart size. Injection of the pulmonary veins fills the portal system and opacifies the hepatic sinusoids.

2. Term gestation excludes surfactant deficiency. Venous edema implies left-sided cardiac obstruction. Normal heart size suggests that the obstruction lies before the left atrium.

3. Atrial septal defect (ASD) is necessary for survival.

4. With feeding, the full esophagus compresses the aberrant pulmonary veins still further in the esophageal hiatus.

Reference

Kirks DR, Griscom NT, editors: *Practical pediatric imaging*, ed 3, Philadelphia, 1998, Lippincott-Raven, pp 562–566.

Cross-Reference

Blickman JG, Parker BR, Barnes PD: *Pediatric radiology— the requisites*, ed 3, Philadelphia, 2009, Mosby, pp 54–55.

Comment

Normally, oxygenated blood returns from the lungs to the left atrium through the pulmonary veins so that it can be pumped out to the rest of the body by the left ventricle. However, persistence of fetal vessels can result in abnormal connections of the pulmonary veins to structures feeding back to the *right* side of the heart. This can be partial (which can be difficult to detect and can include Scimitar syndrome and pulmonary sequestration in its spectrum) or complete (which is described here). This is usually in conjunction with an ASD, but the oxygenated blood is diluted with deoxygenated blood. The end result is hypoxemia, which is immediately apparent at birth.

The abnormal connection can be above or below the diaphragm. In the first instance, the connection can be to the superior vena cava or the coronary sinus and results in volume overload of the right atrium and pulmonary arterial system. Plain film findings mimic those of left-to-right shunts. The moderate hypoxemia would be a differentiating point, however, from those other shunts. When the pulmonary drainage passes below the diaphragm through the esophageal hiatus (to the ductus venosus or portal venous system), obstruction occurs at the diaphragm. The pulmonary veins leak with the increased pressure and pulmonary edema ensues, worsening the hypoxemia.

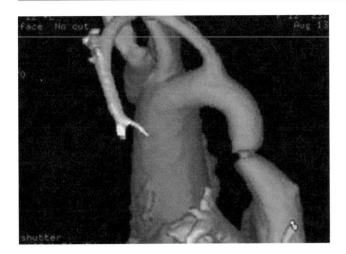

1. The magnetic resonance image (MRI) is from a 2-year-old boy with elevated blood pressure in the arms but not in the legs. His chest radiograph was normal. What does the image show?

2. What is this condition called?

3. What vessels supply the distal aorta?

4. What is the treatment for this condition?

Diagnosis: Coarctation of the Aorta

1. Focal narrowing of the aorta after the take off of the left subclavian artery.

2. Coarctation of the aorta.

3. Collateral blood flows though the intercostal, superior epigastric, and mediastinal vessels.

4. Surgical repair with either resection and direct anastomosis or subclavian patch or balloon dilatation of the narrowing.

Reference

Kuhn JP, Slovis TL, Haller JO: *Caffey's pediatric diagnostic imaging*, Philadelphia, 2004, Elsevier, pp 1292–1294.

Cross-Reference

Blickman JG, Parker BR, Barnes PD: *Pediatric radiology— the requisites*, ed 3, Philadelphia, 2009, Mosby, pp 58–59.

Comment

Coarctation of the aorta is classified into two types. One is the juxtaductal type, which is usually seen in young infants and children and is associated with transverse arch and isthmus hypoplasia. Closure of the ductus arteriosus may result in significant acute narrowing of the aorta and acute heart failure. The second type, post-ductal coarctation, tends to present later in life and may be asymptomatic, discovered by the finding of abnormal blood pressure or heart murmur.

Coarctation constitutes 5% of congenital heart disease, with a male predominance (2:1). Associated anomalies include patent ductus arteriosus (66%), ventricular septal defect (33%), other heart lesions, Shone complex (left heart obstructions), and Turner syndrome.

In the early presentation, the infant may have cardiomegaly and pulmonary edema. In the older patient, mild or no cardiomegaly may be present. The "Figure 3" sign in the left upper mediastinum may be seen, and the notch is the site of coarctation with poststenotic dilatation of the aorta. Rib notching from the dilated intercostal arteries is most common, involving the inferior surface of the third to fifth ribs; however, it does not usually occur until the patient is 5 years old.

Diagnosis in the young infant is usually confirmed by echocardiography. In the older child, the distal arch may be difficult to visualize by echocardiography. In these cases, either computed tomography (CT) or MRI is useful. CT is a fast, easy study to perform but requires iodinated contrast and radiation. MRI may require sedation because it is a longer test, but no radiation is involved and flow quantification is possible.

The prognosis is excellent for isolated coarctation, with either a surgical or catheter approach to repair. However, mortality may be higher if the patient has more complex heart disease. Postoperative complications include aneurysm or pseudoaneurysm, recurrent coarctation, and persistent hypertension.

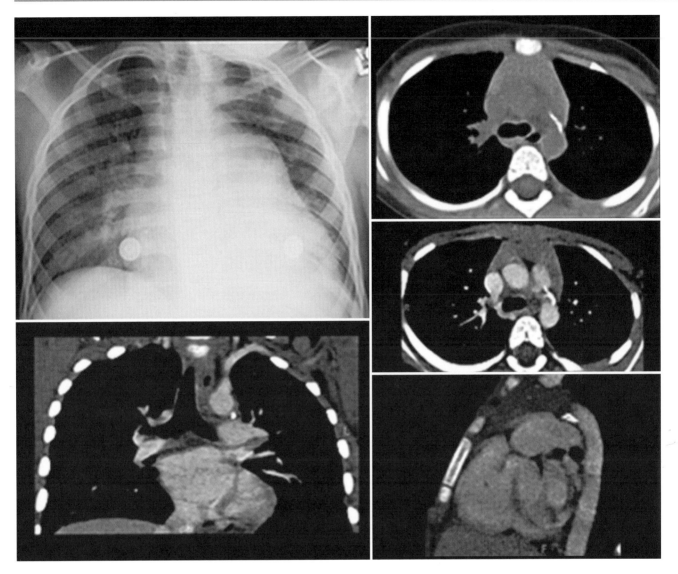

1. Images of two infants are shown here. One has had an anteroposterior (AP) chest radiograph; the other has had multiple computed tomography (CT) images. Both have findings related to the same structure. What is this structure?

2. What are the findings on the chest radiograph? What is the likely cause?

3. What is the finding on the CT images?

4. How common is the CT finding in children?

Diagnosis: Ductus Arteriosus

1. Ductus arteriosus.

2. On the chest radiograph, the heart and aorta are enlarged; the pulmonary vessels are enlarged and indistinct. The likely cause is left-to-right shunting secondary to patent ductus arteriosus (PDA).

3. Linear calcification between the aorta and pulmonary artery.

4. Calcification of the ligamentum arteriosum on noncontrast CT is seen in 13% of children.

Reference

Bisceglia M, Donaldson JS: Calcification of the ligamentum arteriosum in children: a normal finding on CT, *AJR Am J Roentgenol* 156:351–352, 1991.

Cross-Reference

Blickman JG, Parker BR, Barnes PD: *Pediatric radiology— the requisites*, ed 3, Philadelphia, 2009, Mosby, p 52.

Comment

The ductus arteriosus is derived from the sixth aortic arch. It connects the pulmonary artery to the aorta. After week 6 of fetal life, most of the right ventricular outflow passes through the ductus to the aorta rather than to the lungs. Only about 5% to 10% of the right ventricular outflow passes through the lungs. The ductus arteriosus is an important structure in fetal development; it diverts blood from the fluid-filled, high-resistance lungs to the aorta, which contributes to the development of the fetal organs and other structures. Closure of the ductus before birth may lead to right heart failure. After birth the ductus normally undergoes closure by day 10 of life.

Persistence of the PDA represents 5% to 10% of all congenital heart diseases, excluding PDA seen in premature infants. It occurs in approximately 8 of 1000 live premature births. In term infants the incidence is about 1 in 2000 births. The female-to-male ratio is 2:1. This lesion is diagnosed by the combination of its clinical presentation and echocardiography.

When the defect is large, heart failure with tachypnea and poor weight gain or failure to thrive are the main presentations. Patients who present with heart failure need medical therapy followed by a definitive procedure to close the PDA by either surgery or catheterization.

When the ductus closes normally, the ligamentum arteriosum is formed; it calcifies in some patients. This finding is relatively common on chest radiograph (although the calcification may be quite small and unapparent). The calcification is readily apparent on CT imaging, especially when no contrast is used. Awareness of this appearance is important for the clinician not to mistake the calcification for evidence of a significant condition manifesting as calcified lymphadenopathy or mass.

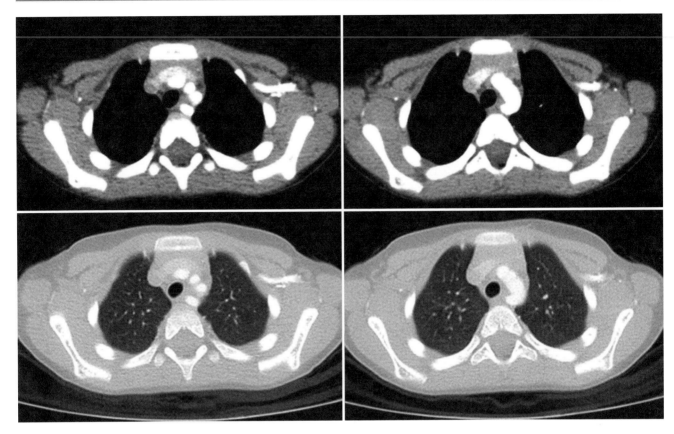

1. What are the imaging findings on the computed tomography (CT) for this 2½-year-old boy with failure to thrive?

2. What is the most frequently occurring symptomatic vascular ring?

3. Which symptoms are most common with vascular rings?

4. Which nerve may show an aberrant course?

Diagnosis: Dysphagia Lusoria

1. Vascular sling with aberrant right subclavian artery and left aortic arch.

2. Vascular sling with aberrant left subclavian artery and right aortic arch.

3. Airway obstruction and dysphagia.

4. The recurrent nerve.

Reference

Hermans R, Dewandel P, Debruyne F, et al: Arteria lusoria identified on preoperative CT and nonrecurrent inferior laryngeal nerve during thyroidectomy: a retrospective study, *Head Neck* 25:113–117, 2003.

Comment

Vascular rings or slings become clinically symptomatic because of tracheal compression in combination with symptoms of dysphagia and/or recurrent episodes of aspiration. Airway compression is usually only present when a complete, tight vascular ring is present. Vascular rings result from an abnormal development of the initially paired aortic arch system. The combination of a right aortic arch with an aberrant left subclavian artery that runs dorsally to the esophagus is most common. A left-sided aortic arch with an aberrant right subclavian artery (originating from the descending aorta) is more unusual (0.5 % of asymptomatic patients). Associated cardiac anomalies are somewhat more frequent, especially when a right aortic arch is present. In addition, frequently an aberrant course of the phrenic nerve exists, which can be of importance for surgical repair. Normally the right recurrent inferior laryngeal nerve passes below the right subclavian artery. If the normal right subclavian artery is absent, the recurrent nerve will move cranially. The aberrant right subclavian artery is also known as the arteria lusoria. Consequently, symptomatic compression of the esophagus by an aberrant right subclavian artery is also known as dysphagia lusoria.

Conventional radiography frequently fails to identify the aberrant right subclavian artery. Diagnosis is easily made on contrast-enhanced CT of the chest. Three-dimensional reconstruction may be helpful in the preoperative setting.

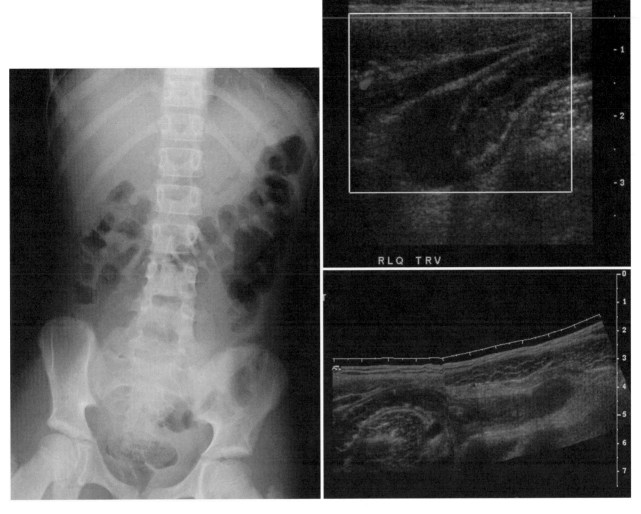

RLQ TRV

1. What are the plain film findings in this 8-year-old patient (first image)?

2. What pros and cons should be weighed when choosing between computed tomography (CT) and ultrasound for the follow-up cross-sectional examination?

3. What should be apparent in both modalities (as demonstrated in ultrasound images, (second and third images)?

Diagnosis: Appendicitis

1. A soft tissue mass and paucity of gas in the right lower quadrant, calcified fecalith, and localized ileus.

2. No operator dependence (pro: CT; con: ultrasound); no radiation (pro: ultrasound; con: CT); finds interloop abcesses (pro: CT; con: ultrasound); works even for large body size (pro: CT; con: ultrasound); reliably visualizes the normal appendix (pro: CT; con: ultrasound); easily excludes gynecologic disease (pro: ultrasound; con: CT); localizes pain to palpation (pro: ultrasound; con: CT); sensitive to free air—an unusual complication (pro: CT; con: ultrasound).

3. Appendix enlarged more than 6 mm in diameter, fecalith, free fluid, and fluid collection.

Reference

Pitt S, Reid J: Appendicitis, 2005: In Reid J, editor: *Pediatric radiology curriculum*, Cleveland, 2005, Cleveland Clinic Center for Online Medical Education and Training. Available from: https://www.cchs.net/pediatricradiology.

Cross-Reference

Blickman JG, Parker BR, Barnes PD: *Pediatric radiology—the requisites*, ed 3, Philadelphia, 2009, Mosby, pp 99-101.

Comment

Impaction of the appendix, with inspissation of secretions and superinfection, can occur at any age. Because the appendix and the cecal tip to which it is attached are quite mobile in early life, the eventual location of the appendix and the way it will express its inflammation are extremely variable: locations like retrocecal, subhepatic, alongside the bladder, or in the pouch of Douglas might result in symptoms mimicking renal stone, cholelithiasis, cystitis, or pelvic inflammatory disease.

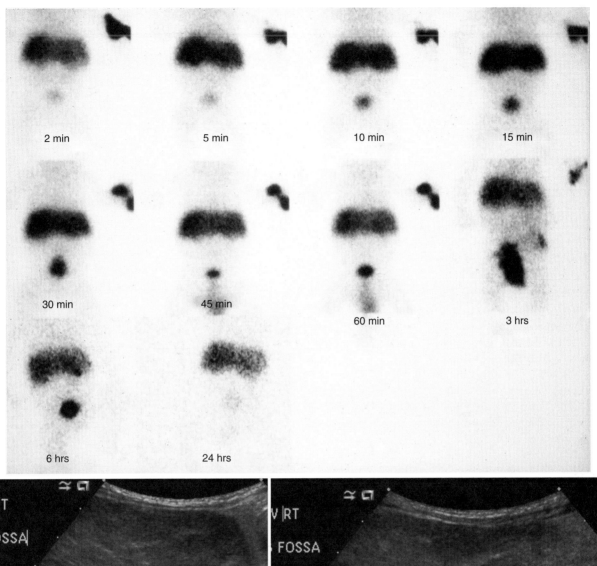

2 min 5 min 10 min 15 min

30 min 45 min 60 min 3 hrs

6 hrs 24 hrs

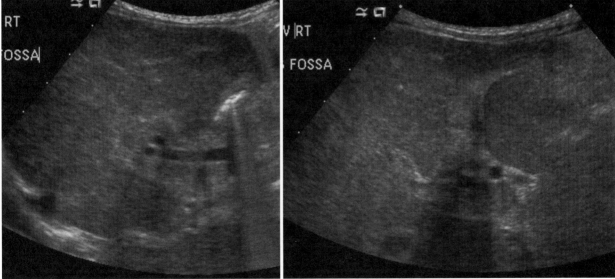

1. When is neonatal jaundice considered a pathologic condition?

2. What entities are in the differential list?

3. How do these imaging findings help diagnose the problem? (Patient A, first image; patient B, second image [longitudinal along portal vein] and third image [transverse through porta hepatis])

4. Why is it important to find this entity before 8 weeks of age?

Diagnosis: Biliary Atresia

1. Persistence of jaundice past the first 2 weeks of life is a pathologic condition, particularly if direct (conjugated) hyperbilirubinemia exists.

2. Idiopathic hepatitis, inherited metabolic syndromes (galactosemia, α1-antitrypsin deficiency), cystic fibrosis, sepsis, gallstones, bile plug syndrome (caused by dehydration and inanition), biliary atresia (BA), and choledochal cyst.

3. Patient A has no excretion of isotope to the bowel in over 24 hours (only to the bladder), liver is transverse, suggesting heterotaxy.

   Findings shows that Patient B has liver parenchyma that is coarsely echogenic, consistent with cirrhosis, no choledochal cyst, and echogenic cord that takes the place of the common duct.

4. In many cases of BA, an ongoing inflammatory aspect exists that progressively eradicates the bile ducts unless halted by surgery.

References

Cassady C: Newborn jaundice. In Reid J, editor: *Pediatric radiology curriculum*, Cleveland, 2005, Cleveland Clinic Center for Online Medical Education and Training. Available from: https://www.cchs.net/pediatricradiology.

Siegel MJ, editor: *Pediatric sonography*, ed 3, Philadelphia-Baltimore, 2002, Lippincott Williams & Wilkins, pp 290-291.

Cross-Reference

Blickman JG, Parker BR, Barnes PD: *Pediatric radiology—the requisites*, ed 3, Philadelphia, 2009, Mosby, pp 103-105.

Comment

The cause of BA is unclear. In some infants it may represent a true atresia—nonformation of the biliary tree in fetal life. In others it appears to be an autoimmune inflammatory reaction to a virus contracted after birth. In any case the blockage of bile flow leads to hepatocyte injury, fibrosis, and cirrhosis. Early diagnosis is essential, both in an attempt to remove the inflamed bile ducts, if present, and to decompress the hepatocytes and save them. Bile duct absence can occur at any level; surgically approachable disease is confined to abnormality at the level of the right and left hepatic ducts and below.

Ultrasound can detect abnormalities highly associated with BA, although no sign is absolutely specific. At the organ level, heterotaxy (transverse liver, polysplenia or asplenia) should raise suspicion that BA is also present. A gallbladder should be carefully searched for (but only after the infant has received nothing by mouth for 3 to 4 hours to maximize distension). The presence of a gallbladder does not exclude BA; if it appears small and irregular, or if a thick, echogenic cord is found in the gallbladder bed, then BA may well be present. A gallbladder that does not contract after a milk feeding suggests obstruction by BA. Another echogenic cord paralleling the portal vein (triangular in cross-section) is thought to represent the fibrosed common duct. No proximal duct dilatation occurs within the liver, although irregular bile lakes adjacent to portal triads may be seen.

Lack of isotope excretion into the bowel on nuclear medicine (technetium-99m iminodiacetic acid [99mTc-IDA]) scan can be helpful, if sufficient hepatic parenchymal functioning exists for adequate uptake. Biopsy looks for bile duct proliferation, periportal fibrosis, and giant cell proliferation, but this also overlaps with neonatal hepatitis.

In the Kasai procedure, the surgeon cuts back through the porta hepatis to expose patent bile ducts. A small bowel loop is then brought up to this hepatic plate to funnel the bile into the gastrointestinal tract. This procedure has its best chance of success if it is performed before the infant is 8 weeks old.

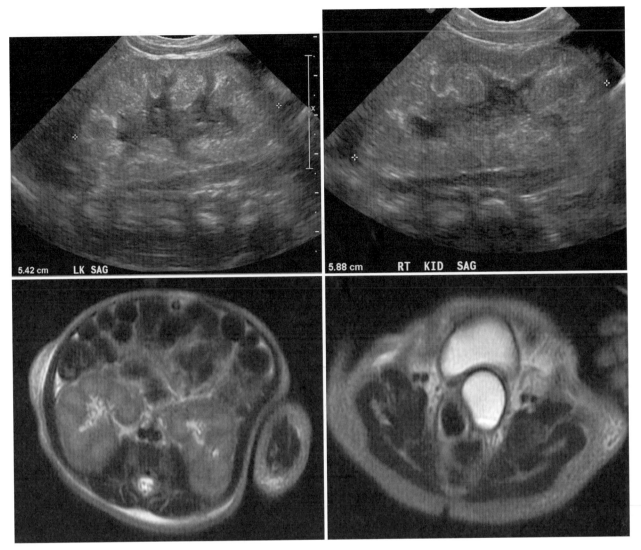

5.42 cm   LK SAG

5.88 cm   RT KID SAG

1. This 1-month-old infant with ambiguous genitalia (46, XY) has renal failure. The kidneys are imaged by ultrasound (first and second images) and magnetic resonance imaging (MRI) (repetition time [TR] 4500; echo time [TE] 180, postgadolinium) (third image). What is the most important thing to exclude?

2. Why were the kidneys removed surgically 1 month later?

3. This syndrome shares attributes with what two other, related syndromes?

4. What is the cystic structure in the pelvis on the fourth image?

Diagnosis: Denys-Drash Syndrome

1. Wilms tumor.

2. The kidneys were failing, and the child needed to be prepared for transplant. In addition, near-universal occurrence of nephroblastomatosis with this disorder makes the probability of Wilms tumor 90%.

3. WAGR (Wilms tumor, aniridia, genitourinary [GU] anomalies, mental retardation) and Frasier syndrome (chronic renal failure, XY gonadal dysgenesis, increased risk of gonadoblastoma).

4. A utricular cyst—a müllerian duct remnant.

References

Taybi H, Lachman RS: *Radiology of syndromes, metabolic disorders and skeletal dysplasias*, ed 4, Baltimore, 1996, Mosby, pp 130–131.

Shapiro O, Welch TR, Sheridan M, et al: Mixed gonadal dysgenesis and Denys-Drash syndrome: urologists should screen for nephrotic syndrome, *Can J Urol* 14(6):3767–3769, 2007.

Cross-Reference

Blickman JG, Parker BR, Barnes PD: *Pediatric radiology— the requisites*, ed 3, Philadelphia, 2009, Mosby, pp 140–142.

Comment

Mutation in the Wilms tumor suppressor gene results in abnormalities in fetal development of the GU system. Among the disorders mediated by this gene, Denys-Drash syndrome consists of a triad of medullary glomerulosclerosis, Wilms tumor, and ambiguous genitalia. In this infant, pathologic examination of the kidneys found severe glomerulosclerosis but no definite nephroblastomas. The testes were intraabdominal.

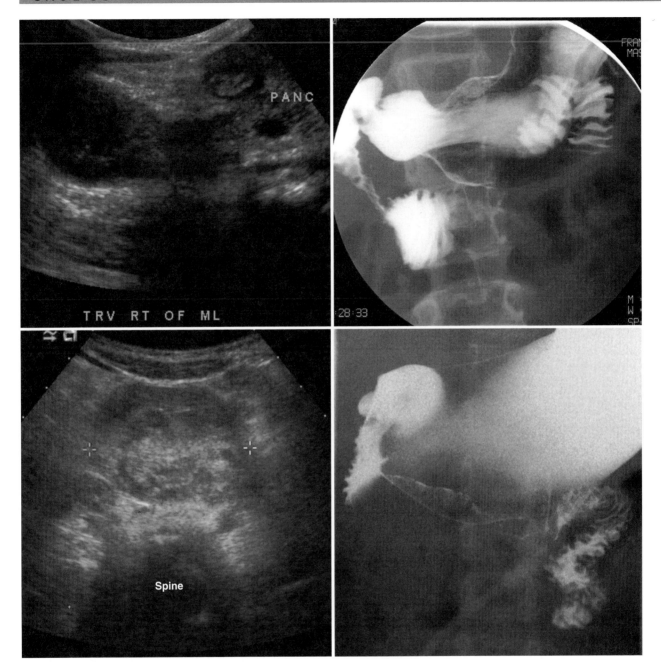

1. Patient 1 is an 8-year-old girl who had abdominal pain and vomiting after a deceleration injury caused by a sledding accident (first and second images). Patient 2 (6 years old, third and fourth images) began vomiting after duodenoscopy and biopsy.
   What do they have in common?

2. Under what other circumstances can this condition be found?

3. What is the treatment?

4. What complications can occur?

Diagnosis: Duodenal Hematoma

1. Fluid collection in the region of the duodenum on ultrasound (patient 1, second portion of duodenum; patient 2, third portion) and deformation of the barium column on fluoroscopy consistent with intramural collection.

2. Child abuse, lap belt injury, crush injury, anticoagulant agent overdose, thrombocytopenia, and Henoch-Schönlein purpura.

3. Usually conservative, although computed tomography–guided and laparascopic drainage have been reported if prolonged duodenal obstruction exists.

4. Early infection; delayed stricture.

Reference

Stringer DA, Babyn PS: *Pediatric gastrointestinal imaging and intervention*, ed 2, Hamilton-London, 2000, BC Decker Inc, pp 400–408.

Cross-Reference

Blickman JG, Parker BR, Barnes PD: *Pediatric radiology— the requisites*, ed 3, Philadelphia, 2009, Mosby, p 119.

Comment

The duodenum is uniquely vulnerable to crush injury as it passes across the spine to reach the ligament of Treitz. Unlike the rest of the small bowel, which is mobile in the peritoneum and can move away from the force, the duodenum is retroperitoneal and fixed. If duodenal injury is found in a trauma victim, then associated injuries of the spine and gallbladder should be excluded.

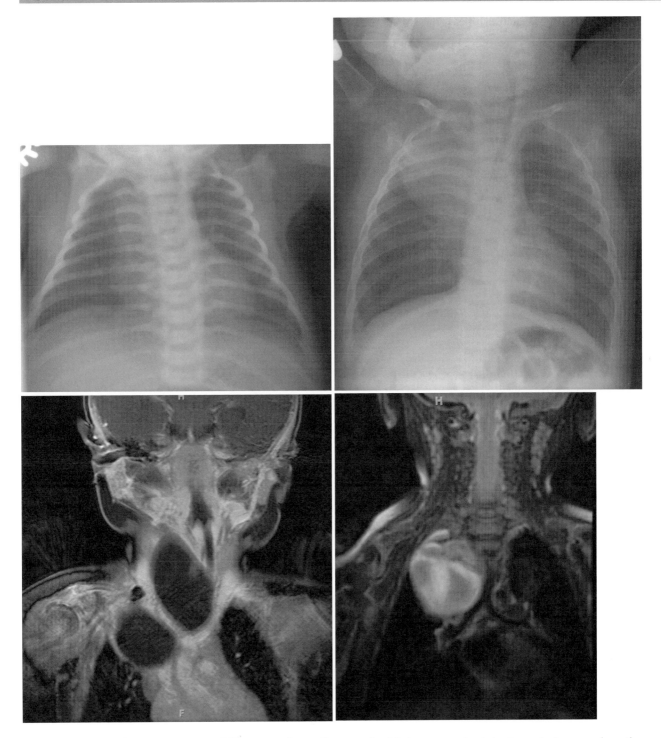

1. This child was having a routine follow-up echocardiogram for his known patent ductus arteriosus, when the sonographer saw a fluid collection above the heart. A chest radiograph was obtained (first image). What are some differential possibilities?

2. Five months later, the child returned, now in respiratory distress. What are the chest radiographic findings (second image)? How do they help you with your differential list?

3. A magnetic resonance imaging (MRI) scan was obtained (third image repetition time [TR] 310, echo time [TE] 2.5 postcontrast; fourth image TR 2900, TE 77, precontrast]). What does it show? How does this scan help you?

Diagnosis: Foregut Duplication Cyst

1. Differential possibilities include bronchogenic cyst, neuroenteric cyst, lateral meningocele, abscess, pericardial cyst, and cervical radicular cyst.

2. A large right-sided mass pushes the trachea toward the left. The gradual clinical course excludes abscess. No vertebral anomaly exists, making a neuroenteric cyst less likely. The child has no clinical signs of neurofibromatosis type 1 and no widened neural foramina are visible; however, the lateral meningocele is best imaged with MRI.

3. The study was able to show that the cyst did not communicate with the spinal canal. The cyst fluid is different from cerebrospinal fluid. This scan is helpful because lateral meningocele is excluded.

References

Stringer DA, Babyn PS: *Pediatric gastrointestinal imaging and intervention*, ed 2, Hamilton-London, 2000, BC Decker Inc, pp 191–195.

Barkovich AJ, Moore KR, Jones BV, et al, editors: *Diagnostic imaging: neuroradiology*, Amirsys, III, 2007, Salt Lake City, pp 6–49.

Cross-Reference

Blickman JG, Parker BR, Barnes PD: *Pediatric radiology—the requisites*, ed 3, Philadelphia, 2009, Mosby, pp 43–77.

Comment

The pathologic examination revealed an undifferentiated foregut duplication cyst. The primitive foregut divides in the fourth gestational week with budding of the trachea; the tracts then continue parallel development. Rests of pluripotent cells can persist anywhere along both tracts and form cysts. They are lined with secretory epithelium that may show differentiation toward gastrointestinal tissue, respiratory tissue, or both in the same cyst or in neither cyst. They may or may not be associated with other foregut malformations, such as esophageal atresia, or communicate with either tract. Their slow growth and gentle deformation of surrounding structures often allows them to achieve great size before they come to clinical attention.

Of all the differential possibilities, excluding lateral meningocele before surgery is the most important. The lack of neurologically important signs or symptoms is also reassuring.

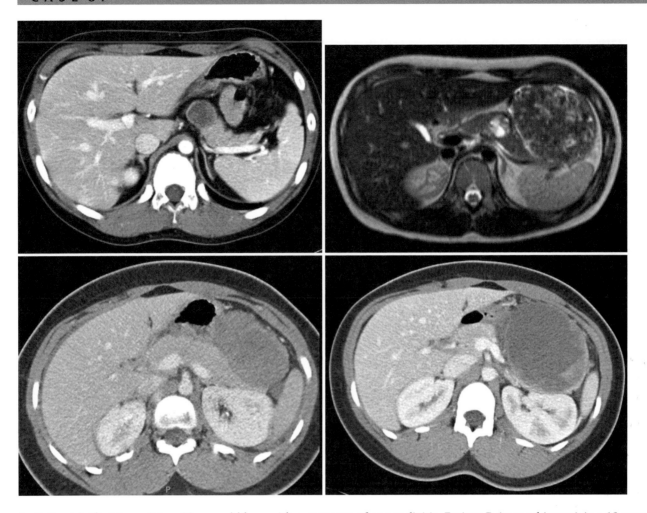

1. Patient A (first image) is a 10-year-old boy with symptoms of appendicitis. Patient B (second image) is a 13-year-old girl who was involved in a motor vehicle accident. Each got a computed tomography (CT) scan. Patient 1's appendicitis was confirmed, but both he and patient B had unexpected findings in the upper abdomen. What unexpected findings are present?

2. What are the differential diagnoses?

3. Patient A had a magnetic resonance imaging (MRI) follow-up after 18 months (third image repetition time 323, echo time 80, postgadolinium). Patient B had a CT follow-up after 10 months (fourth image). How does that help you with your differential list?

Diagnosis: Solid and Papillary Epithelial Neoplasm

1. Well-circumscribed cystic-appearing tumors in the pancreas body (patient A) and tail (patient B); no infiltration or fluid accumulation in surrounding mesentery and no adenopathy.

2. Cystic tumor, congenital cyst, pseudocyst, lymphangioma, and necrotic lymphoma.

3. Both tumors have increased in size (making congenital cyst less likely), and patient B's tumor looks even more cystic. No inflammation is evident (probably not pseudocyst), and no splenomegaly or adenopathy is seen (lymphoma unlikely). Congenital cysts are often seen in combination with renal cysts and hepatic cysts (not present here) and can be part of the von Hippel-Lindau complex that includes renal and cerebellar lesions. Cystic tumor versus lymphangioma seems the most likely diagnosis.

Reference

Siegel MJ: *Pediatric body CT*, Philadelphia, 1999, Lippincott Williams & Wilkins, pp 273-274.

Cross-Reference

Blickman JG, Parker BR, Barnes PD: *Pediatric radiology— the requisites*, ed 3, Philadelphia, 2009, Mosby, p 115.

Comment

This rare tumor has many names (solid and papillary epithelial carcinoma, solid and papillary epithelial neoplasm (SAPEN), epithelial carcinoma, papillary carcinoma, papillary-cystic carcinoma, Hamoudi tumor, Frantz tumor, solid pseudopapillary tumor), reflecting the varying proportions of its tissue elements, but all agree on its low grade of malignancy and good prognosis when surgically resected. The majority is seen in young women in their teens and 20s, but can be seen in younger patients of either gender. The most common site of origin is the pancreatic tail.

The reader may be puzzled as to why such a long delay occurs before resection of these tumors. In the case of patient A, the tumor was small and well-localized to the pancreas, the patient was postoperative from emergency surgery, and confidence existed in both the diagnosis of SAPEN and the likelihood of the patient's coming in for follow-up. When the tumor began to enlarge, the decision was made to electively resect it. In the case of patient B, the patient's presentation after trauma led to the erroneous diagnosis of hematoma. When she presented again later with nonspecific abdominal pain, the fresh look with no preconceived ideas resulted in the correct diagnosis of SAPEN.

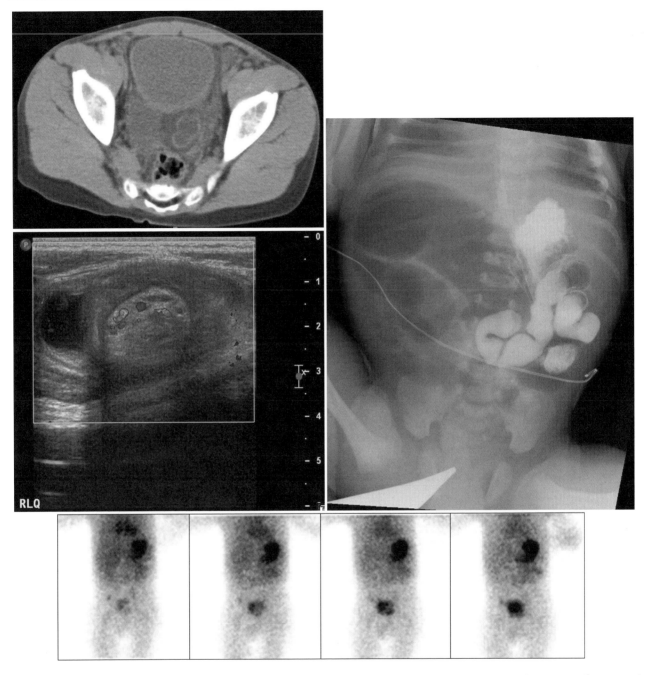

1. This 8-year-old boy had symptoms indicating possible appendicitis and had this computed tomography scan (first image). What is the finding?

2. This 2-day-old infant had feeding intolerance. This is an image from the upper gastrointestinal tract (second image). What condition does it suggest?

3. This Doppler ultrasound image (third image) was obtained on a 13-year-old boy with several days of crampy abdominal pain who finally came to the emergency department when he began to vomit. What could this be?

4. This 2-year-old boy had a 2-week history of painless melena with a single episode of bright-red blood in the diaper. Here are four images taken 15 minutes apart from a Tc-99m sodium pertechnetate scan (fourth image). What is seen from the image?

Diagnosis: Meckel Diverticulum/ Omphalomesenteric Duct Remnant

1. A fluid collection exists in the pouch of Douglas that surrounds a cystlike structure with an enhancing wall. The differential diagnoses include duplication cyst with torsion or infection, abscess, and appendicitis (patient could be malrotated). The pathologic condition can be identified as infected Meckel diverticulum with acute perforation.

2. The image suggests localized dilatation of the middle-to-distal small bowel with no contrast (the study also showed no malrotation). The proximal bowel has been decompressed, so apparently these loops are not in continuity. The differential diagnosis would include internal hernia with torsion. At operation: small bowel torqued around a persistent omphalomesenteric duct remnant.

3. An echogenic mass is seen with Doppler flow inside a bowel loop shown in cross-section. This is the usual presentation for an intussusception. An uncomplicated intussusception, it must be remembered, is uncommon in this age group. However, a fluid-filled structure appears next to the intussusceptum that looks to be paired with it. At operation: Meckel diverticulum acting as lead point for ileocolic intussusception.

4. A focus of isotope uptake appears in the right lower quadrant at the same time as uptake in the stomach. The pathologic condition can be identified as Meckel diverticulum with gastric mucosa.

References

Kuhn JP, Slovis TL, Haller JO: *Caffey's pediatric diagnostic imaging*, ed 10, Philadelphia, 2004, Mosby, pp 140, 160, 1430-1432.

Moore KM: *The developing human*, ed 2, Philadelphia, 1977, Saunders, pp 206-207, 214-215.

Cross-Reference

Blickman JG, Parker BR, Barnes PD: *Pediatric radiology— the requisites*, ed 3, Philadelphia, 2009, Mosby, pp 90-91.

Comment

The omphalomesenteric (or vitelline) duct connects the yolk sac to the primitive midgut and nourishes the developing fetus through week 8 of gestation. Normally the duct closes and disappears after that time. It can persist, however, as a true diverticulum from the antimesenteric border of the distal ileum, containing all four intestinal layers, which Johann Friedrich Meckel described in 1809.

A memory aid is the rule of twos: 2% of the population have it, and 2% of these patients are symptomatic. It is usually found within 2 feet (from the ileocecal valve); it is 2 inches (in length); two types of ectopic tissue are most commonly present (gastric and pancreatic), the most common age at clinical presentation is 2 years old, and male patients are two times as likely to be affected. The secretions from the ectopic tissue can ulcerate the diverticulum and cause bleeding, which can be profuse in infants. A 99mTc scan will detect the gastric mucosa in the diverticulum; because this is present in only 15% of the diverticula, the anomaly can still be present despite a negative scan. The diverticulum can also become impacted and inflamed; enteroliths can be seen on plain films. The diverticulum can invert and become the lead point of an intussusception.

The duct itself can persist, either in total as a fistulous tract from the small bowel to the umbilicus (with thick secretions, not the clear fluid seen with persistent urachus) or segmentally as a cyst. The duct may close but persist as a fibrous band. The connection to the base of the umbilicus acts as an axis around which the small bowel can volvulize.

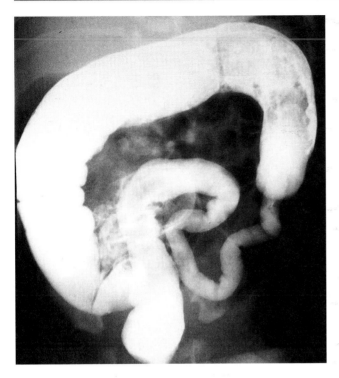

1. This infant failed to pass meconium for 24 hours and had progressive abdominal distension. What entities are in the clinical differential diagnoses?

2. A water-soluble contrast enema has been performed. What does this image of the full colon show?

3. Based on this image and the fact that the infant passed some meconium when the enema tip was removed, what are the differential diagnoses?

4. What other maternal history would be helpful?

Diagnosis: Neonatal Small Left Colon Syndrome

1. Diagnoses include low ileal atresia and stricture, meconium ileus, colonic atresia and stricture, megacystis microcolon intestinal hypoperistalsis syndrome, Hirschprung disease, small left colon syndrome. (High intestinal obstruction usually results in passage of a small amount of succus entericus from the patent distal bowel.)

2. This image shows an abrupt transition from distended cecum, ascending and transverse colon to a much smaller descending and sigmoid colon; the rectum appears close to normal diameter; the cecum is in the right lower quadrant; the meconium is seen proximal to the transition; and reflux into the terminal ileum is seen.

3. Differential diagnoses are colonic stricture, Hirschprung disease, or small left colon syndrome.

4. If the mother was diabetic (small left colon), drug addicted (ischemic strictures), or if she was toxemic and got magnesium sulfate therapy (ileus and functional hypoperistalsis).

Reference

Stringer DA, Babyn PS: *Pediatric gastrointestinal imaging and intervention*, ed 2, Hamilton-London, 2000, BC Decker Inc, pp 493-494.

Cross-Reference

Blickman JG, Parker BR, Barnes PD: *Pediatric radiology—the requisites*, ed 3, Philadelphia, 2009, Mosby, pp 92-94.

Comment

The basic decision that must be made is between surgical and functional disease. In this case the enema was able to exclude ileal pathologic condition. The passage of meconium and the knowledge that the mother was diabetic point the diagnosis more toward neonatal small left colon syndrome, a self-limiting functional condition in which the colon slowly acquires a normal peristaltic pattern. However, even the reassuring appearance of the rectum cannot entirely exclude Hirschprung disease. The patient should be closely monitored for feeding or stooling problems and reexamined if needed.

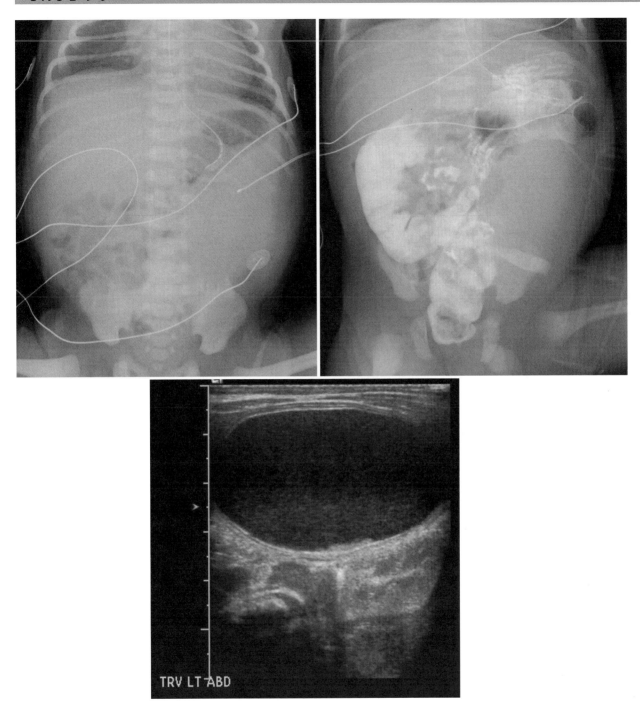

TRV LT ABD

1. What are the differential diagnoses of an abdominal mass in the newborn infant?

2. What are the radiographic (first image), sonographic (second image), and fluoroscopic (third image) findings in this case?

3. How do these studies help narrow the differential diagnoses?

Diagnosis: Small Bowel Duplication Cyst

1. Hydronephrosis, multicystic dysplastic kidney, mesenteric cyst, duplication cyst, meconium cyst, neuroblastoma, and hemangioepithelioma.

2. Left-sided mass, no calcifications, bowel loops draped around the mass, clear fluid with little debris, and smooth wall with discernable layers.

3. These tests reveal that the mass is more likely to be intraperitoneal than retroperitoneal and less likely a meconium cyst or tumor.

Reference

Kirks DR, Griscom NT, editors: *Practical pediatric imaging*, ed 3, Philadelphia, 1998, Lippincott-Raven, p 926.

Cross-Reference

Blickman JG, Parker BR, Barnes PD: *Pediatric radiology—the requisites*, ed 3, Philadelphia, 2009, Mosby, p 90.

Comment

In fetal life the bowel begins as a solid cord of endodermal cells that hollows out to form a tube. In some places the hollowing out process goes slightly awry and a second lumen can form parallel to the first. This might open onto the main channel at both ends or at one end, or it might pinch off and form an enclosed space. The epithelial lining of mucous-producing cells forms, no matter what the lumen size or configuration. If the secondary lumen is pinched off, the mucus produced by the lining accumulates and distends, forming a cyst. The wall contains smooth muscle. These two layers help in diagnosis by ultrasound: the epithelial layer is echogenic, whereas the smooth muscle layer is hypoechoic.

The most common sites of formation are the terminal ileum (one third of cases), distal esophagus, stomach, and jejunum. Presentation depends on size: larger cysts result in distension, pain, palpable mass, and obstruction, whereas smaller cysts can be the lead points of intussusception. In a toddler or older child, Meckel diverticulum (omphalomesenteric duct remnants) must be included in the differential diagnoses.

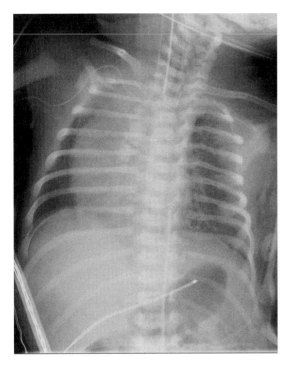

1. What are the two salient observations in this newborn's image?

2. What associated anomalies must be excluded, and how is this done?

3. When do most repairs take place?

4. What complications can occur, and how are they diagnosed?

Diagnosis: Esophageal Atresia and Tracheoesophageal Fistula

1. The blind-ending pharyngeal pouch (nasogastric tube) does not reach the stomach and air in the bowel.

2. All of these infants must be screened for the skeletal, renal, anal, and cardiac anomalies that can coexist with esophageal atresia and tracheoesophageal fistula (EA-TEF) in the VATER or VACTERL associations in about half of the patients (VATER/VACTERL = vertebrae, anus, cardiac, trachea, esophagus, renal, limb) (in about half of the patients). Plain film can be used to diagnose vertebral and limb abnormalities, whereas ultrasound is the most efficient screen for the brain, kidneys, and heart. Anorectal malformations may be apparent clinically.

3. Most repairs take place shortly after birth.

4. Postoperative follow-up must be alert for early anastomotic leaks, late anastomotic strictures, and recurrent fistulas. Pneumothorax, pneumomediastinum, or pleural effusion might be a sign on plain films of developing complications. Leaks may be seen with water-soluble contrast swallow.

Reference

Benson JE: The pediatric esophagus. In Ekberg O, editor: *Radiology of the pharynx and the esophagus*, Berlin-Heidelberg, 2004, Springer-Verlag, pp 195-206.

Cross-Reference

Blickman JG, Parker BR, Barnes PD: *Pediatric radiology—the requisites*, ed 3, Philadelphia, 2009, Mosby, pp 76-78.

Comment

Incomplete differentiation of the presumptive trachea from the esophagus and/or failure of the esophagus to recanalize during fetal weeks 4 to 8 results in a spectrum of abnormalities that usually comes to clinical attention immediately, when the infant cannot swallow oral secretions, has profound respiratory distress, and a tube cannot be passed to the stomach. The largest group (82%) has esophageal atresia (EA) with a tracheoesophageal fistula (TEF) connecting the trachea to the distal esophageal remnant. This is visible on plain film, with an air-filled sac projecting in the neck (perhaps with a coiled tube) and air in the stomach and gut. A few infants in this spectrum (6%) have an isolated TEF. A few others not considered part of this group have laryngeal cleft (a high defect at the level of the aditus that can be confused clinically and fluoroscopically with TEF).

The surgeon may wish the radiologist to more extensively study a smaller group before surgery—the 10% that have EA without TEF or with a TEF from the proximal esophageal segment. These infants will have no air distally in the gastrointestinal tract. The timing of the surgery may depend on the growth of the proximal and distal esophageal segments. The smaller the distance is between the ends, as demonstrated by the approximation of radioopaque catheters under fluoroscopy, the more successful is the repair.

Repair of the TEF may not relieve all respiratory symptoms; tracheomalacia almost always occurs when TEF exists, and the residual tracheal weakness may demand its own surgical intervention. Embryonic remnants in the esophageal wall can cause luminal narrowing. These can take the form of respiratory tract traces, such as cartilage, which will stiffen the wall and interfere with peristalsis. This can occur in conjunction with TEF and EA, and it may be overlooked because of the magnitude of these other abnormalities.

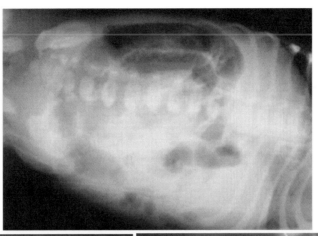

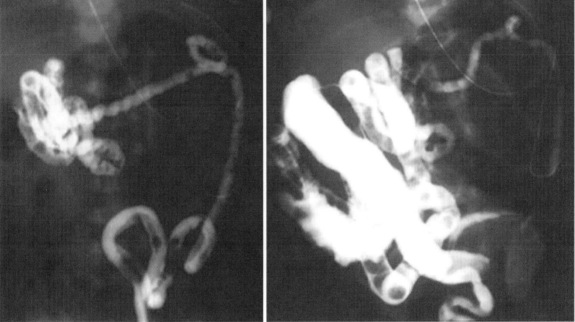

1. How would the patient in these images present?

2. What do the films show?

3. What contrast media would you use for the enema?

4. What test should be ordered later for this patient?

Diagnosis: Meconium Ileus

1. This newborn presents with abdominal distention, bilious emesis, and failure to pass meconium.

2. The left lateral decubitus view shows dilated bowel loops with bubbly-appearing material within the air-filled loops. No air fluid levels exist. The enema shows a microcolon and reflux of contrast into the meconium-filled ileum and more proximally into dilated empty small bowel. These findings are typical of meconium ileus.

3. Many prefer slightly diluted gastrograffin for its hypertonic and slippery qualities as a contrast media.

4. A sweat test should be ordered later to detect cystic fibrosis (CF).

References

Leonidas JC, Berdon WE, Baker DH, et al: Meconium ileus and its complication: a reappraisal of plain film roentgen diagnostic criteria, *AJR Am J Roentgenol* 108(3):598–609, 1970.

Kao SCS, Franken EA: Nonoperative treatment of simple meconium ileus: a survey of the Society for Pediatric Radiology, *Pediatr Radiol* 25(2):97–100, 1995.

Cross-Reference:

Blickman JG, Parker BR, Barnes PD: *Pediatric radiology—the requisites*, ed 3, Philadelphia, 2009, Mosby, pp 92-93.

Comment

Meconium ileus is almost always a complication of CF and is seen in the newborn. It is a distal ileal obstruction caused by inspissated meconium. This occurs because of abnormal composition of meconium because of the enzyme deficiencies seen in CF. In its simple form, the obstruction is functional rather than structural. Plain film findings include dilated bowel loops with bubbly appearance of the bowel contents and lack of air-fluid levels. The absence of air-fluid levels is due to thick meconium filling the distal small bowel.

Meconium ileus can be diagnosed and treated with a contrast enema. In longstanding and distal fetal ileal obstruction, the colon is small (microcolon) from lack of antegrade meconium passage. In many cases of meconium ileus, contrast does pass the level of obstruction into the dilated proximal bowel (as in this example). Many advocate using gastrograffin as the contrast agent when this diagnosis is suspected, because it is hypertonic, causes increased small bowel secretion, and has a slippery quality that will allow the tenacious meconium to pass into the colon. Caution in the use of nondiluted gastrograffin is advised because its hypertonicity may cause fluid loss through the bowel and significant electrolyte disturbances.

Stenosis, atresia (or atresias) of the ileum, volvulus of the ileum, pseudocyst formation, and bowel perforation may complicate meconium ileus. Meconium peritonitis is the term used for in utero bowel perforation. Calcifications may be seen in the abdomen. These calcifications occur in the meconium that enters the peritoneal cavity after perforation. Complications of meconium ileus almost always require surgical intervention.

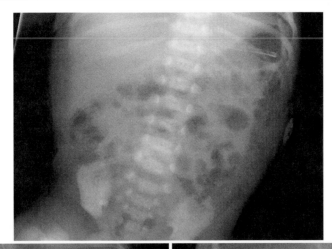

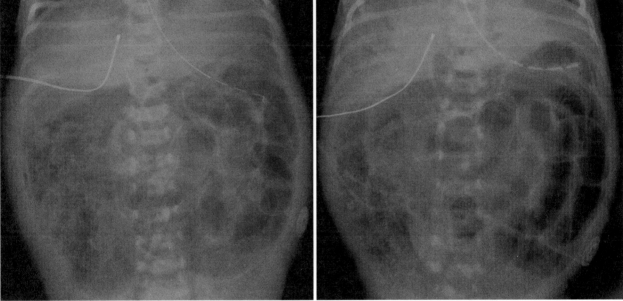

1. What are the findings in these three films of two patients (both neonates)?

2. In a premature infant, what is the diagnosis?

3. What is the presumed cause of this condition?

4. How would this patient be treated?

C A S E 9 3

Diagnosis: Necrotizing Enterocolitis

1. Dilated featureless bowel loops, extensive intestinal pneumatosis, and air in the portal venous system and in the peritoneal cavity.

2. Necrotizing enterocolitis (NEC).

3. Ischemia and infection.

4. Bowel rest, antibiotic agents, and general support.

Reference

Bin-Nun A, Bromiker R, Wilschanski M, et al: Oral probiotics prevent necrotizing enterocolitis in very low birth weight neonates, *J Pediatr* 147(2):192-196, 2005.

Cross-Reference

Blickman JG, Parker BR, Barnes PD: *Pediatric radiology— the requisites*, ed 3, Philadelphia, 2009, Mosby, pp 70-71.

Comment

NEC is a common affliction of the neonate; the exact cause is unknown. Risk factors include prematurity, enteral feeds, ischemic and/or reperfusion mucosal injury, and the presence of bacteria. Normal gut microflora is vital for bowel health, and recent studies (animal models and clinical trials) have shown that probiotic agents may decrease the incidence of NEC. The age of onset of this disease is inversely proportional to the gestational age. In other words, the extremely premature infant is more likely to develop NEC several weeks after birth, whereas in a term infant the onset may be at 1 to 3 days.

The presentation of NEC is often nonspecific: feeding intolerance, abdominal distention, increasing apnea and bradycardia, lethargy, and temperature instability. However, rapid deterioration may occur. In addition to abdominal distention, palpable bowel loops may be present, and most patients experience abdominal tenderness, abdominal wall erythema, and hematochezia.

Radiographs may show diffuse or localized dilated air-filled bowel loops (a nonspecific finding). Intestinal pneumatosis and portal venous air are diagnostic of NEC. The air in the bowel wall may be linear or rounded and is secondary to bacterial invasion of the bowel wall. The portal venous air occurs when air in the bowel wall enters the veins draining the bowel. Intraperitoneal air is secondary to bowel perforation and requires intervention—either open surgery or simple drain placement when the patient cannot tolerate laparotomy. Sonography has been used to evaluate infants with possible NEC; air in the bowel wall, air in the portal venous system, peritoneal air or fluid, abscess, or fixed loop can be seen. The arterial blood supply to the small bowel may demonstrate extremely high peak systolic velocity in early NEC; this finding may help differentiate a more benign cause of feeding intolerance from early NEC.

The medical treatment of NEC is bowel rest, antibiotic administration, and general support. Bell has described the stages of NEC; this categorization allows therapy to be tailored to the individual patient and helps determine prognosis.

NEC, whether medically managed or after surgery, may result in bowel strictures. If symptoms suggest such a complication, then appropriate contrast studies are necessary, including enema and/or small bowel study.

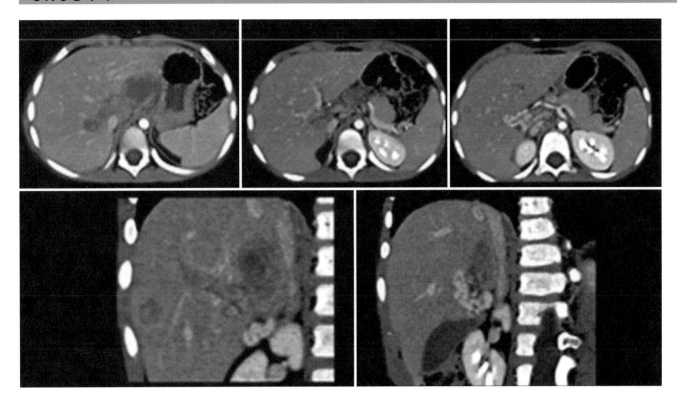

1. What are the vascular findings in this 5-year-old boy?

2. What are the causes of this abnormality?

3. In this example, what other finding is the likely cause?

4. What is the natural history of the vascular finding?

Diagnosis: Portal Vein Thrombosis and Multifocal Hepatoblastoma

1. Vague lucency in the location of the main portal vein and multiple serpiginous vessels around the area.

2. Portal vein thrombosis (PVT) and its cavernous transformation.

3. Multiple low-density masses appear in the liver and in the porta hepatis area consistent with the tumor. In this 5-year-old patient, the masses are due to multifocal hepatoblastoma with metastasis to the lymph nodes of the porta hepatis. Adjacent or invasive tumor may cause PVT.

4. In some cases the PVT can resolve without specific treatment.

Reference

Novick SL, Fishman EK: Portal vein thrombosis: spectrum of helical CT and CT angiographic findings, *Abdom Imaging* 23:505–510, 1998.

Cross-Reference

Blickman JG, Parker BR, Barnes PD: *Pediatric radiology—the requisites*, ed 3, Philadelphia, 2009, Mosby, pp 110–111.

Comment

Sepsis, hypercoagulable states, myeloproliferative disorders, severe dehydration, umbilical vein catheterization, ascending cholangitis, cirrhosis, portal hypertension, and adjacent or invasive neoplasm may cause PVT. Besides hepatoblastoma, other neoplasms associated with PVT are hepatocarcinoma, cholangiocarcinoma, and pancreatic carcinoma. In most cases it is not possible to differentiate a tumor within the portal vein from thrombosis alone. Sometimes, however, the tumor thrombus may enhance with contrast. Cavernous transformation of the portal vein is the development of periportal venous collaterals; this may occur with slowly occurring or long-standing PVT. PVT may extend into the superior mesenteric vein and the splenic vein. Over time, the portal vein may recanalize. This is especially true in patients with sepsis.

In many patients, PVT is asymptomatic. Symptoms may be present because of the underlying cause of the PVT or in some cases, gastrointestinal bleeding from varices may occur. When the mesenteric veins are also involved, abdominal pain may be present.

Because of the widespread use of ultrasound, PVT is recognized with increasing frequency. It is well characterized by duplex sonography. Multidetector computed tomography (CT) is a simple, fast, and exquisite modality for analysis of the portal vein. Dual-phase CT arteriography and three-dimensional reconstruction allow complete vascular analysis and definitive evaluation of the other abdominal organs. Magnetic resonance imaging is a valuable alternative imaging modality.

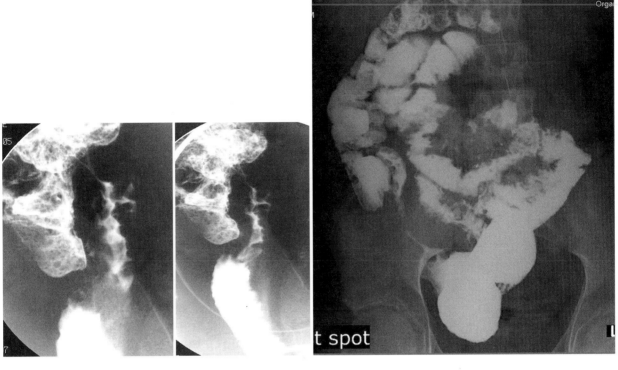

1. List the imaging findings on the upper gastrointestinal (GI) barium study in this 10-year-old girl who presented with abdominal pain and weight loss. What is the likely diagnosis?

2. List three presenting features.

3. List three possible serious intraabdominal complications.

4. Is surgery a recommended form of treatment?

Diagnosis: Crohn Disease

1. Spot views of the ileocecal region obtained during this upper GI series with small bowel follow-through demonstrate luminal narrowing of the terminal ileum with thickening of the mucosal folds, as well as linear and transverse ulceration resulting in "cobblestoning." No evidence of obstruction is seen with oral contrast opacifying the cecum and ascending colon. Findings are most consistent with Crohn disease.

2. Diarrhea, colicky abdominal pain, weight loss, and malabsorption.

3. Enteroenteric fistulas, sinus tracts, and abscesses.

4. No. Surgical resection of the affected bowel is not typically recommended in Crohn disease because 30% to 50% recur after resection.

Reference

Parker BR: Small intestine. In Kuhn JP, Slovis TL, Haller JO, editors: *Caffey's pediatric diagnostic imaging*, ed 10, Philadelphia, 2004, Mosby, pp 1631–1633.

Cross-Reference

Blickman JG, Parker BR, Barnes PD: *Pediatric radiology—the requisites*, ed 3, Philadelphia, 2009, Mosby, pp 96–98.

Comment

Crohn disease, also known as regional enteritis, is characterized by segmental transmural granulomatous inflammation of the intestine. Peak incidence is in young adulthood, but 25% present before teenage years. The terminal ileum is the most frequently involved segment, but it may occur anywhere in the GI tract from the mouth to the anus. Clinical presentation may include diarrhea, colicky abdominal pain, weight loss, and malabsorption. Upper GI and small bowel follow-through with barium demonstrates thickening of the mucosal folds, linear and transverse ulceration resulting in cobblestoning, "rose thorn" ulcers, pseudopolyps, luminal narrowing, and fistulas. Computed tomography findings are similar but more sensitive for mesenteric thickening and abscess formation. Magnetic resonance imaging with contrast is most helpful to distinguish active disease from fibrosis and to evaluate anal fistulas. Major intraabdominal complications include enteroenteric fistulas, sinus tracts, and abscesses. Other complications include toxic megacolon, gallstones, sclerosing cholangitis, ankylosing spondylitis, and a 20-fold increase in adenocarcinoma. Differential diagnosis includes ulcerative colitis (not transmural, continuous from anus advancing in a retrograde fashion and not skip lesions), lymphoma, and infectious colitis (*Yersinia* typically affects the terminal ileum, tuberculosis).

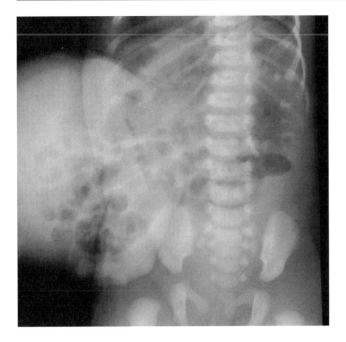

1. What is the most likely diagnosis?

2. What are the differential diagnoses, and what can help differentiate each?

3. Are associated congenital anomalies common?

4. What is the prognosis?

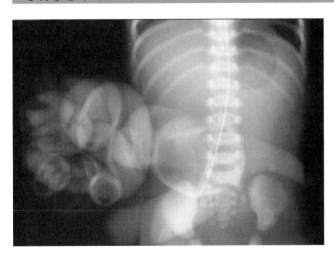

1. What are the imaging findings in this newborn, and what are the differential diagnoses?

2. How does the insertion of the umbilical cord aid in narrowing the differential diagnosis?

3. Do most cases have associated anomalies?

4. Does maternal α-fetoprotein help narrow the differential?

CASE 96

Diagnosis: Omphalocele

1. Omphalocele.

2. Omphalocele, which is a midline defect in the anterior abdominal wall that most commonly contains liver and small bowel; gastroschisis is off-midline, usually in the right paraumbilical region.

3. In newborns with omphalocele, 50% to 70% have associated abnormalities (e.g., genitourinary [GU], gastrointestinal [GI], cardiac, skeletal).

4. The prognosis for survival in patients with omphalocele is high (near 90%) if the chromosomes are normal and no life-threatening associated anomalies exist.

References

Schlesinger AE, Parker BR: Abdominal wall abnormalities. In Kuhn JP, Slovis TL, Haller JO, editors: *Caffey's pediatric diagnostic imaging*, ed 10, Philadelphia, 2004, Mosby, p 1429.

Farmer DL: Abdominal wall defects. In Kuhn JP, Slovis TL, Haller JO, editors: *Caffey's pediatric diagnostic imaging*, ed 10, Philadelphia, 2004, Mosby, pp 112–113.

Cross-Reference

Blickman JG, Parker BR, Barnes PD: *Pediatric radiology— the requisites*, ed 3, Philadelphia, 2009, Mosby, pp 88–89.

Comment

Omphalocele is a herniation of abdominal contents, usually liver and small bowel, into the umbilical cord. The umbilical cord inserts onto the sac, and the defect is at midline; most are sporadic. Associated structural abnormalities are seen in 50% to 70% of patients, including GU (ureteropelvic junction obstruction, ectopia, cloacal exstrophy), GI (tracheoesophageal fistula, imperforate anus, malrotation, omphalocele), cardiac (septal defects, transposition, absent inferior vena cava), musculoskeletal (dysplasia, clubfoot, vertebral anomalies), and central nervous system (encephalocele, holoprosencephaly, cerebellar hypoplasia). Most are diagnosed in utero with elevated α-fetoprotein in the mother and midline abdominal wall defect seen on fetal ultrasound. Differential diagnosis includes gastroschisis (off-midline) and umbilical hernia. Because the abdominal contents are covered by peritoneal membrane, surgical correction need not be performed immediately. Nearly all cases of omphalocele have an intestinal malrotation with resultant increased risk of midgut volvulus.

CASE 97

Diagnosis: Gastroschisis

1. An anterior abdominal wall defect exists that contains bowel loops. Differential diagnoses include gastroschisis, omphalocele, and cloacal exstrophy.

2. Normal insertion of the umbilical cord exists with gastroschisis; insertion is abnormal with omphalocele and exstrophy variants.

3. Only about 15% of patients with gastroschisis have associated anomalies, and they are usually much less severe than with omphalocele.

4. Maternal α-fetoprotein is elevated in both gastroschisis and omphalocele.

References

Schlesinger AE, Parker BR: Abdominal wall abnormalities. In Kuhn JP, Slovis TL, Haller JO, editors: *Caffey's pediatric diagnostic imaging*, ed 10, Philadelphia, 2004, Mosby, p 1429.

Farmer DL: Abdominal wall defects. In Kuhn JP, Slovis TL, Haller JO, editors: *Caffey's pediatric diagnostic imaging*, ed 10, Philadelphia, 2004, Mosby, p 112.

Cross-Reference

Blickman JG, Parker BR, Barnes PD: *Pediatric radiology— the requisites*, ed 3, Philadelphia, 2009, Mosby, pp 88–89.

Comment

Gastroschisis is a right paraumbilical abdominal wall defect that involves all three layers of the abdominal wall. Small bowel is always involved and is, by definition, nonrotated. Gastroschisis is rarely associated with other anomalies; the associated anomalies tend to be less severe than those seen with omphalocele and include hypoplastic gallbladder, hiatal hernia, and Meckel diverticulum. The umbilical cord insertion is in the normal location with gastroschisis (abnormal with omphalocele). Postoperative complications almost always include motility disorders. In gastroschisis the herniating bowel loops are exposed without membranous coverage as in omphalocele. Intestine exposed to amniotic fluid becomes edematous, matted, and inflamed. Differential diagnosis includes omphalocele (midline, associated anomalies, umbilical cord inserts onto hernia sac) and exstrophy (umbilical cord inserts above the defect, absent bladder).

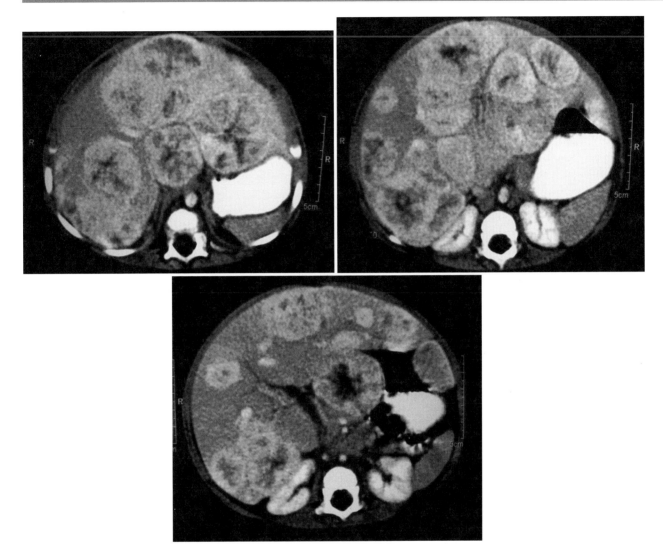

1. What are the imaging findings in this 2-month-old girl with a palpable liver edge on a routine well-child visit? What are the differential diagnoses?

2. What is the most common clinical presentation with this disorder?

3. What are some possible clinical symptoms?

4. What should be the first imaging modality used in an infant with hepatomegaly or a palpable abdominal mass?

Diagnosis: Hemangioendothelioma

1. Contrast-enhanced axial computed tomography (CT) scans through the liver demonstrate multiple, well-defined enhancing masses within both liver lobes. Differential diagnoses include hemangioendothelioma, hepatoblastoma, and neuroblastoma metastases.

2. The most common clinical presentation of infants with hemangioendothelioma is incidentally noted hepatomegaly at a well-child visit.

3. Possible clinical symptoms include abdominal distention and congestive heart failure.

4. Ultrasound should be the first imaging done in an infant with hepatomegaly. On ultrasound, hemangioendotheliomas appear as high-flow vascular lesions that are well-defined and predominantly hypoechoic.

Reference

Roos JE, Pfiffner R, Stallmach, Stuckmann G, Marincek B, Willi U: Infantile hemangioendothelioma, *Radiographics* 23:1649–1655, 2003.

Cross-Reference

Blickman JG, Parker BR, Barnes PD: *Pediatric radiology— the requisites*, ed 3, Philadelphia, 2009, Mosby, pp 108–109.

Comment

Hemangioendothelioma is the third most common hepatic tumor in children (12% of all childhood hepatic tumors), the most common benign vascular tumor of the liver in infancy, and the most common symptomatic liver tumor during the first 6 months of life. A 2:1 female predilection exists, and 45% to 50% of patients also have cutaneous hemangiomas. Hemangioendotheliomas are usually benign. Most tumors continue to grow during the first year of life and then spontaneously regress, probably as a result of thrombosis and scar formation.

The tumor may be asymptomatic and discovered incidentally. Most patients with hemangioendothelioma present with hepatomegaly, abdominal distention, or a palpable upper abdominal mass. In addition, extensive arteriovenous shunting exists within the lesion, which may lead to high cardiac output and congestive heart failure in 50% to 60% of patients.

On ultrasound, single or multiple lesions are well demarcated from the surrounding liver parenchyma. Sometimes calcifications are seen.

On noncontrast-enhanced CT, they are usually well-defined and hypodense to the normal liver parenchyma. With intravenous contrast-enhanced CT, *nodular* peripheral puddling of contrast material in the early phase is characteristic, with subsequent peripheral pooling and central enhancement with variable delay. Small lesions tend to be multifocal and frequently enhance completely.

Differential diagnosis includes hepatoblastoma, which is a malignant embryonic tumor and the most common primary hepatic neoplasm in infants and children younger than 5 years old. A 3:2 male predilection exists, and the tumor is more commonly located in the right hepatic lobe (> 60% of cases). The serum α-fetoprotein level is elevated in up to 90% of patients with hepatoblastoma but is typically normal in cases of hemangioendothelioma. The lesions are usually large and solitary but may also be multifocal. Differentiation from hemangioma is challenging.

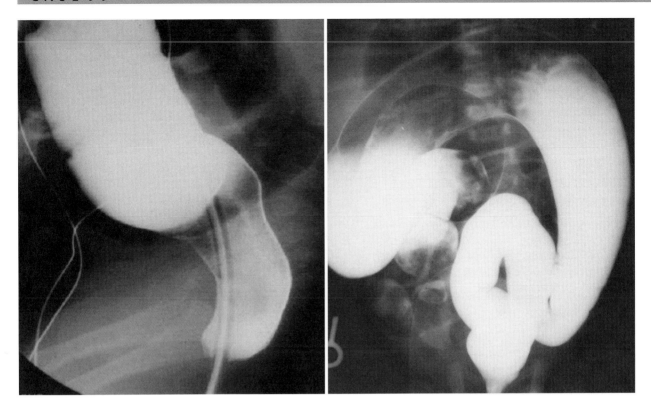

1. What is the diagnosis in this newborn male infant with a failure to pass meconium in the first 48 hours of life?

2. What is the normal rectosigmoid index, and how is it measured?

3. What is the typical clinical presentation?

4. What are the pathologic findings?

Diagnosis: Hirschsprung Disease

1. A lateral view of the rectosigmoid region on this contrast enema demonstrates a sigmoid colon larger than the rectum, which is consistent with the diagnosis of Hirschsprung disease.

2. The normal rectosigmoid index should be greater than 1. The transverse measurement of the rectum should be greater than the transverse measurement of the sigmoid.

3. A failure to pass meconium in the first 24 hours of life accompanied by increasing bowel distention.

4. The pathologic findings on rectal biopsy in Hirschsprung disease is an absence of ganglion cells, hypertrophy and hyperplasia of nerve fibers, and an increase in acetylcholinesterase-positive nerve fibers in the lamina propria and muscularis mucosa of the affected portion of the colon.

Reference

Swischuk LE: *Imaging of the newborn, infant and young child*, ed 5, Philadelphia, 2004, Lippincott Williams & Wilkins, pp 445–453.

Cross-Reference

Blickman JG, Parker BR, Barnes PD: *Pediatric radiology— the requisites*, ed 3, Philadelphia, 2009, Mosby, pp 94–95.

Comment

Hirschsprung disease, or colonic aganglionosis, is characterized by the absence of myenteric and submucosal ganglion cells, which results in decreased motility of the affected bowel segment, a lack of propagation of peristaltic waves into the aganglionic colon, and an abnormal or absent relaxation of this segment and of the internal anal sphincter. It most typically occurs in full-term male newborns and is diagnosed in the first weeks of life. Failure to pass meconium in the first 24 hours accompanied by increasing bowel distention is the classic presentation. Aganglionosis most commonly involves the distal colon, with greater than 80% involving the rectum or rectosigmoid regions. Plain-film findings include increasing gaseous distention of the bowel. A contrast enema typically identifies a transition zone at the level of aganglionosis with dilation of the colon proximally. The normal rectosigmoid index is greater than 1. If the transverse measurement of the rectum is less than the transverse measurement of the sigmoid, Hirschsprung disease should be suggested. Suction rectal biopsy is required for a definitive diagnosis. The classic pathologic findings include an absence of ganglion cells, hypertrophy and hyperplasia of nerve fibers, and an increase in acetylcholinesterase-positive nerve fibers in the lamina propria and muscularis mucosa.

Short segment distal rectal aganglionosis and total colonic aganglionosis are two subtypes that are extremely difficult to diagnosis with a contrast enema.

In older children, Hirschprung disease presents as chronic constipation and may be complicated by toxic megacolon.

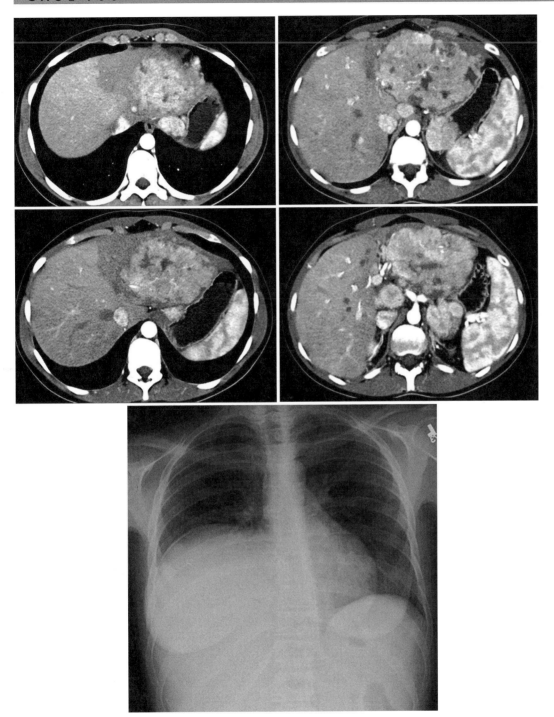

1. A 14-year-old female adolescent presents with abdominal distention and difficulty breathing. What are the findings on the frontal radiograph of the chest?

2. What is the differential diagnosis based only on the chest radiograph?

3. What are the findings on the contrast enhanced computed tomographic (CT) scan of the abdomen and pelvis?

4. List some predisposing factors observed in approximately 50% of these patients.

C A S E 1 0 0

Diagnosis: Hepatocellular Carcinoma

1. An elevated right hemidiaphragm.

2. A differential diagnosis includes both intrathoracic and intraabdominal processes that may cause diaphragm elevation such as phrenic nerve paralysis, atelectasis (less likely because no mediastinal shift has developed), right subphrenic effusion, and a large right upper-quadrant mass.

3. Large heterogeneously enhancing mass in the left lobe of the liver.

4. Approximately 50% of children with hepatocellular carcinoma (HCC) have underlying liver disease, often associated with hereditary tyrosinemia, biliary atresia, infantile cholestasis, Alagille syndrome, glycogen storage diseases, and chronic hepatitis.

Reference

Schlesinger AE, Parker BR: Tumors and tumor-like conditions. In Kuhn JP, Slovis TL, Haller JO, editors: *Caffey's pediatric diagnostic imaging*, ed 10, Philadelphia, 2004, Mosby, pp 1502–1503.

Cross-Reference

Blickman JG, Parker BR, Barnes PD: *Pediatric radiology—the requisites*, ed 3, Philadelphia, 2009, Mosby, pp 111–112.

Comments

HCC is uncommon in the pediatric population but is the second most common hepatic malignancy in children after hepatoblastoma. Two age peaks exist: (1) 2 to 4 years of age and (2) 12 to 14 years of age. Approximately 50% of children with HCC have underlying liver disease, often associated with hereditary tyrosinemia, biliary atresia, infantile cholestasis, Alagille syndrome, glycogen storage diseases, and chronic hepatitis; however, many arise without any known underlying liver abnormality. Most patients with HCC present with a slowly enlarging, right upper-quadrant mass that may be found by the patient, by the patient's parents, or during a routine physical examination. Many children present with right upper-quadrant pain, nausea, vomiting, and weight loss. Nearly 25% of patients demonstrate jaundice.

Laboratory evaluations reveal an elevated α-fetoprotein (AFP) level in 40% to 50% of patients and, to a lesser extent, abnormal levels of beta–human chorionic gonadotropin (β-hCG).

Sonography typically demonstrates a heterogeneous liver mass with increased size of the portal vein and increased velocity of blood flow. A CT scan will demonstrate a tumor that is typically lower attenuation than the liver on noncontrast-enhanced scans but may be isodense to the liver. With intravenous contrast, enhancement is typically heterogeneous, and invasion into the portal vein, inferior vena cava, and hepatic veins and arteries can be appreciated, if present.

If surgical resection is under consideration, magnetic resonance imaging with magnetic resonance angiography will best demonstrate tumor margins and vasculature.

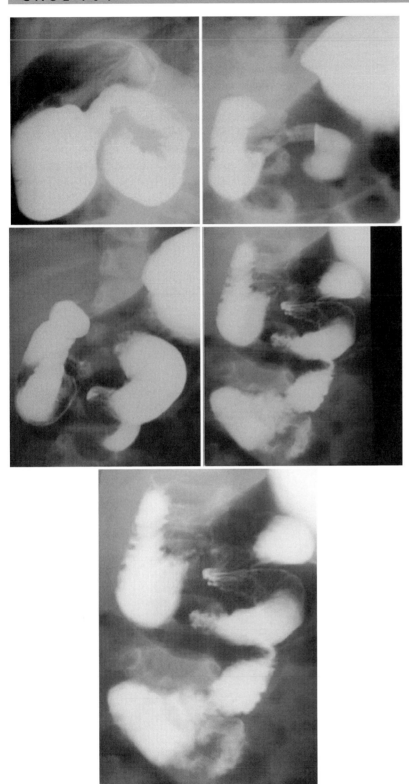

1. What are the imaging findings in the infant with bilious emesis? What is the diagnosis?

2. What is the classic clinical presentation?

3. What is demonstrated on a plain radiograph of the abdomen?

4. What is the treatment?

Diagnosis: Midgut Volvulus

1. Images from an upper gastrointestinal (GI) series demonstrate a dilated proximal duodenum with thickened folds and the classic *corkscrew* pattern (i.e., proximal jejunum spiraling downward in the right- or middle-upper abdomen), which are characteristic of midgut volvulus.

2. Bilious emesis is the classic presentation of midgut volvulus, but most cases of bilious emesis are not the result of midgut volvulus.

3. On plain abdominal radiographs, a high-grade obstruction is classic, but the bowel gas pattern can be normal because of intermittent twisting and obstruction.

4. Midgut volvulus is a surgical emergency. Surgical correction with the Ladd procedure is the treatment of choice.

Reference

Ortiz-Neira CL: The corkscrew sign: midgut volvulus, *Radiology* 242:315–316, 2007.

Cross Reference

Blickman JG, Parker BR, Barnes PD: *Pediatric radiology— the requisites*, ed 3, Philadelphia, 2009, Mosby, pp 70–72.

Comments

In normal embryos at approximately 6 weeks gestation, the midgut herniates through the umbilical stalk and ultimately undergoes a 270-degree counterclockwise rotation around the superior mesenteric artery before returning to the abdomen at 10 to 12 weeks gestation. At this time the normal small bowel mesentery should have a broad attachment, stretching diagonally from the duodenojejunal junction (DJJ) in the left upper quadrant to the cecum in the right lower quadrant. Incomplete rotation of the intestine results in malrotation. Peritoneal bands (Ladd bands) fix the malpositioned high-riding cecum to the posterior abdominal wall, and more proximal bands often surround the duodenum and jejunum. Because of the shortened mesenteric root, malrotation predisposes patients to two problems: (1) midgut volvulus and (2) small bowel obstruction. If the gut twists around the shortened mesenteric root, the accompanying superior mesenteric vascular compromise (first venous, then arterial) can lead to life-threatening ischemia of the small bowel and gangrenous necrosis. In neonatal patients, malrotation with midgut volvulus classically presents with bilious vomiting and radiographic findings consistent with high intestinal obstruction. In suspected malrotation with midgut volvulus, an upper GI series should be performed. Barium is administered either orally or through a nasogastric tube. The normal DJJ lies to the left of the left-sided spinal pedicle at the level of the duodenal bulb on a true frontal view. The duodenal C-sweep courses posteriorly, inferiorly, anteriorly, and then superiorly. In approximately 60% of patients with malrotation, associated anomalies are demonstrated and include congenital heart disease with heterotaxy, diaphragmatic hernia, and anterior abdominal wall defects. Other associated anomalies include imperforate anus, duodenal atresia, duodenal web, annular pancreas, and biliary atresia. On upper GI series in the patient with malrotation, the downward displacement of the DJJ is typically demonstrated, which is also displaced to the right on the frontal view with an abnormal course on the lateral view. In malrotation with midgut volvulus, the findings also include a dilated, fluid-filled duodenum, proximal small bowel obstruction, the corkscrew pattern, mural edema, and thickened duodenal folds. Malrotation with midgut volvulus is a surgical emergency.

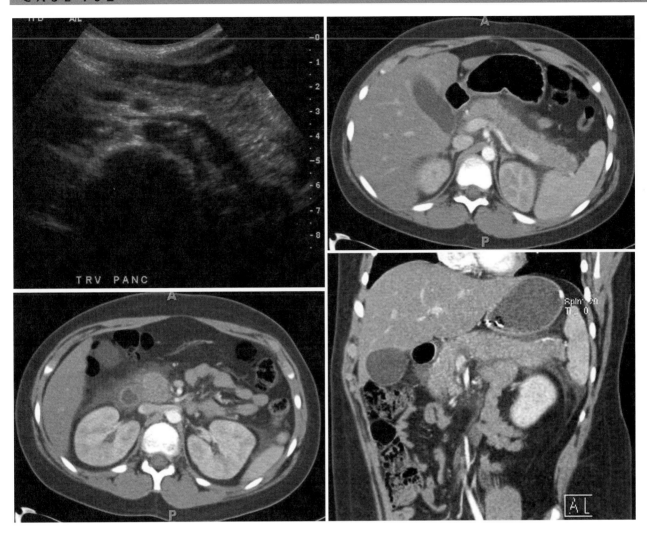

TRV PANC

1. What are the imaging findings in this 6-year-old boy with abdominal pain?

2. What is the diagnosis?

3. What is the differential diagnosis?

4. What are the complications?

Diagnosis: Acute Pancreatitis

1. Ultrasonography (US) shows increased thickness and hypoechogenicity of the pancreatic body and tail. In addition to US, computed tomography (CT) demonstrates peripancreatic fluid and dilation of the common bile duct at the level of the pancreatic head. The duodenal loop adjacent to the pancreatic head is dilated.

2. Acute pancreatitis is the diagnosis.

3. Acute pancreatitis is essentially the only diagnosis, considering the imaging findings.

4. Complications include fluid collections, pseudocyst formation, pancreatic necrosis, chronic pancreatitis, fat necrosis, thrombosis of the splenic vein, abscess formation, and fistula.

Reference

Balthazar EJ, Freeny PC, Van Sonnenbergh E: Imaging and intervention in acute pancreatitis, *Radiology* 193:297–306, 1994.

Benifla M, Weizman Z: Acute pancreatitis in childhood: analysis of literature data, *J Clin Gastroenterol* 37:169–172, 2003.

Cross-Reference

Blickman JG, Parker BR, Barnes PD: *Pediatric radiology—the requisites*, ed 3, Philadelphia, 2009, Mosby, pp 113–114.

Comment

Acute pancreatitis occurs less frequently in children when compared with adults. Alcohol use, gallstones, and drugs are the leading causes of acute pancreatitis in those who are idiopathic (23%), experience trauma (22%), have structural and anatomic abnormalities (e.g., pancreatic divisum, annular pancreas) (15%), are on drug regimens (e.g., chemotherapeutic agents) (12%), have developed viral infections (10%), or have hereditary and metabolic disorders (e.g., hypercholesterolemia) (2%). In addition, acute pancreatitis occurs more commonly in children with human immunodeficiency virus (HIV) and cystic fibrosis. The most common clinical symptoms and signs are abdominal pain with vomiting and abdominal tenderness with abdominal distention.

Increased level of amylase, lipase, and trypsinogen, along with typical abdominal pain and vomiting, are highly suggestive of this diagnosis. Imaging is helpful in confirming and limiting differential diagnoses and to exclude complications.

Plain films obtained in the upright position are helpful to exclude bowel perforation. US is the first cross-sectional imaging modality to be performed, because ionizing radiation is not involved. It can show increased thickness of the organ, increased echogenicity secondary to inflammation, fluid collections and necrosis, if any; however, increased bowel gas can easily obscure visualization of the pancreas in the midline view. CT performed with oral (water) and intravenous contrast is found to be the most reliable imaging modality. Balthazar has classified the findings of CT imaging in acute pancreatitis to define the severity and to predict the outcome in terms of morbidity and mortality. Balthazar constructed a CT severity index (CTSI) for acute pancreatitis that combines the grade of pancreatitis with the extent of pancreatic necrosis. The CTSI assigns points to patients according to the grade of acute pancreatitis and the degree of pancreatic necrosis. More points are given for a higher grade of pancreatitis and for more extensive necrosis. Patients with a CTSI of 0 to 3 had a mortality of 3% and a complication rate of 8%. Patients with a CTSI of 4 to 6 had a mortality rate of 6% and a complication rate of 35%. Patients with a CTSI of 7 to 10 had a 17% mortality rate and a 92% complication rate. Defining the presence of necrosis is most important because it significantly affects morbidity and mortality.

Pancreas divisum is the most common congenital anomaly of the pancreatic ductal system. This anomaly results when the ventral and dorsal pancreatic ducts fail to fuse. The ventral duct (Wirsung duct) drains only the ventral pancreatic anlage, whereas the majority of the gland empties into the minor papilla through the dorsal duct (Santorini duct). Annular pancreas is another rare congenital anomaly in which the incomplete rotation of the ventral anlage leads to a segment of the pancreas encircling the second part of the duodenum. A definitive diagnosis of these anatomic abnormalities can be made with endoscopic retrograde pancreatography. Magnetic resonance (MR) pancreatography has been shown to be highly sensitive and specific for pancreas divisum. MR cholangiopancreatography with secretin stimulation helps identify pancreas divisum.

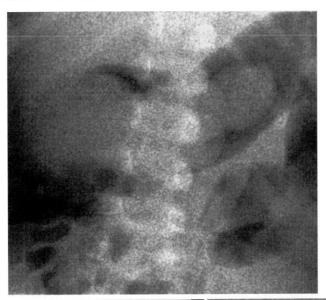

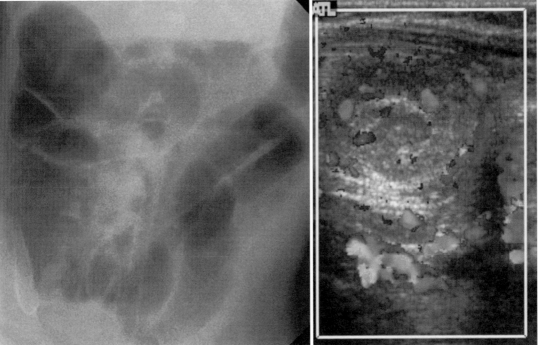

1. What is the most common location for this entity?

2. What are the common presenting clinical symptoms?

3. What is the most common age?

4. What is the most common cause?

Diagnosis: Acute Ileocecal Intussusception

1. Terminal ileum and ileocecal valve.

2. Alternating lethargy and irritability, colic abdominal pain, palpable right abdominal mass, jellylike stool, ileus, and vomiting.

3. Between 3 months and 1 year of age. After 3 years of age, a lead point should be investigated such as Meckel diverticulitis, polyps, lymphoma, and bowel wall hemorrhage.

4. Idiopathic. A seasonal occurrence (winter, spring) has been found with a viral infection, particularly with adenovirus but also with enterovirus, echovirus, and human herpes virus.

Reference

Kimberly E: Applegate intussusception in children: imaging choices, *Semin Roentgenol* 43(1):15-21, 2008.

Cross-Reference

Blickman JG, Parker BR, Barnes PD: *Pediatric radiology— the requisites*, ed 3, Philadelphia, 2009, Mosby, pp 73-75.

Comment

After pyloric stenosis, intussusception is the most common cause of acute bowel obstruction in young children. Most cases are idiopathic because the cause of the intussusception is due to hypertrophied lymphoid tissue in the terminal ileum, which results in ileocolic intussusception. The classic triad of colicky abdominal pain, vomiting, and bloody stools is present in fewer than 25% of children. Abdominal radiographs have a sensitivity of 45% for the detection of intussusception; however, they do play an important role in screening for other causes such as constipation, masses, stones, volvulus, and bowel perforation with free peritoneal air. The presence of a curvilinear mass within the course of the colon (crescent sign), particularly in the transverse colon just beyond the hepatic flexure, is a nearly pathognomonic sign of intussusception. Ultrasonography is the first modality of choice in diagnosing intussusception with high accuracy, approaching 100% in experienced hands with a sensitivity of 98% to 100% and a specificity of 88% to 100%. Pseudokidney or bullseye appearance is often diagnostic. Air or barium enema is the most common approach in reducing the intussusceptum.

Pneumatic reduction of intussusception is an effective and safe procedure in children. The patient is placed in the lateral decubitus position, and a rectal tube is placed. After securing the rectal tube to avoid air leakage, air insufflation of the colon is performed under manometric (less than 120 mm Hg) and fluoroscopic control.

The examination is complete when air reflux into the cecum and terminal ileum is visualized. Absolute contraindications to an enema include intestinal perforation or peritonitis. Recurrent cases after three attempts of unsuccessful reduction with air or patients with peritonitis and intestinal perforations are treated with surgery.

The duration of symptoms is the most important factor that decreases the reduction success of an enema. Duration of symptoms beyond 24 to 48 hours will significantly reduce the success of reduction.

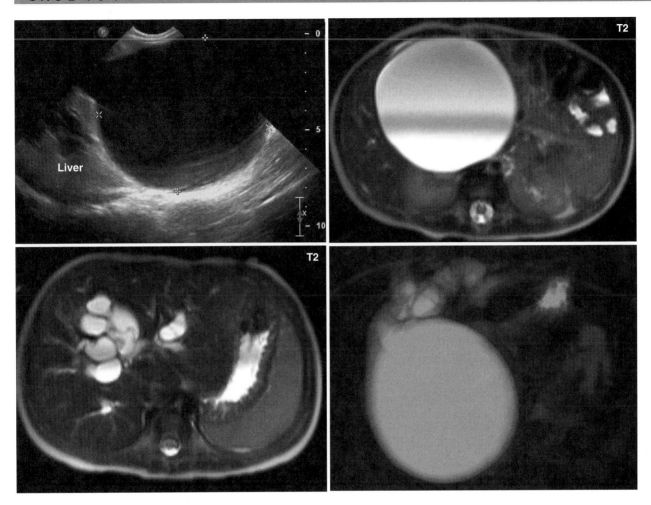

1. What are the imaging findings with ultrasonography (US) in this 2-year-old girl?

2. In addition, what does magnetic resonance imaging (MRI) and magnetic resonance cholangiopancreatography (MRCP) show?

3. What are the differential diagnoses?

4. What is the cause?

Diagnosis: Choledochal cyst

1. Dilation of the common bile and the intrahepatic bile ducts.

2. Axial T2-weighted MRI and MRCP performed in the coronal plane reveal the length of the involved duct, the pancreaticobiliary junction (PBJ), and the length of the common channel and intrahepatic ducts. Background stomach and bowel loops are visualized in the MRCP image.

3. The diagnosis is type I choledochal cyst. The differential diagnoses include chronic cholangitis, obstructing cholelithiasis, pancreatic pseudocyst, and hydatid cyst of the liver.

4. Anomalous junction of the common biliary and pancreatic ducts, which provides a conduit, mixing pancreatic secretions and bile.

References

Chavhan GB, Babyn PS, Manson D, et al: Pediatric MR cholangiopancreatography: principles, technique, and clinical applications, *Radiographics* 28(7):1951–1962, 2008.

Todani T, Watanabe Y, Narusue M, Tabuchi K, Okajima K: Congenital bile duct cysts: classification, operative procedures, and review of thirty-seven cases including cancer from choledochal cyst, *Am J Surg* 134:263–269, 1977.

Cross-Reference

Blickman JG, Parker BR, Barnes PD: *Pediatric radiology—the requisites*, ed 3, Philadelphia, 2009, Mosby, pp 103–106.

Comment

Choledochal cysts are rare and observed in 1 in 100,000 to 150,000 live births in the United States versus 1 in 1000 live births in Japan. Choledochal cysts are rare anomalies that appear as cystic or fusiform dilations of the extrahepatic or intrahepatic biliary tree or both. Approximately two thirds of the patients are diagnosed before 10 years of age. Todani and associates have classified choledochal cysts based on the cholangiographic morphologic location and the number of intrahepatic and extrahepatic bile duct cysts. Todani describes five types of choledochal cysts. Type I cysts consist of a cystic dilation of the common bile duct (type IA), a focal segmental dilation of the distal common bile duct (type IB), or a fusiform dilation of both the common hepatic duct and the common bile duct (type IC). Type II cysts are true diverticula of the common bile duct. Type III cysts, or choledochoceles, are cystic dilations involving only the intraduodenal portion of the common

bile duct. Type IV cysts consist of multiple intrahepatic and extrahepatic cysts (type IVA) or multiple extrahepatic cysts only (type IVB). Type V cysts comprise single or multiple cystic dilation of the intrahepatic bile ducts. The prevalence of choledochal cysts is higher among female patients; in most series, 70% to 84% of the patients are women. Abdominal pain, jaundice, and an abdominal mass make up the classic triad of signs and symptoms in one third of the patients. US is the best initial screening modality. MRCP is a fast, accurate, non-invasive alternative to endoscopic retrograde cholangiography (ERCP) in the evaluation of biliary tract disease. The diagnosis of choledochal cyst is usually made with US. However, information about the type of cyst, the length of the involved duct, the presence and location of protein plugs or calculi, the PBJ, and the length of the common channel is required for preoperative planning. ERCP is traditionally used to obtain this information. However, MRCP has been shown to be 100% accurate in the evaluation of choledochal cysts. Hepatobiliary scintigraphy with technetium-99m disofenin provides physiologic information on hepatic uptake and the accumulation of radionuclide in the dilated biliary tree.

Complications include cholelithiasis, choledocholithiasis, cirrhosis and portal hypertension, malignant transformation (usually adenocarcinoma), and pancreatitis. To reduce the risk complications, a complete cyst excision without compromising the pancreatic duct and common pancreaticobiliary channel should be performed as soon as the diagnosis is made.

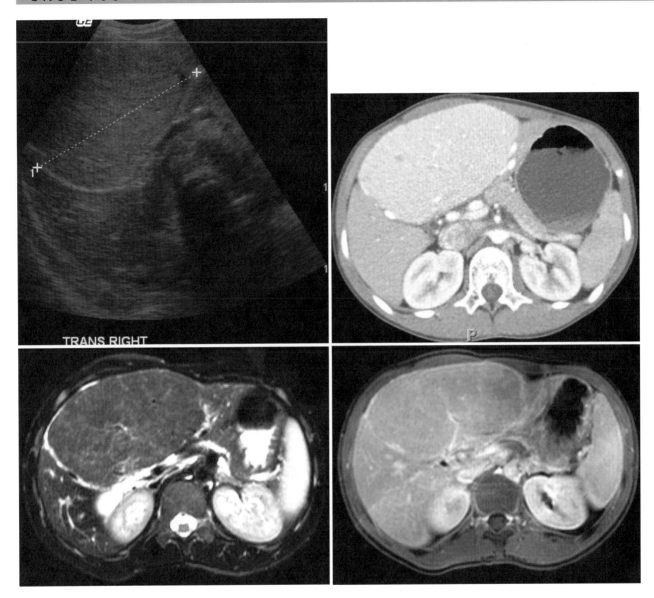

1. What are the imaging findings in this 12-year-old asymptomatic girl?

2. What is the most likely diagnosis, and is this entity common in children?

3. What is the prognosis?

4. What are the differential diagnoses?

Diagnosis: Focal Nodular Hyperplasia

1. Ultrasonography (US) of the liver shows a well-circumscribed, large mass in the liver with a relatively high echo signal, compared with normal liver parenchyma. Contrast-enhanced computed tomographic (CT) examination shows a large homogeneous-enhancing hypervascular mass that is partially involving the left and right lobes of the liver without evidence of calcification, necrosis, or central scarring. A T2-weighted axial image of the liver shows that the mass reveals relatively similar signal intensity to the liver with different architecture of the parenchyma. A postcontrast T1-weighted image shows homogenous enhancement of the mass, again similar to normal liver parenchyma.

2. Focal nodular hyperplasia is the most likely diagnosis and is rare in children. This entity is most commonly seen in women in the third and fourth decades of life.

3. The prognosis is excellent. Surgery is performed in patients who are symptomatic or whose imaging findings are equivocal.

4. Giant hemangioma, hepatocellular carcinoma (fibrolamellar type), hepatic adenoma, metastasis, and hepatoblastoma in young children.

Reference

Hussain SM, et al: Focal nodular hyperplasia: findings at state-of-the-art MR imaging, US, CT, and pathologic analysis, *Radiographics* 24:3–17, 2004.

Cross-Reference

Blickman JG, Parker BR, Barnes PD: *Pediatric radiology— the requisites*, ed 3, Philadelphia, 2009, Mosby, pp 109–110.

Comment

Focal nodular hyperplasia (FNH) is one of the most common benign liver tumors, second only to hemangioma. FNH is most commonly found in women (80% to 95% of patients) in their third and fourth decades of life; however, FNH is rarely seen in children.

FNH is a hyperplastic process in which all the normal constituents of the liver are present but in an abnormally organized pattern. Liver function tests in these patients are usually within the reference range.

FNH is classified into two types: (1) classic (80% of patients) and (2) nonclassic (20% of patients). The gross appearance of classic FNH consists of lobulated contours and parenchyma that is composed of nodules surrounded by radiating fibrous septa originating from a central scar. Distinction between FNH and other hypervascular liver lesions, such as hepatocellular adenoma, hepatocellular carcinoma, and hypervascular metastases, is critical to ensure proper treatment. The asymptomatic patient with FNH does not require biopsy or surgery.

US is often the initial imaging modality that identifies a focal liver lesion. Only a subtle change in echogenicity may be demonstrated, compared with the surrounding normal liver parenchyma. The conspicuity of the lesions with US may improve when a central scar is present. The lesions may be slightly hypoechoic, isoechoic, or slightly hyperechoic. Magnetic resonance imaging (MRI) has a higher sensitivity and specificity for FNH than do US or CT. Typically, FNH is isointense or hypointense on T1-weighted images, is slightly hyperintense or isointense on T2-weighted images, and has a hyperintense central scar on T2-weighted images. FNH demonstrates intense homogeneous enhancement during the arterial phase of contrast administration and delayed enhancement of the central scar during later phases. A central scar is present at imaging in most patients with FNH. The amount of scar tissue within FNH and the size of the central scar may vary. The central scar is typically high in signal intensity on T2-weighted images (unlike hepatocellular carcinoma) and low in signal intensity on T1-weighted images.

Typical FNH can be diagnosed with confidence with CT or MRI. Atypical FNH may appear as a large lesion, which is sometimes multiple in location. The tumor may show less intense enhancement, unusual appearance or nonenhancement of the central scar, and pseudocapsular enhancement on delayed images. With these patients, differentiating atypical FNH from benign and malignant lesions such as hepatic adenoma, hepatocellular carcinoma, fibrolamellar carcinoma, and hypervascular hepatic metastases may be difficult.

The best imaging modalities for characterizing FNH are those that can delineate the lesion's central scar or can show Kupffer cell activity. The best modalities for identifying the central scar are CT and MRI, and Kupffer cell activity is best demonstrated by radionuclide scans. Hepatocellular neoplasms such as hepatic adenoma and hepatocellular carcinoma can also reveal increased uptake. In the future, however, MRI superparamagnetic contrast agents or liver-specific contrast agents may challenge radionuclide scanning.

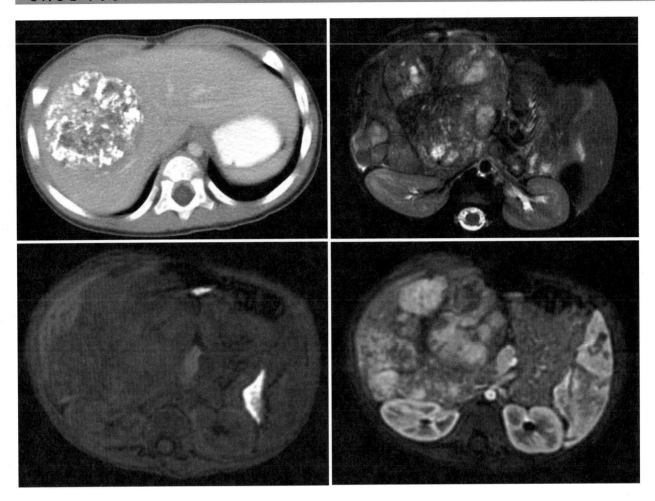

1. What are the imaging findings in these infants with a palpable right upper quadrant mass?

2. What is the diagnosis?

3. What are the differential diagnoses?

4. A prior infection such as hepatitis is a predisposing factor. Is this statement *true* or *false*?

Diagnosis: Hepatoblastoma

1. Patient 1: An axial contrast-enhanced computed tomographic (CT) image of the liver shows a large, well-circumscribed, densely calcified mass in the right lobe of the liver. Patient 2: A large, well-defined, slightly exophytic mass is observed arising from the right lobe of the liver. The T2-weighted signal characteristics and contrast enhancement are heterogeneous.

2. Hepatoblastoma.

3. Hemangioendethelioma, neuroblastoma metastasis, mesenchymal hamartoma, and hepatocellular carcinoma.

4. The statement is false. Hepatoblastoma is a congenital hepatic malignancy. It can either be familial, or short-arm chromosome 11 deletions may be present.

Reference

Sallam A, Paes B, Bourgeois J: Neonatal hepatoblastoma: two cases posing a diagnostic dilemma, with a review of the literature, *Am J Perinatol* 22:413–419, 2005.

Cross-Reference

Blickman JG, Parker BR, Barnes PD: *Pediatric radiology— the requisites*, ed 3, Philadelphia, 2009, Mosby, pp 110–111.

Comment

Hepatoblastoma is the most common hepatic tumor in very young children and, after Wilm tumor and neuroblastoma, one of the most common abdominal malignancies in older children. Although most commonly found in infants, hepatoblastoma can be seen in children up to 15 years of age. A painless abdominal mass and hepatomegaly describe the most common clinical presentation. Incidences of hepatoblastoma increase in Beckwith-Wiedemann syndrome, hemihypertrophy, and familial adenomatous polyposis. The five histologic subtypes are (1) pure fetal, (2) embryonal, (3) mixed epithelial, (4) mesenchymal or macrotrabecular, and (5) small-cell undifferentiated. The fetal type carries the most favorable prognosis, and the small-cell undifferentiated type presents the worst. Serum alpha-fetoprotein (AFP) levels are elevated in more than 90% of the patients, and tumors that fail to express AFP at diagnosis are biologically more aggressive. Metastatic disease is common; lungs and periaortic lymph nodes are commonly affected, whereas brain metastasis is rare. The right lobe of the liver is affected in 60% of the patients, and approximately 50% of the patients show calcification. Hepatoblastomas are usually well-demarcated heterogeneous tumors and are likely secondary to tumor necrosis or hemorrhage.

Ultrasonography (US) with Doppler imaging is the first modality of choice in defining the presence of the mass and the extent of disease. Further cross-sectional imaging with CT or magnetic resonance imaging is indicated because of the anatomic extent of the disease, which involves the hepatic veins, portal veins, and inferior vena cava; it is also indicated because the relationship to the hepatic lobar anatomy is crucial for preoperative planning and for monitoring the response to chemotherapy. Chemotherapy is helpful in downstaging the tumor, allowing for either surgical resection of the tumor or liver transplantation. Hepatoblastomas can metastasize to the lungs, periaortic lymph nodes, and rarely to the brain.

US can show a solid mass with a heterogeneous signal from hemorrhage or necrosis or calcification. Color-coded duplex sonography shows hypervascularity. CT imaging may show heterogeneous mass, predominantly hypoattenuating, compared with normal liver parenchyma. Contrast enhancement is nonuniform and less than normal liver parenchyma. Hepatoblastomas may appear as a low-signal mass on T1-weighted images. On T2-weighted images, the signal is typically high but may be variable, secondary to the degree of hemorrhage and necrosis. Contrast enhancement is heterogenous.

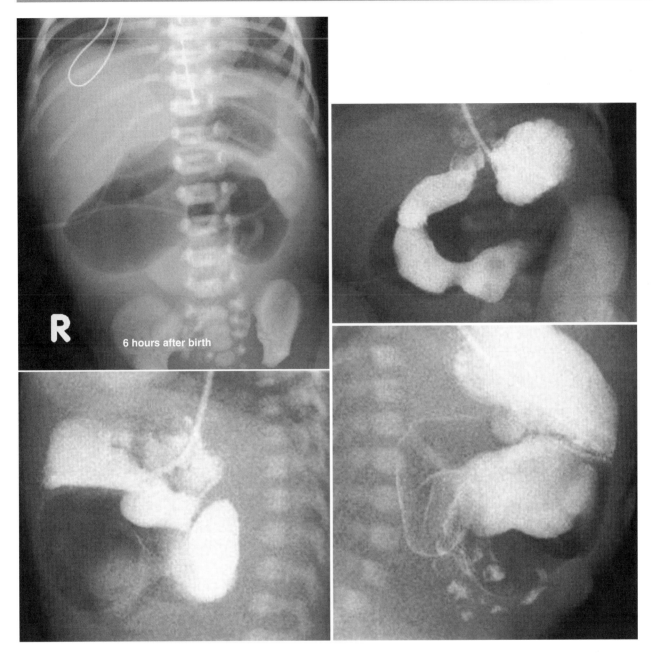

6 hours after birth

1. What are the imaging findings in this newborn with bilious vomiting?

2. What is the diagnosis?

3. What are the differential diagnoses?

4. What is the cause?

Diagnosis: Jejunal Atresia

1. In a plain anteroposterior view of the abdomen, few air-filled, dilated proximal bowel loops are visible, which suggests an upper intestinal obstruction. No air-filled bowel loops are noted in the distal intestine. An upper gastrointestinal (GI) barium study confirms the near complete obstruction in the proximal jejunum, as evidenced by an apparent dilation of the duodenum and only a small trickle of barium passing into the remainder of the small bowel.

2. Jejunal atresia.

3. In a neonate, the differential diagnoses would include extrinsic versus intrinsic obstructions, which include duodenal atresia, jejunoileal atresia, meconium ileus, meconium plug syndrome, Hirschprung disease, ileal duplication cyst, malrotation, and volvulus.

4. The most commonly accepted theory is in utero ischemia, resulting from volvulus, occlusion of superior mesenteric artery, and intussusception.

Reference

Berrocal T, et al: Congenital anomalies of the upper gastrointestinal tract, *Radiographics* 19(4):855–872, 1999.

Cross-Reference

Blickman JG, Parker BR, Barnes PD: *Pediatric radiology—the requisites*, ed 3, Philadelphia, 2009, Mosby, p 90.

Comment

Patients with jejunoileal atresia present with bilious emesis, a failure to pass meconium, or abdominal distension, based on the level of atresia. Proximal jejunal involvement would present with bilious emesis, whereas distal jejunal or ileal location would present with a failure to pass meconium. Patients with delayed partial or incomplete jejunal atresia may present with a failure to thrive. The radiologic work-up starts with plain radiographic films of the abdomen. Plain films reveal dilated small bowel loops proximal to the level of atresia. Jejunal or proximal ileal obstruction presents with few severely dilated loops of bowel. Distal ileal obstruction generally presents with diffuse similarly dilated multiple loops of bowel proximal to the level of obstruction. The presence of a soft tissue mass or curvilinear calcification suggests complicated obstruction such as perforation with meconium peritonitis, pseudocyst formation, and segmental volvulus.

In the presented case, an upper GI study was performed because the radiologic findings and clinical symptoms suggested a proximal obstruction. The passage of contrast from the duodenum to the proximal jejunum was delayed, and only a small amount of contrast passed through. Sometimes the atresias that allow passage of contrast material are incomplete.

Water-soluble enema studies are performed when distal bowel obstruction is suspected. The size of the colon is helpful in determining a differential diagnosis. Microcolon can be seen in distal obstructions such as ileal atresia, meconium ileus, or total colonic Hirschprung disease. A normal- or near normal–sized colon can be seen in jejunal or proximal ileal atresias or ileal duplications. The earlier the timing of the insult in utero, the smaller the caliber of the colon. The reflux of the contrast material to a normal-sized terminal ileum indicates a distal ileal atresia. Jejunal atresias can be multiple, and additional distal atresias may be seen.

Enema studies should be avoided if any sign of perforation is revealed. Prognosis depends on the amount of residual functional small bowel. Potential complications include dysmotility, functional obstruction, and delayed ileus as a result of bands.

Ileal atresia is associated with several syndromes and chromosomal aberrations such as trisomy 21.

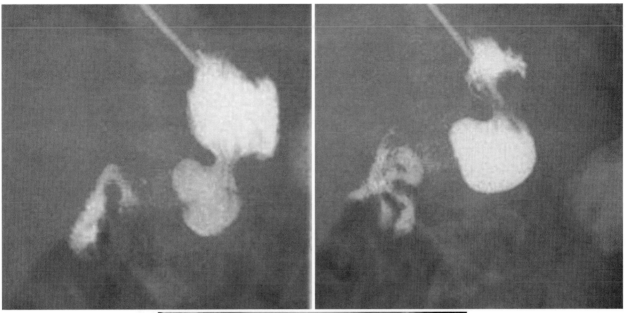

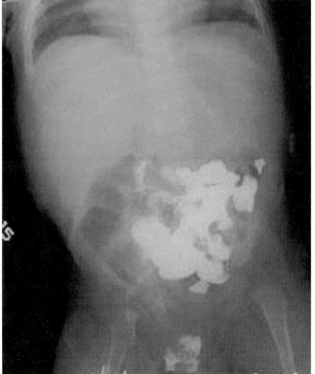

1. What are the imaging findings in this newborn infant with bilious vomiting?

2. What is the diagnosis?

3. Does ultrasonography (US) play a role in the diagnosis?

4. Name associated syndromes.

Diagnosis: Malrotation

1. An upper gastrointestinal (GI) examination shows that the duodenum is redundant and the duodenojejunal junction (DJJ) is to the right of the spine. Follow-up plain radiographic films of the abdomen 8 hours after the upper GI examination show that the colon is in the left upper and lower quadrants.

2. Malrotation without volvulus.

3. The accuracy of US has been found higher in patients who are symptomatic and can be used as a screening tool. Reversal of the normal anatomic relation of the superior mesenteric artery (SMA) and the superior mesenteric vein (SMV) (i.e., the SMA is to the right of the SMV) can be seen in malrotation; however, this abnormal relation can be seen in cases with normal rotation of the midgut.

4. Apple-peel intestinal atresia, Cornelia de Lange syndrome, Cantrell pentalogy, cat-eye syndrome, chromosomal abnormalities (e.g., trisomies 13, 18, 21), Marfan syndrome, and prune-belly syndrome.

Reference

Applegate KE, Anderson JM, Klatte EC: Intestinal malrotation in children: a problem-solving approach to the upper gastrointestinal series, *Radiographics* 26 (5):1485-1500, 2006.

Cross-Reference

Blickman JG, Parker BR, Barnes PD: *Pediatric radiology— the requisites*, ed 3, Philadelphia, 2009, Mosby, pp 87-88.

Comment

Intestinal malrotation is defined as the failure of the embryologic midgut to rotate 270 degrees counterclockwise on its return from the omphalocele into the abdominal cavity. This results in abnormal mesenteric attachments and a shortening of the base of the mesentery, which may lead to midgut volvulus, a potentially life-threatening condition. Malrotation occurs in approximately 1 in 500 births and is usually diagnosed in newborns and young infants with up to 75% occurring in symptomatic newborns and up to 90% occurring in symptomatic infants within the first year of life.

The classic clinical presentation is bilious vomiting with or without abdominal distension associated with either duodenal obstructive bands or midgut volvulus.

Malrotation of the bowel can be associated with a syndrome and other anomalies. Malrotation can be seen in the patient with omphalocele and gastroschisis or congenital diaphragmatic hernia in whom the normal embryologic development and resulting positioning of the developing gut were disrupted. Malrotation is very common in children with heterotaxy syndrome.

In malrotation the mesenteric attachment of the midgut, particularly the portion from the DJJ to the cecum, is abnormally short; therefore the gut is prone to twist counterclockwise around the SMA and SMV.

The modality of choice in radiologic evaluation of malrotation is an upper GI series. The initial passage of barium through the duodenum should be observed directly with fluoroscopy to confirm the course of the duodenum and the position of the DJJ. The normal position of the DJJ is to the left of the left-sided pedicles of the vertebral body at the level of the duodenal bulb on frontal views and posterior (retroperitoneal) on lateral views. However, variations of the normal location that mimic malrotation may appear, particularly on frontal views in the upper GI series. Inferior displacement of the normal DJJ can be seen as a variation, which may be caused by the displacement of the relatively mobile ligament of Treitz by the adjacent distended stomach or bowel.

True AP positioning of the child is important because oblique views may result in a misinterpretation of the location of the DJJ. Redundancy of the duodenum represents a challenge, making the interpretation of the DJJ difficult. In cases with equivocal findings, delayed images with visualization of the cecum are helpful. The cecum is abnormally positioned in 80% of patients with malrotation, and proximal jejunal loops are seen in the right hemiabdomen. In patients with persisting uncertainty, the upper GI series should be repeated.

In acutely symptomatic patients, the upper GI tract examination should be performed urgently because the treatment for acute volvulus is immediate surgery with the Ladd procedure, during which the bands are cut to eliminate any obstruction and the small bowel is placed and fixed in the right abdomen and the colon in the left abdomen.

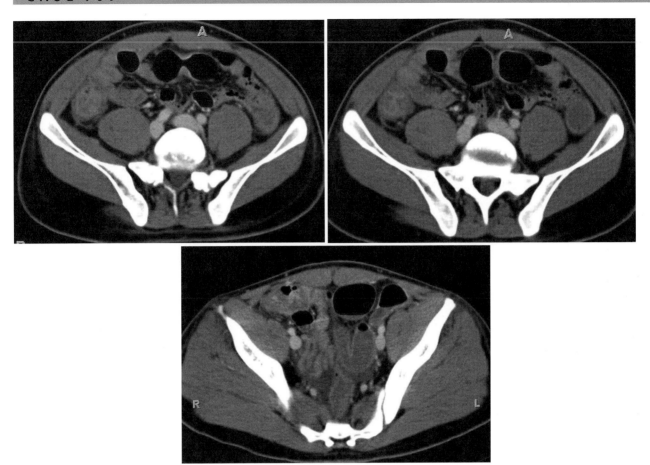

1. What are the imaging findings?

2. What is the clinical presentation?

3. What are the differential diagnoses?

4. What is the cause?

Diagnosis: Typhilitis

1. Thickening of the colonic wall with increased contrast enhancement that is limited to the ascending colon and cecum, as well as free fluid in the pelvis.

2. Distension, right lower quadrant pain, bloody stools, fever, and vomiting.

3. Benign and malignant tumors, inflammatory processes (e.g., appendicitis, diverticulitis, Crohn disease), infectious diseases, and congenital conditions (e.g., cecal volvulus, duplication cyst).

4. Typhilitis is a necrotizing enterocolitis that affects the right colon and ileum in patients with neutropenia that can be seen secondary to leukemia, lymphoma, anaplastic anemia, acquired immunodeficiency syndrome, chemotherapy, or transplantation.

Reference
Davila ML: Neutropenic enterocolitis: current issues in diagnosis and management, *Curr Infect Dis Rep* 9(2):116–120, 2007.

Cross-Reference
Blickman JG, Parker BR, Barnes PD: *Pediatric radiology— the requisites*, ed 3, Philadelphia, 2009, Mosby, pp 99–101.

Comment
Neutropenic enterocolitis or typhilitis (from the Greek word *typhlon*, which means *cecum*) is a clinical syndrome that occurs in the setting of disease or chemotherapy-induced neutropenia. The disease is characterized by an inflammatory process involving the ascending colon or small bowel or both and can result in ischemia, necrosis, bacteremia, hemorrhage, and perforation.

At present, computed tomography (CT) is considered a first-line imaging modality for the evaluation of the ileocecal area. Massively thickened wall of the colon is limited to the ascending segment of the right colon in the right appropriate clinical setting and is pathognomonic. Ultrasonography (US) of the right lower quadrant will demonstrate a target sign that represents the thickened bowel with an echogenic mucosa.

Radiographically, small bowel obstruction, ileus, paucity of the right lower quadrant air, thickened wall of the right colon, and intestinal pneumatosis can be seen. The diagnosis is supported by the findings of bowel wall thickening on US or CT imaging.

The management of neutropenic enterocolitis is controversial. Neither prospective nor high-quality retrospective studies concerning medical or surgical therapies are available. Most authors recommend initial conservative management with bowel rest, intravenous fluids, total parenteral nutrition, and broad-spectrum antibiotics. Surgical intervention is recommended in the setting of obstruction, perforation, persistent gastrointestinal bleeding, and clinical deterioration.

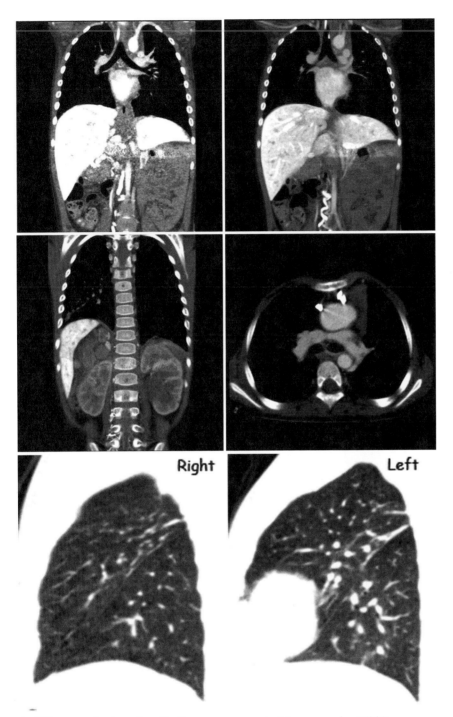

Right Left

1. What are the imaging findings on computed tomography (CT)?

2. What is the diagnosis?

3. What kind of additional malformations should be excluded?

4. What could be a reason for an acute abdomen?

Diagnosis: Polysplenia in Left Isomerism (Heterotaxia)

1. Symmetrical, hypoarterial mainstem bronchi, multiple spleens, and two left lungs.

2. Polysplenia in left isomerism.

3. Cardiac anomalies, azygous continuation, bilateral superior vena cava (SVC), preduodenal portal vein, and intestinal malrotation.

4. Midgut volvulus.

Reference

Borenstein SH, Langer JC: Heterotaxia syndromes and their abdominal manifestations, *Curr Opin Pediatr* 18:294–297, 2006.

Cross-Reference

Blickman JG, Parker BR, Barnes PD: *Pediatric radiology—the requisites*, ed 3, Philadelphia, 2009, Mosby, p 116.

Comment

The two major heterotaxia variations are asplenia syndrome (right isomerism) and polysplenia (left isomerism). The asplenia syndrome is characterized as bilateral right sidedness with a centrally located liver, an absence of the spleen, and two morphologic right lungs. The polysplenia syndrome is characterized as bilateral left sidedness with multiple spleens and two morphologic left lungs.

In addition to the multiple spleens, several other anomalies can be observed in polysplenia syndrome. Azygos continuation of the inferior vena cava is common. The hepatic veins may drain separately into a common atrium and bilateral SVC may connect to the coronary sinus. Next to an increased incidence of congenital heart diseases, the transposition of the great vessels, and pulmonary valvulary stenosis, children with heterotaxia syndrome often have gastrointestinal abnormalities that may include preduodenal portal veins, biliary atresia, and gastric volvulus. A potentially life-threatening acute abdomen caused by midgut volvulus can result from abnormalities of intestinal rotation.

Polysplenia syndrome or left isomerism can be demonstrated on chest radiography by symmetrical mainstem bronchi with a left-sided morphology that is characterized by a wide carinal angle and a hyparterial course of the mainstem bronchi. These findings can be easily confirmed with CT. In addition, both lungs will only show a major fissure and no minor fissure. The multiple spleens can be located anywhere within the upper abdomen.

Prognosis is variable, and treatment is frequently symptomatic.

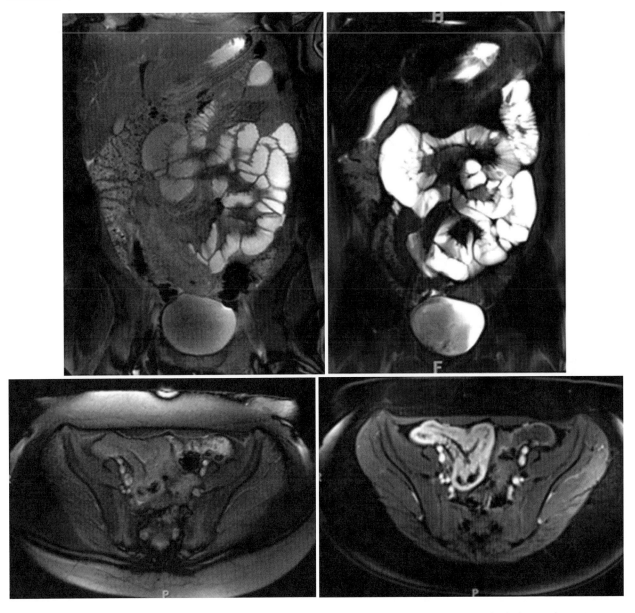

1. What are the magnetic resonance imaging (MRI) findings in this 13-year-old girl with abdominal pain?

2. Which sequences are used?

3. What is the most likely diagnosis?

4. What are characteristic imaging findings that may be seen in this disease?

CASE 111

Diagnosis: Crohn Disease

1. Diffuse contrast enhancing bowel wall thickening that affect a distal ileal loop.

2. T2-weighted fat saturated sequence (first image); long-echo, heavily T2-weighted sequence (second image); T1-weighted precontrast sequence (third image); and T1-weighted postcontrast with fat saturation and intravenous glucagon sequence (fourth image).

3. Crohn disease (CD).

4. Bowel wall thickening (ileum >4 to 5 mm), T2-weighted hyperintensity of the bowel wall, contrast enhancement of affected loops, wall stratification, ulcers, cobblestone appearance of mucosa, single or multiple stenosis, prestenotic dilation, skip lesions, transmural extension with extraluminal abscesses, fistulae, comb sign, fibrofatty proliferation of mesentery, and mesenteric lymphadenopathy.

Cross-Reference
Blickman JG, Parker BR, Barnes PD: *Pediatric radiology— the requisites*, ed 3, Philadelphia, 2009, Mosby, pp 96-98.

Comment
CD is named after Dr. Burril Crohn who described this autoimmune and likely chronic, recurrent inflammatory disease of the gastrointestinal (GI) tract as early as 1932. CD may affect the entire GI tract from the mouth to the anus. The small bowel is affected in 30% to 40% of patients, ileocolonic disease is seen in 40% to 55% of patients, and 90% of the patients with small bowel CD have terminal ileum involvement. Clinically, patients present with relapsing and remitting episodes of abdominal cramps, fever, diarrhea, and weight loss. Frequently, the patients are young and will suffer for many years from CD. The disease typically involves all bowel wall layers and may extend extramurally. Locally, cryptitis and crypt abscesses may be seen. In chronic cases, the relapsing inflammation frequently results in fibrosis with thickened, stenotic bowel loops. Frequently, multiple segments are affected with nonaffected segments in between (skip lesions). Because these patients have chronic symptoms, MRI with the use of biphasic hyperosmolar endoluminal contrast is the imaging method of choice. The use of intravenous contrast and glucagon increases the diagnostic sensitivity. Imaging findings include focal or segmental bowel wall thickening with matching transmural contrast enhancement. The affected segments are frequently stenotic with dilation of more proximal bowel loops. In addition, because the disease may extend transmurally, the demarcation of the outer bowel wall may be lost with extraluminal fluid collections or abscess formation. Progressive transmural disease should be suspected if the comb sign is observed, which is the result of proliferating mesenteric vessels surrounded by fat. Chronic infection also results in a fibrofatty proliferation of the adjacent mesentery with creeping fat that may displace and separate adjacent bowel loops. Finally, multiple mesenteric lymph nodes are frequently observed. Differential diagnosis includes ulcerative colitis, which is, however, typically limited to the mucosa and rarely extends transmurally. Moreover, ulcerative colitis (UC) typically extends without interruption retrograde from the anus to the cecum.

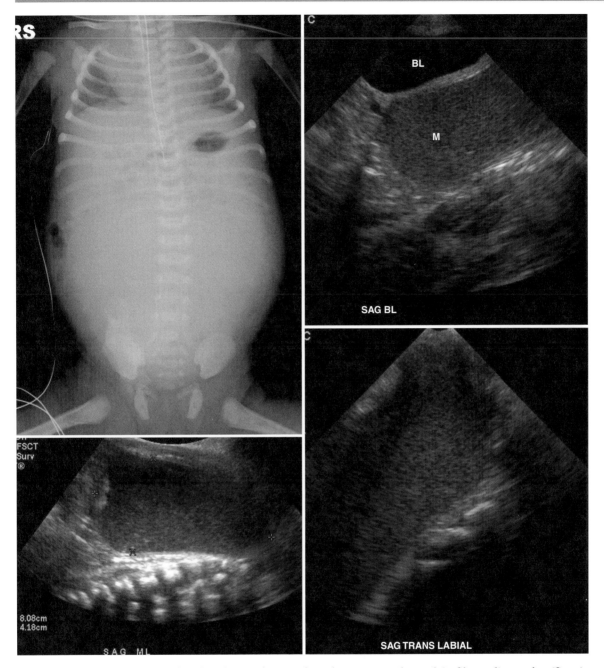

1. What are the findings in this female newborn infant demonstrated on plain-film radiography (first image)?

2. What possible differential diagnoses come to mind?

3. What is the best imaging modality for diagnosis? What are the differentiating features on transabdominal (second and third images) and transperineal (fourth image) images?

4. When is this entity usually detected?

Diagnosis: Hydrometrocolpos

1. A smooth mass rising from the pelvis, displacing bowel gas upward.

2. Overdistended bladder, ovarian cyst, gastrointestinal (GI) duplication cyst, mesenteric cyst, enlarged uterus, and teratoma.

3. Ultrasonography (US) can characterize the mass and show its cystic character and intrauterine and intravaginal location. Internal debris suggests the presence of old blood products. The third image, shows the indentation of the cervix into the vaginal fluid. Transperineal sonography confirms the location of the cystic collection in the vagina and may visualize the curving contour of the bulging hymen.

4. In the newborn period or at puberty.

Reference

Kuhn JP, Slovis TL, Haller JO, editors: *Caffey's pediatric diagnostic imaging*, ed 10, Philadelphia, 2004, Mosby, pp 1946-1947.

Cross-Reference

Blickman JG, Parker BR, Barnes PD: *Pediatric radiology— the requisites*, ed 3, Philadelphia, 2009, Mosby, p 151.

Comment

Even before menarche occurs, the uterus and cervix produce secretions that drain through the vagina. Secretion surges in the immediate newborn period and again at puberty under the influence of female hormones— maternal in the first instance and endogenous in the second. If the egress from the vagina is blocked, then secretions build up, distending the vagina and uterus. Amenorrhea may bring the patient to clinical attention at puberty. In this infant, abdominal distension and discomfort are demonstrated.

The main differential point is determining whether the obstruction is caused by an intact hymen or if segmental vaginal or cervical atresia exists. The former situation is a benign condition, although it deserves treatment to alleviate the obstruction to prevent hematosalpinx and endometriosis from reflux of blood products and endometrial cells into the fallopian tubes and peritoneum. Such a development may eventually predispose the patient to ectopic pregnancy and infertility. In patients with extreme vaginal distension, urethral obstruction can develop.

The presence of a vaginal septum or segmental atresia is associated with urogenital sinus, ambiguous genitalia, renal anomalies, GI atresias, and congenital heart disease.

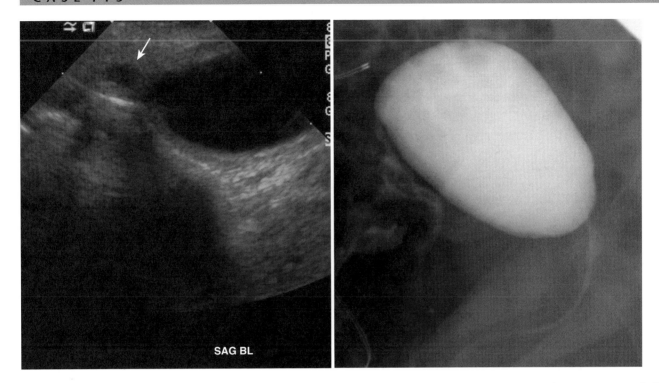

SAG BL

1. The mother of this full-term infant complains that his umbilicus is always wet. An ultrasound image is provided (first image). What are the findings?

2. A pediatric voiding cystourethrogram is also provided (second image). What does it show?

3. What is usually done about this?

Diagnosis: Patent Urachus

1. The bladder extends cephalad in a point. A channel goes to the base of the umbilicus (*arrow*).

2. Leakage of contrast from the umbilicus through a channel from the bladder. The bladder and urethra are otherwise normal.

3. Surgical excision.

Reference

Fotter R, editor: *Pediatric uroradiology*, ed 2, Berlin-Heidelberg-New York, 2008, Springer, pp 133–330.

Comment

The urachus is a normal structure that connects the fetal bladder with the placenta and helps the fetus rid itself of wastes. The present case represents a persistence of that connection in an unusually patent state. More often, a diverticulum at the dome of the bladder is found incidentally. The urachal channel can still be present, sealed off at each end, but containing a cyst. These cysts can become infected and form abcesses. Rare carcinomatous degeneration of these cysts in adulthood has been reported; consequently, excision is usually warranted.

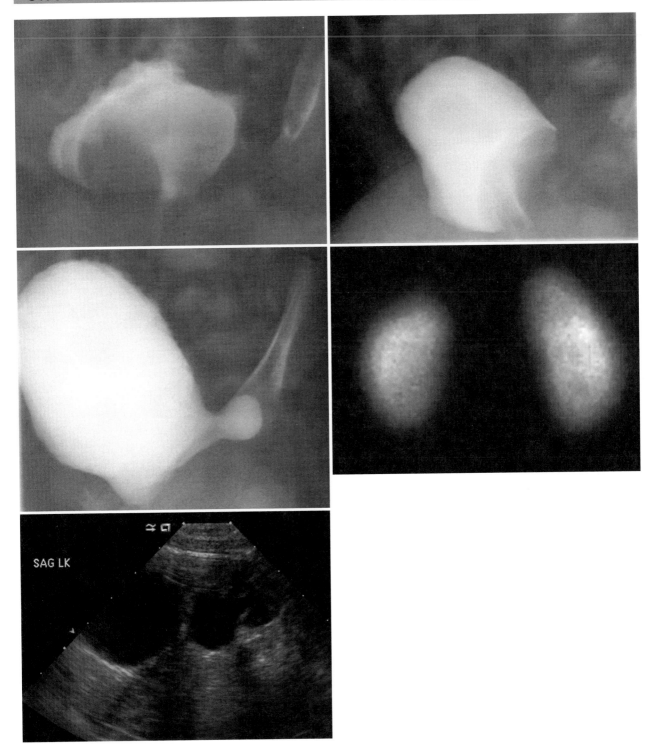

1. What is the diagnosis?

2. How might the clinical presentation be described?

3. Do all patients have symptoms?

4. What is the treatment for this patient?

Diagnosis: Everting Ureterocele with Duplication of the Renal Collecting System

1. Duplication of the renal collecting system with obstruction of the upper pole by an everting ureterocele is the diagnosis. The lower pole may also be partially obstructed.

2. In utero diagnosis includes urinary tract infection or incontinence in the female patient later in life.

3. No, especially the patient with duplication without obstruction of the upper pole or reflux into the lower pole. In this situation, the finding is considered a normal variant.

4. Incision of the ureterocele initially, followed by upper pole resection, as long as no significant function of the upper pole exists.

Reference

Grattan-Smith J, Jones R: MR urography in children, *Pediatr Radiol* 22:1679–1688, 2006.

Cross-Reference

Blickman JG, Parker BR, Barnes PD: *Pediatric radiology— the requisites*, ed 3, Philadelphia, 2009, Mosby, pp 128–129.

Comment

Complete duplication of the renal collecting system is a common anomaly seen in girls more than boys (2:1) and is frequently complicated by the obstruction of the upper pole moiety either by ureterocele or stenosis at its ectopic insertion. The upper pole ureter inserts ectopically, medial and inferior to the trigone (Weigert-Meyer rule). The ectopic ureter inserts anywhere from quite close to the trigone to as far away as the lower bladder, urethra, vagina, or perineum in a girl. The ectopic insertion in a boy is always above the external urethral sphincter. This difference explains why incontinence is not a sign of complicated duplication in the male patient; the lower pole inserts normally.

To evaluate patients with this anomaly, multiple studies may be necessary. Careful attention to the bladder, especially during early filling when performing a voiding cystourethrogram, should show a ureterocele if it is within the bladder. It is effaced and may evert as the bladder is filled or as the patient voids. Reflux, when present, usually involves the lower pole moiety. Ultrasound examination is usually able to demonstrate the amount of dilation of the upper pole and its ureter and provide some idea of the amount of parenchyma in the upper pole moiety. The ureterocele may be seen in the bladder. Functional nuclear medicine studies will allow quantitative analysis of the overall function of the upper pole. Occasionally in difficult cases, especially where the upper pole is dysplastic without a dilated collecting system, magnetic resonance (MR) urography or computed tomography or both may be useful. MR urography is gaining more widespread use as its utility is demonstrated.

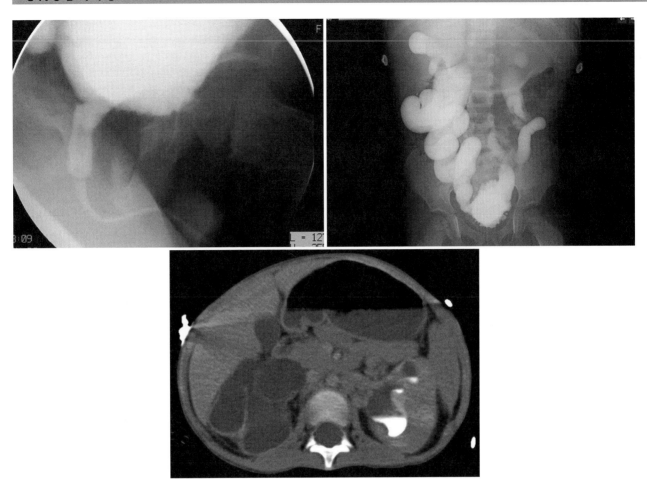

1. What are the findings in this male newborn infant?

2. What causes these findings?

3. Describe the possible consequences of this condition.

4. What is the treatment?

Diagnosis: Posterior Urethral Valves

1. Findings include a posterior urethra dilated above the level of the verumontanum and a trabeculated and small bladder with bilateral grade V vesicoureteral reflux (VUR). Computed tomography (CT) shows no renal cortex on the right.

2. Bladder outlet obstruction by posterior urethral valves (PUVs).

3. This obstruction can lead to VUR, an abnormal thick-walled noncompliant bladder from longstanding obstruction, upper tract obstruction, and renal insufficiency and failure.

4. Ablation or resection of the valve tissue and close follow-up of the condition, secondary to the obstruction.

Reference

Bloom DA: Dilation of the neonatal urinary tract. In Kuhn JP, Slovis TL, Haller JO, editors: *Caffey's pediatric diagnostic imaging*, Philadelphia, 2004, Mosby, pp 206–213.

Cross-Reference

Blickman JG, Parker BR, Barnes PD: *Pediatric radiology—the requisites*, ed 3, Philadelphia, 2009, Mosby, pp 133–135.

Comment

The patient whose images are shown presented at 6 years of age after a motor vehicle accident. The urinary tract abnormalities were incidental findings on a CT scan, and the diagnosis of PUVs was confirmed by the voiding cystourethrogram shown. No significant right renal function was found by nuclear scintigraphy. He has early-stage chronic renal disease with a decreased glomerular filtration rate and is being followed expectantly after the transurethral resections of the valves.

PUVs are fused mucosal folds at the bottom of the verumontanum not normally found but probably related to the normal folds called *plicae colliculi*. These valves result in a varying amount of obstruction and its sequela. The bladder may become thickened, trabeculated, and small with diverticula. The noncompliant bladder may cause obstruction of the distal ureters. When dilation of the ureters is seen in utero or afterward by ultrasound, it may be the result of this obstruction or VUR, as in this case. Renal dysplasia is often present in severe cases and is most significant in kidneys that are subject to VUR. This dysplasia is the cause of renal insufficiency or frank renal failure and may progress, even after the valves have been resected.

PUVs are the most common cause of renal failure in infants. When findings suggesting PUVs are found in utero, maternal oligohydramnios and resulting lung hypoplasia may be revealed. Potter sequence may occur. If perinephric collections (urinomas) or urinary ascites develop, this *pop-off* phenomenon may be protective of renal function. Fetal surgery has been advocated by some and usually consists of the placement of a shunt between the bladder and the amniotic cavity.

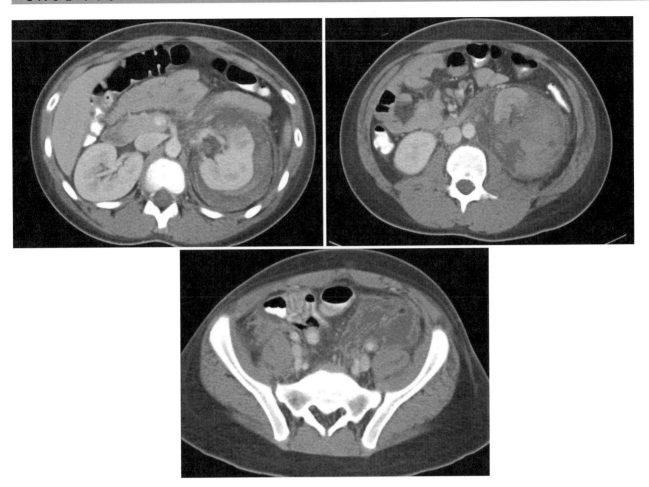

1. What are the findings in this school-age child?

2. How is this renal lesion graded?

3. Is intervention indicated?

4. What is the prognosis?

Diagnosis: Renal Laceration

1. A fracture of the left kidney with perinephric and retroperitoneal hematoma and a disruption of the collecting system with a small amount of contrast noted in the perinephric collection.

2. Severe lacerations with extensive hematoma and a disruption of the collecting system is a grade IV renal lesion.

3. If the patient is clinically stable and the hematoma or urinoma (or both) are not growing, nonsurgical conservative management is recommended.

4. Without vascular pedicle injury, the prognosis is excellent for healing without significant sequela.

Reference

Casale AJ: Urinary tract trauma. In Gearhart JP, Rink RC, Mouriquand PDE, editors: *Pediatric urology*, Philadelphia, 2001, Mosby, pp 923-931.

Cross-Reference

Blickman JG, Parker BR, Barnes PD: *Pediatric radiology—the requisites*, ed 3, Philadelphia, 2009, Mosby, pp 149-150.

Comment

Children are more vulnerable to renal trauma in part because of their body proportions. The kidney is relatively larger than in the adult, and the rib cage is more flexible and does not afford as much protection. Musculature is not as developed. Children are more likely to be struck by a motor vehicle, which is the most common cause of renal laceration (35%). Other causes include being a passenger in a motor vehicle accident, falling, and assaults. Boys are more likely to suffer blunt renal trauma than girls (2:1). Abnormal kidneys are more vulnerable to blunt injury. Hydronephrosis (38%), tumors (7%), and malposition (7%) are three of the most common abnormalities seen underlying trauma. Renal injury is most often associated with other injuries such as trauma to the liver or spleen (46%), head (35%), and bone (21%). For this reason, when renal injury is suspected, imaging the complete abdomen and pelvis and other parts of the body for multisystem injury is reasonable, and using computed tomographic (CT) scans is widely accepted in this country. Ultrasound examination is more useful in following perinephric collections after the extent and severity of the injury is defined by CT examination.

The grading system is useful for categorizing the injury; however, it does not correlate well with outcome and the need for intervention. Grade I is a renal parenchymal contusion; Grade II is a small parenchymal laceration and perinephric hematoma; Grade III is a larger parenchymal laceration and hematoma; Grade IV may have collecting system disruption and minor vascular tears; and Grade V is extensive laceration and collecting system and vascular pedicle disruption.

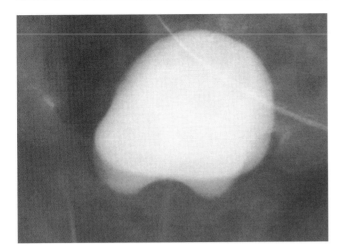

1. This image shows a normal finding. What is it?

2. In what age group does the bladder have this appearance?

3. Is there a differential diagnosis for this finding?

4. Is there any associated abnormality in the patient?

Diagnosis: Bladder Ears

1. This image is from a voiding cystourethrogram (VCUG). The bladder is not distended, and symmetrical protrusions of the contrast-filled bladder are demonstrated inferiorly toward the inguinal region. These protrusions are called *bladder ears*.

2. In infants and young children.

3. This appearance should be differentiated from a diverticulum.

4. An inguinal hernia.

Reference

Fernbach SK, Feinstein KA: Normal findings and anatomic variants. In Kuhn JP, Slovis TL, Haller JO, editors: *Caffey's pediatric diagnostic imaging*, Philadelphia, 2004, Mosby, p 1747.

Cross-Reference

Blickman JG, Parker BR, Barnes PD: *Pediatric radiology—the requisites*, ed 3, Philadelphia, 2009, Mosby, pp 125–126.

Comment

The symmetrical appearance of these outpouchings and their broad necks and location are typical of the bladder ear—a normal variant. The bladder ear or ears are not seen when the bladder is distended. The bladder ear may be unilateral and generally occurs because the processus vaginalis is patent in this age group, allowing for the herniation of the bladder into the inguinal canal. Of course this finding is associated with a true inguinal hernia, which can be detected by physical examination. This normal variant is not seen in the older patient.

Although a diverticulum can be similar in appearance, attention to the timing of its appearance on the VCUG, the age of the patient, and the broad communication with the bladder lumen make the bladder ear normal variation more likely.

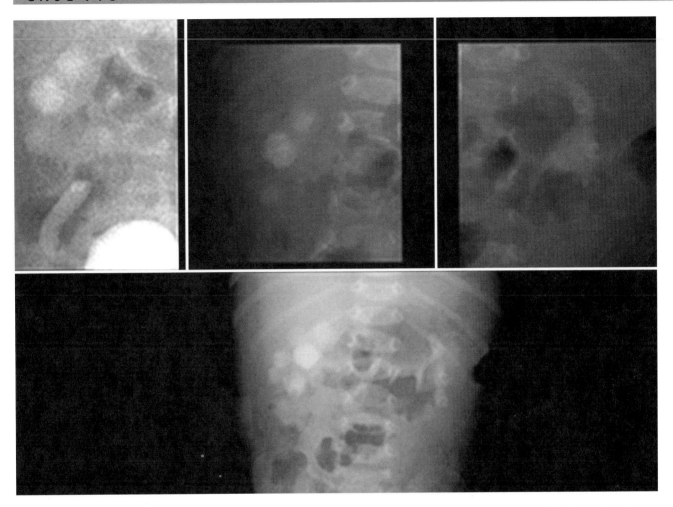

1. What examination is shown in this male infant? Ultrasound examination had shown bilateral hydronephrosis greater on the right than the left.

2. What are the findings?

3. One process is demonstrated on the left and two processes are seen on the right. What are they?

4. Which process must be addressed first if surgery is necessary?

Diagnosis: Ureteropelvic Junction Obstruction with Vesicoureteral Reflux

1. A voiding cystourethrogram.

2. Bilateral vesicoureteral reflux (VUR).

3. Simple grade II VUR is visualized on the left. The VUR on the right is seen with delayed filling and emptying of the upper tract and dilation greater than that of the ureter, which suggests coexisting ureteropelvic junction (UPJ) obstruction.

4. If severe enough, the UPJ obstruction should be corrected first; the VUR may spontaneously resolve.

Reference

Churchill BM, Feng WC: Ureteropelvic junction anomalies: congenital UPJ problems in children. In Gearhart JP, Rink RC, Mouriquand PDE, editors: *Pediatric urology*, Philadelphia, 2001, Elsevier, pp 328–333.

Cross-Reference

Blickman JG, Parker BR, Barnes PD: *Pediatric radiology— the requisites*, ed 3, Philadelphia, 2009, Mosby, pp 130–131.

Comment

The hydronephrosis indicating UPJ obstruction is almost always found on routine maternal ultrasound screening. Before 1978 when screening fetal ultrasound became routine, UPJ obstruction presented in many ways including febrile urinary tract infection, abdominal mass, abdominal pain, and hematuria after minor trauma.

Realizing that UPJ obstruction in the young child is not complete and the condition is not static is important. Complete obstruction in utero is known to be the cause of the multicystic dysplastic kidney. The severity of the UPJ obstruction varies; mild obstruction may not be clinically significant. When diagnosed early in life, the degree of obstruction remains the same in approximately one third of patients; the obstruction improves in one third and worsens in one third. After determining the severity of the obstruction, devising a plan of timely follow-up is important to determine if and when to surgically intervene.

Two main causes of childhood UPJ obstruction exist: (1) The most common cause of intrinsic obstructions is a short hypoplastic adynamic ureteral segment at the UPJ, which results in a patent but narrowed ureter. (2) The most common cause of extrinsic obstructions is vessels crossing the UPJ, either the renal artery or the vein. These vessels can best be shown with computed tomographic or magnetic resonance (MR) imaging. Preoperatively determining the cause in all cases is not necessary because open rather than endoscopic surgery is the most common approach to treating UPJ obstruction in the infant and young child, and these vessels may be directly visualized during the procedure. In the case of extrinsic obstruction, a dismembered pyeloplasty is performed.

UPJ obstruction is seen in less than 1% of patients with VUR. This coexistence limits the grading of the VUR because dilation of the intrarenal collecting system has already occurred.

Ultrasound examination is a reasonable way to follow the amount of dilation immediately after birth and thereafter. The quantitative degree of functional obstruction is best determined by nuclear diuretic urography using technetium-99m mercaptoacetyltriglycine (99mTc-MAG3). Alternatively, MR urography is gaining popularity.

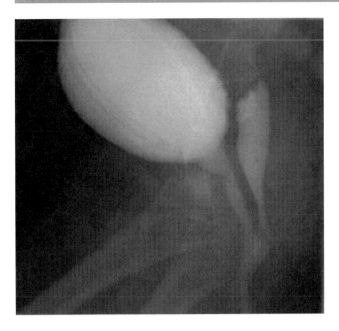

1. What are the findings in this newborn?

2. What study was performed?

3. Why was the study performed?

4. What is the sex of the patient?

Diagnosis: Urogenital Sinus

1. The findings include a short urogenital (UG) sinus. The vagina is normal in size, and a cervical impression is revealed.

2. A catheter has entered the bladder; consequently, in effect, the study is a voiding cystourethrogram (VCUG). In this case, the modality can also be called a *genitogram*.

3. The study is usually performed in patients with ambiguous genitalia.

4. The patient is female. The presence of a cervical impression indicates a uterus is present.

Reference

Cohen HL, Haller JO: Anomalies of sex differentiation. In Kuhn JP, Slovis TL, Haller JO, editors: *Caffey's pediatric diagnostic imaging*, Philadelphia, 2004, Mosby, pp 1976-1978.

Cross-Reference

Blickman JG, Parker BR, Barnes PD: *Pediatric radiology— the requisites*, ed 3, Philadelphia, 2009, Mosby, pp 134-135.

Comment

For social reasons, infants born with ambiguous genitalia require emergency evaluation. This evaluation includes physical examination, hormonal assays, chromosomal determination, and imaging to determine the internal genital anatomy. Detailed radiography of the lower genitourinary tract is useful not only for diagnostic purposes but also for guiding the surgical approach to reconstruction.

Most patients have a UG sinus, which is a common channel for the anterior urethra and posterior vagina. The sinus usually terminates at the base of the phallus. This sinus should be suspected whenever a single perineal opening or any degree of genital ambiguity exists.

A VCUG, as in this case, may demonstrate all the anatomy. The catheter may preferentially enter the bladder or the vagina; filling either with contrast may be helpful. If the anatomy is not clearly delineated with these techniques, then a catheter should be placed in the UG sinus as close to the perineal opening as possible and contrast gently instilled. This procedure may opacify the UG sinus and the vagina. The longer the UG sinus, the more masculinized the patient will be. The vagina may be small or normal in size. The vaginal opening to the UG sinus may be stenotic or completely obstructed, resulting in hydrocolpos at birth or hematocolpos at puberty. The cervical impression on the vagina ensures that a uterus is present. If the uterus is not seen, ultrasound examination may be useful to examine the internal gonads and uterus.

This patient had congenital adrenal hyperplasia, which is the most common cause of ambiguous genitalia in female patients.

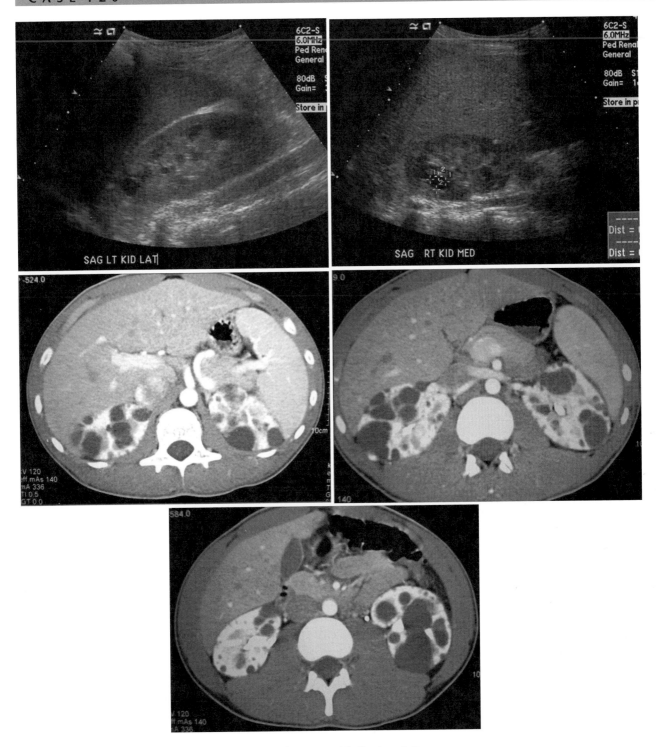

SAG LT KID LAT

SAG RT KID MED

1. What is the diagnosis in this 12-year-old adolescent with flank pain?

2. What are the common long-term complications?

3. What are the common short-term complications?

4. List three or more common imaging findings.

Diagnosis: Autosomal Dominant Polycystic Kidney Disease

1. Autosomal dominant polycystic kidney disease (ADPKD).

2. Renal insufficiency or failure and hypertension.

3. Hemorrhage and infection.

4. Enlarged kidneys, innumerable macrocysts (>1 cm), possible pancreatic cysts, heart valve disorders, and berry aneurysms.

References

Zerin JM: Computed tomography and magnetic resonance imaging of the kidneys in children. In Gearhart JG, Rink RC, Mouriquand PDE, editors: *Pediatric urology*, Philadelphia, 2001, Saunders, pp 135-136.

Fernbach SK: Congenital renal anomalies. In Kuhn JP, Slovis TL, Haller JO, editors: *Caffey's pediatric diagnostic imaging*, ed 10, Philadelphia, 2004, Mosby, p 1772.

Cross-Reference

Blickman JG, Parker BR, Barnes PD: *Pediatric radiology—the requisites*, ed 3, Philadelphia, 2009, Mosby, pp 136-137.

Comment

ADPKD occasionally develops in childhood. The cysts are typically small and few in number early in life. As the child grows, however, the cysts get larger and increase in number. The kidneys are affected in 100% of patients with liver cysts and in 50% of patients or less with pancreatic cysts. ADPKD is associated with heart valve disorders, hernias, and berry aneurysms. In infants, the kidneys are usually normal in size with few or no cysts identified. In older children, the kidneys are enlarged with innumerable cysts that usually measure >1 cm. Prognosis declines in adulthood with renal insufficiency and hypertension. Ultrasonography and computed tomography or magnetic resonance imaging (MRI) are useful for follow-up imaging. Differential diagnoses include autosomal recessive polycystic kidney disease, multiple simple cysts, and tuberous sclerosis (in combination with angiomyolipomas).

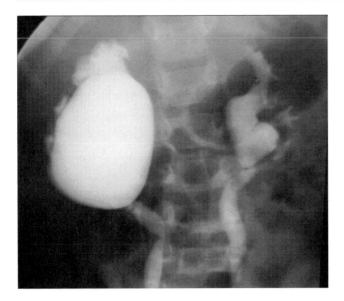

1. What are the findings on ultrasound, and what are the differential diagnoses?

2. What are the findings on intravenous pyelogram (IVP), and what are the differential diagnoses?

3. Are both sides affected?

4. What is the most common cause of an abdominal mass in the newborn?

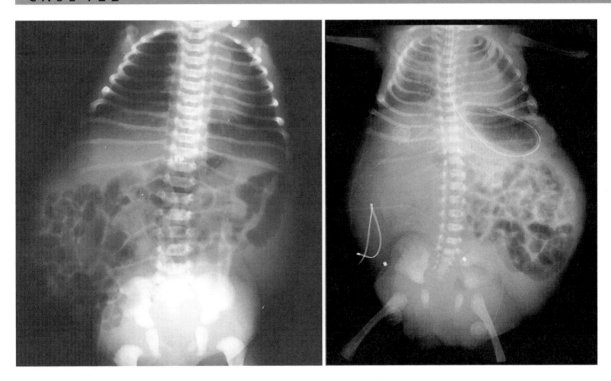

1. What is the likely diagnosis in this male newborn infant?

2. What organ systems are affected in this condition?

3. What is Potter syndrome?

4. Can this disorder occur in female newborn infants?

CASE 121

Diagnosis: Ureteropelvic Junction Obstruction

1. On ultrasound, dilation of the renal pelvis, which is disproportionate to the caliectasis, is demonstrated. Differential diagnoses include ureteropelvic junction (UPJ) obstruction and multicystic dysplastic kidney.

2. On IVP, good renal function with symmetrical excretion is seen. Dilation of the renal pelvis is disproportionate to the calyces, and the ureter is normal in caliber. Differential diagnoses include UPJ obstruction, high-grade reflux, and megacalycosis.

3. UPJ obstruction is bilateral in 10% of patients. The left kidney is more commonly affected. In this patient, bilateral disease exists with the right side worse than the left.

4. UPJ obstruction.

Reference

Fernbach SK: Congenital renal anomalies. In: Kuhn JP, Slovis TL, Haller JO, editors: *Caffey's pediatric diagnostic imaging*, ed 10, Philadelphia, 2004, Mosby, pp 1778-1784.

Cross-Reference

Blickman JG, Parker BR, Barnes PD: *Pediatric radiology—the requisites*, ed 3, Philadelphia, 2009, Mosby, p 131.

Comment

UPJ obstruction occurs more often in boys than in girls and more often on the left side than the right. Between 10% and 20% of patients are bilateral and may be associated with lower pole duplication. UPJ obstruction is the most common cause of a palpable abdominal mass in the neonate. Many theorize about the cause of this disorder. Some propose that a crossing vessel or fibrous scar at the UPJ is the cause, whereas others propose that an abnormal innervation of the proximal ureter occurs and that the UPJ obstruction may be a Hirschsprung equivalent in the genitourinary tract. Classic findings on ultrasound include significant hydronephrosis that ends abruptly at the UPJ and a disproportionately large renal pelvis compared with the calyces. Nuclear scintigraphy using technetium-99m mercaptoacetyltriglycine (99mTc-MAG3) with diuretic challenge demonstrates hydronephrosis with poor drainage even after administration of diuretic agents. Differential diagnoses include multicystic dysplastic kidney, hydronephrosis secondary to vesicoureteral reflux, and ureterovesicular junction obstruction. Treatment is pyeloplasty. Prognosis is excellent if renal function is not compromised before the surgical repair.

CASE 122

Diagnosis: Prune-Belly Syndrome

1. Prune-belly syndrome.

2. Abdominal wall musculature, genitourinary tract, gastrointestinal (GI) tract, cardiovascular system, respiratory system, and musculoskeletal system.

3. Potter syndrome includes oligohydramnios, secondary to renal disease with associated pulmonary hypoplasia.

4. Yes, though it is extremely rare.

Reference

Bloom DA: Dilatation of the neonatal urinary tract. In Kuhn JP, Slovis TL, Haller JO, editors: *Caffey's pediatric diagnostic imaging*, ed 10, Philadelphia, 2004, Mosby, pp 217-218.

Cross-Reference

Blickman JG, Parker BR, Barnes PD: *Pediatric radiology—the requisites*, ed 3, Philadelphia, 2009, Mosby, pp 133-134.

Comment

Prune-belly syndrome, also called Eagle-Barrett syndrome, is a result of the failure of the anterior abdominal wall musculature to develop. It occurs almost exclusively in male infants and involves the abdominal wall, bladder, ureters, urethra, and kidneys. The abdominal wall is thin or lax. The prostatic urethra is long and dilated as a result of prostatic hypoplasia. Some patients have a utricle diverticulum from the urethra; a large, vertically oriented, thick-walled bladder; an urachal remnant from the dome of the bladder; and tortuous and dilated ureters. Varying amounts of hydronephrosis and varying degrees of renal dysplasia are seen. All have cryptorchism. Occasionally, the corpora of the phallus also fail to develop. Associated abnormalities occur in the GI tract (malrotation, imperforate anus, gastroschisis, Hirschsprung disease), heart (atrial septal defect, ventriculoseptal defect), musculoskeletal system (clubfoot deformity, dislocated hips), and respiratory system (pulmonary hypoplasia). The diagnosis is often made in utero when an enlarged bladder, dilated ureters, and an abnormal abdominal wall are seen on prenatal ultrasound. Cases with in utero urethral obstruction do not survive. All survivors have multiple medical problems, including renal insufficiency and eventual renal failure. Prune-belly syndrome can be confused with a case of severe posterior urethral valves on prenatal ultrasound.

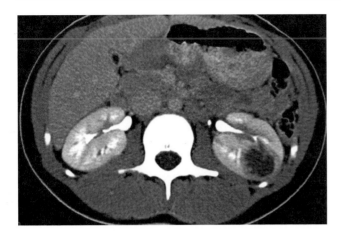

1. What is the diagnosis in this teenage girl with right flank pain?

2. What are the two different mechanisms responsible for the spread of disease?

3. How would this lesion appear on an ultrasound (US) image?

4. How would this lesion appear on a magnetic resonance image (MRI)?

Diagnosis: Renal Abscess

1. Renal abscess.

2. The hematogenous spread of infection and infection ascending from the lower urinary tract.

3. A renal abscess typically appears on US as a round hypoechoic lesion with good through transmission.

4. On an MRI a renal abscess typically demonstrates as high-signal intensity on both T1- and T2-weighted MRIs with restricted diffusion seen on a diffusion-weighted MRI.

Reference

Fernbach SK: Special infections. In: Kuhn JP, Slovis TL, Haller JO, editors: *Caffey's pediatric diagnostic imaging*, ed 10, Philadelphia, 2004, Mosby, pp 1807–1809.

Cross-Reference

Blickman JG, Parker BR, Barnes PD: *Pediatric radiology—the requisites*, ed 3, Philadelphia, 2009, Mosby, pp 148–149.

Comment

Overall, renal abscesses are rare in the pediatric population. Patients with a renal abscess can present with fever, chills, abdominal or flank pain, and occasional weight loss and malaise.

In patients with a cortical abscess, *Staphylococcus aureus* has been identified as the most common causative agent. It is usually the result of the hematogenous spread of infection. Corticomedullary abscesses, however, are usually a result of ascending infection from the urinary bladder and are usually caused by gram-negative organisms.

In patients with a renal abscess, the laboratory study findings will show leukocytosis and an elevated sedimentation rate. Pyuria and bacteriuria will not be evident unless the abscess communicates with the collecting system. Because gram-positive organisms are most commonly blood borne, urine cultures typically show no growth.

Risk factors for renal abscess include recurrent urinary tract infections, renal calculi, genitourinary instrumentation, vesicoureteral reflux, immunosuppression, diabetes mellitus, and sickle cell disease.

In cases of corticomedullary renal abscess, approximately 66% of patients have a history of recurrent urinary tract infections, approximately 30% of patients have nephrolithiasis, and almost two thirds of patients have a history of urinary instrumentation.

On US a round hypoechoic lesion with good through transmission is typically seen. Wall thickness increases as the abscess progresses. With contrast-enhanced computed tomography (CT), a nonenhancing rounded hypoattenuating lesion is characteristic. Typically, a renal abscess has high-signal intensity on both T1- and T2-weighted MRIs with restricted diffusion seen on a diffusion-weighted MRI.

Abscesses less than 3 to 5 cm should be initially treated with appropriate antibiotics for at least 4 weeks. Abscesses greater than 5 cm or those that fail to respond to antibiotic treatment should be considered for CT-guided percutaneous drainage.

The differential diagnosis includes hematoma and hemorrhage into an angiomyolipoma (see fat density on US, CT, and MRI).

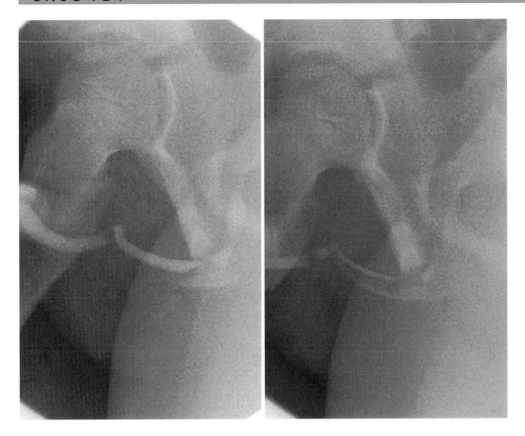

1. What are the most common causes of this abnormality?

2. What is the typical presentation?

3. What is the imaging method of choice?

4. What is the treatment?

Diagnosis: Urethral Fracture

1. Straddle injury and pelvic fractures.

2. Hematuria or difficulty voiding after the injury.

3. Retrograde urethrogram with a catheter placed in the distal urethra is the imaging method of choice with patients suspected of an acute urethral injury.

4. Treatment of a urethral fracture includes placing a urethral catheter and waiting for healing. Only one attempt to pass the site of the tear is advised. If unsuccessful, the urethral catheter must be placed under anesthesia with the aid of a urethroscopic procedure to prevent further injury.

Reference

Casale AJ: Urinary tract trauma. In: Gearhart JP, Rink RC, Mouriquand PDE, editors: *Pediatric urolog*, Philadelphia, 2001, Saunders, pp 937–940.

Cross-Reference

Blickman JG, Parker BR, Barnes PD: *Pediatric radiology—the requisites*, ed 3, Philadelphia, 2009, Mosby, p 150.

Comment

Most anterior urethral injuries are the result of blunt trauma to the perineum (straddle injuries), and many have delayed manifestation, appearing years later as a stricture. A urethral injury should be suspected in the setting of a pelvic fracture, traumatic catheterization, straddle injuries, or any penetrating injury near the urethra. Symptoms include hematuria or an inability to void. Physical examination may reveal blood at the meatus, or a rectal examination may disclose a high-riding prostate gland. Extravasation of blood along the fascial planes of the perineum is another indication of injury to the urethra. The diagnosis is made by retrograde urethrogram, which must be performed before inserting a urethral catheter to avoid further injury to the urethra. Extravasation of contrast demonstrates the location of the tear. Further management depends on the extent of the injury and accompanying fractures or solid organ injuries or both.

The retrograde urethrogram is performed using gentle injection of 20 to 30 ml of contrast into the distal urethra. The presence of extravasation pinpoints the existence and location of the urethral tear. If a urethral tear is identified, the pediatric urologist will make one attempt to pass a urethral catheter past the injury into the bladder. If unsuccessful, the patient is then taken to the surgical department and examined under anesthesia; a urethral catheter is placed during the urethroscopic procedure.

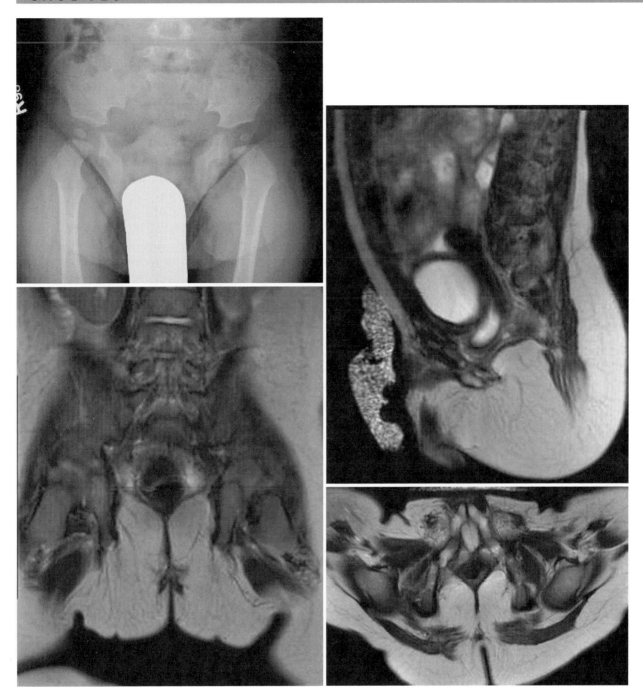

1. What are the imaging findings in this infant with a urogenital anomaly?

2. What is the diagnosis?

3. Is the central nervous system (CNS) involved?

4. What is the cause?

Diagnosis: Classic Bladder Exstrophy

1. Plain radiography of the pelvis reveals pubic diathesis and increased iliac wing angles. Sagittal T1-weighted magnetic resonance imaging (MRI) shows a decreased curvature of the levator ani. T2-weighted images show the decreased curvature of the puborectalis and iliococcygeus muscle groups of the levator ani.

2. Classic bladder exstrophy.

3. No, the CNS is not involved.

4. Exstrophy of the bladder is the result of an abnormal rupture of the cloacal membrane early in the embryonic period. Mesenchymal ingrowth into the abdominal wall is therefore inhibited. Because the pelvis is derived from sclerotomal components of the mesenchyme, the development of the pelvis is also effected.

Reference

Gargollo PC, et al: Magnetic resonance imaging of pelvic musculoskeletal and genitourinary anatomy in patients before and after complete primary repair of bladder exstrophy, *J Urol* 174(4 Pt 2):1559–1566, 2005.

Cross-Reference

Blickman JG, Parker BR, Barnes PD: *Pediatric radiology—the requisites*, ed 3, Philadelphia, 2009, Mosby, pp 134–136.

Comment

Classic bladder exstrophy is a rare developmental defect (1 in 200,000 to 1 in 4000 live births), and boys are affected two to three times more often than girls. Classic bladder exstrophy combines epispadias with a lower defect at the midline of the abdominal wall, exposing an open and protruding bladder.

Classic bladder exstrophy and epispadias result in the abnormal caudad position of the primordial of genital tubercules, combined with a failure of the primordia to migrate ventrally, which prevents the urogenital portion of the cloacal membrane from regressing caudally and results in the anterior placement of the membrane on the abdominal wall. The abnormal position of the cloacal membrane prevents mesenchymal migration into the lower abdominal wall, resulting in a deficiency of mesenchymal-derived tissues in this area. When the cloacal membrane ruptures to form the urogenital and anal orifices in the normal sequence of events, the entire urogenital tract is exposed, producing an exstrophic bladder and associated epispadias.

The exstrophy-epispadias complex of genitourinary malformations can be as simple as a glandular epispadias or an overwhelming multisystem defect such as a cloacal exstrophy. Although transition cases have been reported, this entity can be studied in two major categories: (1) classic bladder exstrophy, and (2) cloacal exstrophy. Cloacal exstrophy is the most severe form of the disease with multisystem involvement.

Classic exstrophic patients have involvement of the genitourinary system and pelvic bones and pelvic floor muscles. The posterior part of the pelvis is externally rotated, the acetabula are retroverted, and pubic rami are shorter than the normal lengths. This results in pubic diastases, a widening of the iliac wings, and a square-shaped pelvic floor. Anatomically, the bladder neck lies more superficial and the anus is anteriorly displaced.

Radiologic evaluation starts with plain-film radiography of the pelvis. Pubic diastases are well visualized on the plain radiography; however, cross-sectional imaging is required to better delineate the anatomy of the pelvic floor. MRI is the modality of choice to study the pelvic floor. The iliac wing angles are increased, and the levator ani muscle group has a decreased curvature that gives a flat look to the pelvic floor. Computed tomography has the disadvantage of radiation and does not show the pelvic floor muscles in detail.

Surgery is the treatment of choice and is designed to (1) secure the initial closure of the bladder, (2) reconstruct a functioning and cosmetically acceptable penis in the male infant and external genitalia in the female infant, and (3) result in urinary continence with the preservation of renal function. The timing of surgery depends on the bladder volume at birth. Single-staged repair or modern-staged reconstruction of the exstrophy (MRSE) is performed, based on the experience and preference of the surgical team. MRSE is designed to close the bladder, posterior urethra, and abdominal wall with or without osteotomy just after birth, and the repair of the epispadias is recommended at ages 6 months to 1 year. Single- or modern-staged surgical correction can be accompanied with iliac wing osteotomies. Pelvic bones are softer early during life, thus the patient with sufficient bladder volume for closure can be surgically treated without osteotomies with sufficient approximation of the pubic bones. However, in selected cases, performance of an osteotomy is expected to improve the shape of the pelvic floor, thus improving functionality—specifically urinary continence.

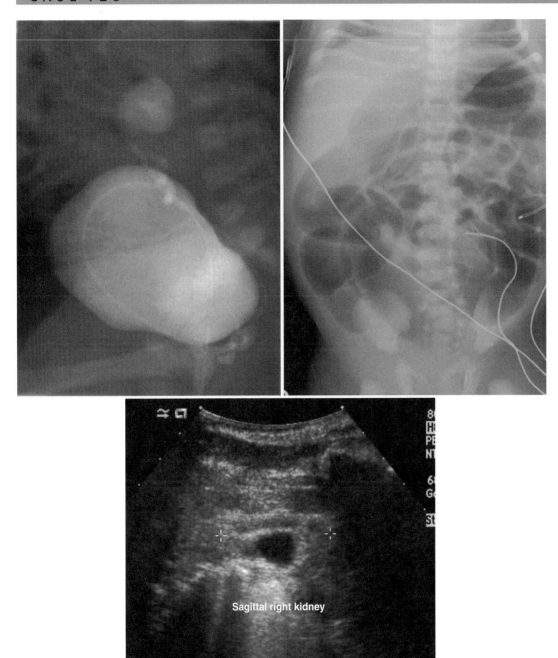

Sagittal right kidney

1. What are the imaging findings in this newborn boy, with abnormal findings in the ultrasound (US) image of the prenatal kidneys?

2. What is the diagnosis?

3. What is the most common anomaly associated with this entity?

4. What is the cause?

Diagnosis: Ectopic Insertion of the Bilateral Ureters

1. Imaging findings include the ectopic insertion of the bilateral ureters to the proximal urethra and superior to the sphincter. A single kidney with reflux is demonstrated. A radiographic image of the abdomen and chest shows the formation abnormality in the T6 vertebra (butterfly vertebra) and sacrum. Air distention of the bowel loops is apparent without the presence of air in the rectum, secondary to anal atresia. US reveals a single small kidney with increased parenchymal echogenicity and dilation of the right renal pelvis.

2. Ectopic insertion of the ureter to the proximal urethra with dilated right renal pelvis with reflux.

3. Hypoplasia or dysplasia of the renal moiety.

4. Failure of differentiation of the bladder and urethra at the sixth gestational week is the cause. Normally, by the end of the sixth gestational week, the ureter and remaining mesonephric duct have separate openings into the urogenital sinus. This absorption of the common excretory duct into the urogenital sinus occurs in such a way that the original meatus of the mesonephric duct migrates in a cephalic and lateral direction. Progressive development of the bladder, bladder neck, and urethra results in continued lateral and cephalic migration of the urethral orifice and more medial and caudal migration of the opening of the mesonephric duct.

Reference

Berrocal T, López-Pereira P, Arjonilla A, et al: Anomalies of the distal ureter, bladder, and urethra in children: embryologic, radiologic, and pathologic features, *Radiographics* 22:1139–1164, 2002.

Cross-Reference

Blickman JG, Parker BR, Barnes PD: *Pediatric radiology— the requisites*, ed 3, Philadelphia, 2009, Mosby, pp 128–129.

Comment

Anomalies of the urogenital tract are among the most common organ system anomalies found in the fetus or neonate. Ectopic insertion of the ureter stems from abnormal ureteral bud migration and usually results in caudal ectopia.

Ectopic insertion of the ureters occurs far more often in girls than it does in boys. In girls, ectopic ureters insert in the embryologic mesonephric duct remnants, which can be found in the vagina, urethra, uterus, vestibule, broad ligaments, and Gartner ducts. In boys, the mesonephric duct remnants include the seminal vesicles, vas deferens, ejaculatory ducts, and prostatic urethra, all of which are also potential sites for ectopic ureteral insertion. As a result, locations for ectopic ureteral insertion are typically sex-specific (i.e., suprasphincteric in boys and often distal to the urethral sphincter in girls); consequently, girls are usually incontinent. However, suprasphincteric urethral insertions can also occur in girls. Because of these differences in ectopic ureteral location, clinical manifestations in boys and girls are usually different. The fundamental difference between ureteral ectopia in girls and boys is that in girls, ectopic ureters can terminate at a level distal to the continence mechanisms of the bladder neck and external sphincter and thus may be associated with incontinence. If symptomatic, boys tend to present signs of epididymitis or orchitis, whereas girls often present signs of urinary incontinence or dribbling. Frequently, the diagnosis is delayed until toilet training.

An ectopic ureter can drain a single kidney, but approximately 70% of cases are associated with complete ureteral duplication. The Weigert-Meyer rule applies in complete ureteral duplication with each segment having its own ureteral orifice in the bladder.

The classic radiologic work-up includes US, voiding cystourethrogram (VCUG), and intravenous pyelogram (IVP). Initial screening must be performed with renal US. In ectopic insertion of the ureter of a single collecting system, the involved kidney is usually small and dysplastic and may not be visible on IVP or US. Renal scintigraphy is required to assess renal function. Scintigraphy is indicated to localize ectopic renal tissue, which is typically dysplastic but may be responsible for continuous dribbling. VCUG is performed to demonstrate reflux into the ectopic ureter and to identify the endpoint of the ureter. However, when an ectopic ureter drains below the bladder sphincter, the ectopic insertion may not be visible on a VCUG. Magnetic resonance urography is a promising imaging modality in selected patients. It has an advantage over US and IVP in that it is capable of demonstrating ectopic extravesical ureteric insertions, thereby providing a global view of the malformation.

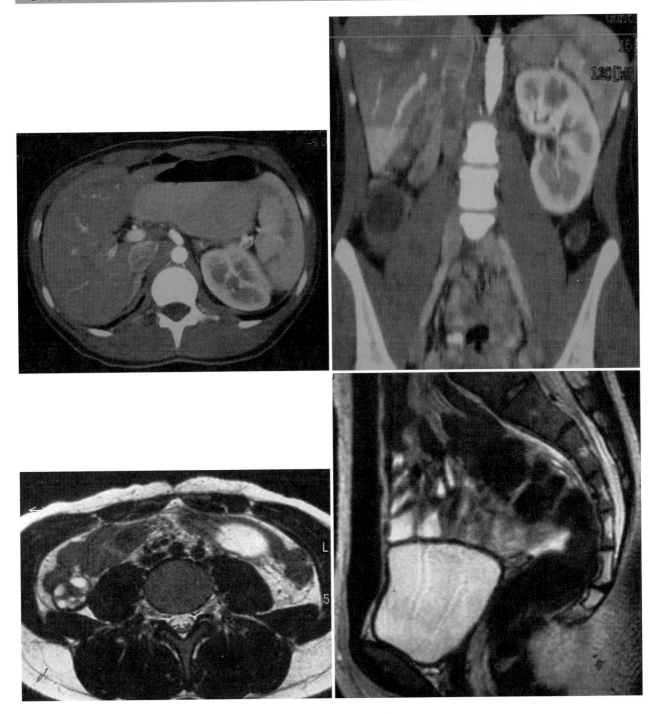

1. What are the imaging findings in this 15-year-old girl?

2. What is the diagnosis?

3. Do secondary sex characteristics normally develop?

4. What is the cause?

Diagnosis: Mayer-Rokitansky-Küster-Hauser Syndrome

1. The absence of a uterus, the partial aplasia of the vagina, and the absence of a right kidney; the ovaries are present.

2. Mayer-Rokitansky-Küster-Hauser syndrome.

3. Yes, the ovaries are present.

4. The cause of this syndrome is unclear, and a multifactorial mode of inheritance has been proposed, involving genetic and environmental factors.

Reference

Morcel K, et al: Mayer-Rokitansky-Küster-Hauser syndrome, *Orphanet J Rare Dis* 14(2):13, 2007.

Cross-Reference

Blickman JG, Parker BR, Barnes PD: *Pediatric radiology—the requisites*, ed 3, Philadelphia, 2009, Mosby, pp 150–151.

Comment

The Mayer-Rokitansky-Küster-Hauser syndrome is defined as the agenesis of the uterus and vagina with normal ovarian function and the development of secondary sex characteristics. Congenital vaginal aplasia, an unusual anomaly of the müllerian ducts, has been estimated to occur in 1 in 4000 to 5000 women. More than 90% of patients with vaginal aplasia are also characterized by the absence of a uterus and amenorrhea. This syndrome is caused by the early arrest in the development of the müllerian ducts. The clinical characteristics of the syndrome may include (1) vaginal aplasia with normal external genitalia; (2) the absence of a uterus or the presence of an extremely rudimentary uterus; (3) normally developed fallopian tubes; (4) normal ovaries; (5) normally developed secondary sex characteristics; and (6) anomalies of the urinary and skeletal systems, middle ear abnormalities and hearing loss, Klippel-Feil syndrome, and a normal set of sex chromosomes. Because patients with the Mayer-Rokitansky-Küster-Hauser syndrome maintain ovarian steroidgenesis, the possibility of developing genital neoplasms dependent on estrogenic actions exists, but uterine leiomyomas of the rudimentary uterus in this syndrome are rare. Patients generally present with amenorrhea and normally developed secondary sex characteristics during the teenage years or when the patient is ready to start sexual activity.

Treatment involves the creation of a neovagina and psychologic support. Reproductive capacity is limited due to the absence of a uterus. Surrogate mothers can be considered.

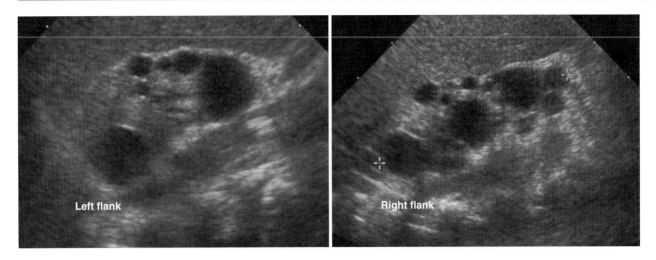

Left flank

Right flank

1. What are the imaging findings in this newborn boy?

2. What is the diagnosis?

3. What are the differential diagnoses?

4. What is the most likely function of the kidneys?

Diagnosis: Multicystic Dysplastic Kidney

1. Numerous noncommunicating hypoechoic cysts of varying sizes with echogenic thinned renal parenchyma. No recognizable corticomedullary differentiation is evident.

2. Multicystic dysplastic kidney (MCDK).

3. Hydronephrosis, multiple cysts in autosomal dominant cystic kidney disease, Wilms tumor, tuberous sclerosis, end-stage renal disease, and congenital mesonephric nephroma.

4. Kidney function is significantly reduced.

Reference

Schreuder MF, Westland R, van Wijk JA: Unilateral multicystic dysplastic kidney: a meta-analysis of observational studies on the incidence, associated urinary tract malformations and the contralateral kidney, *Nephrol Dial Transplant* 24(6):1810–1818, 2009.

Cross-Reference

Blickman JG, Parker BR, Barnes PD: *Pediatric radiology— the requisites*, ed 3, Philadelphia, 2009, Mosby, p 130.

Comment

MCDK is the result of a utero urinary obstruction, secondary to a developmentally atretic or stenosed collecting system. MCDK is the second most common intraabdominal mass in the neonatal period after hydronephrosis. Most of the cases are diagnosed prenatally by ultrasonography (US). Some patients may have delayed presentation and can be diagnosed as an incidental finding when symptoms of contralateral ureteropelvic junction obstruction, urinary tract infection, or traumatic injury is being evaluated. Most commonly, the kidneys are found in the renal fossa; however, ectopic locations such as pelvic and chest kidneys have also been reported. This entity can involve the whole kidney or be segmental in duplicated kidneys. Generally, two major types are identified: (1) pelvoinfundibular and (2) hydronephrotic. The pelvoinfundibular type is more common and is believed to be the result of atresia of ureter or renal pelvis; the cysts represent dilated calyces. The hydronephrotic type is less frequent and is believed to result from atretic segment of ureter, and cysts represent the entire pelvocaliceal system. The work-up should start with US imaging, followed by nuclear medicine scanning. A nuclear medicine scan can reveal a nonfunctioning kidney and help differentiate this entity from hydronephrosis; it could also identify the function of the contralateral kidney. Genetically, MCDK is considered sporadic. Associated abnormalities include genitourinary abnormalities in 25% to 30% of patients including contralateral ureteropelvic or ureterovesical obstruction, megaureter, cystic dysplasia of the testis, vesicoureteral reflux, cardiac and musculoskeletal anomalies, and associated syndromes such as Turner syndrome, trisomy 21, and chromosome 22 deletions. Bilateral MCDK leads to absent fetal and neonatal renal function with associated pulmonary hypoplasia and is therefore generally considered incompatible with extrauterine life. However, unilateral MCDK is a condition that does not lead to any complaints except for potential mechanical problems as a result of a large abdominal mass in rare cases.

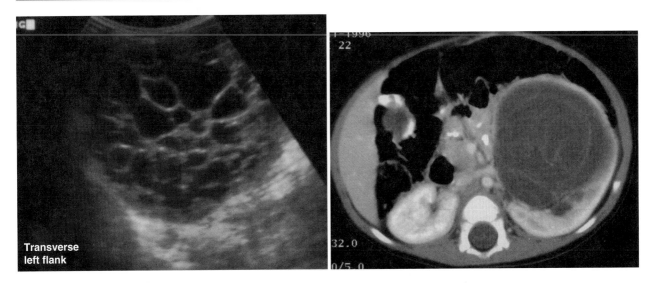

Transverse
left flank

1. What are the imaging findings in this 6-month-old boy with a palpable abdominal mass?

2. What is the diagnosis?

3. What are the differential diagnoses?

4. Is this a hereditary entity?

Diagnosis: Multilocular Cystic Renal Tumor

1. A large multilocular cystic renal mass with honeycombed appearance and mildly enhancing septations.

2. Multilocular cystic renal tumor (MCRT), previously called *multilocular cystic nephroma*.

3. Cortical simple cysts, malignant cystic renal tumors, multicystic dysplastic kidney, and calyceal diverticulum.

4. No.

Reference

Silver IM, Boag AH, Soboleski DA: Best cases from the AFIP: multilocular cystic renal tumor: cystic nephroma, *Radiographics* 28(4):1221–1226, 2008.

Cross-Reference

Blickman JG, Parker BR, Barnes PD: *Pediatric radiology—the requisites*, ed 3, Philadelphia, 2009, Mosby, p 140.

Comment

In the past, MCRTs have been considered to be lesions of developmental origin, hamartomas, or hamartomas with a malignant potential. These are now known to be true neoplasia, characterized by a multicystic tumor lacking blastemal or other embryonal elements.

Cystic nephroma is a rare, nonhereditary benign renal neoplasm that is purely cystic and is lined by an epithelium and fibrous septa that contain mature tubules. Cystic nephroma represents one end of a spectrum. At the other end of this spectrum is cystic partially differentiated nephroblastoma (CPDN), in which the septa contain foci of blastemal cells. Cystic nephroma and CPDN are indistinguishable from one another, based on their gross and radiographic appearances, and can be lumped under the term *multilocular cystic renal tumor*. MCRT has a bimodal age and sex distribution and tends to occur in children, mostly boys with CPDN between 3 months and 4 years of age, and in adults, mostly women with cystic nephroma between 40 and 60 years of age.

MCRT is usually solitary, but bilateral tumors have been described. MCRT is characterized as a solitary, well-circumscribed, multiseptated mass of noncommunicating fluid-filled loculi that are surrounded by a thick fibrous capsule and compressed renal parenchyma. It most frequently manifests itself in children as a painless abdominal mass. Hematuria and urinary tract infections are less common in children.

Plain-film radiographs may reveal a large mass in the kidney bed. Ultrasound (US) is the first modality of choice in children with intraabdominal mass. US may show a renal multicystic mass with no solid or nodular elements and septations. On computed tomography, cystic nephromas typically appear as well-circumscribed, encapsulated multicystic masses with variable-enhancing septa and no excretion of a contrast agent into the loculi. Magnetic resonance imaging reveals hypointense septa in all pulse sequences, which indicates a fibrous nature of the septa. Although renal scintigraphy has been described in the work-up of MCRT, it recently has had no definitive diagnostic value.

Clinical or imaging features of MCRT cannot predict its histologic characteristics; therefore surgery, either nephrectomy or nephron-sparing surgery, is indicated both for diagnosis and treatment. Prognosis is usually excellent with surgery.

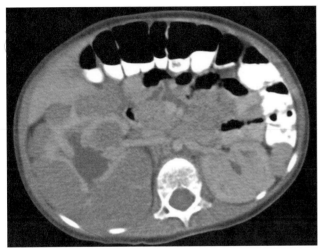

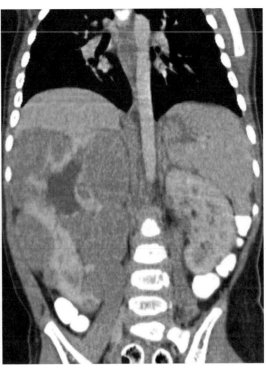

1. What are the imaging findings?

2. What is the diagnosis?

3. What are the differential diagnoses?

4. What is the cause?

Diagnosis: Nephroblastomatosis

1. Homogeneous, multifocal, hypodense, well-demarcated, and mildly enhancing lesions in the renal cortex.

2. Nephroblastomatosis.

3. Lymphoma or leukemia, pyelonephritis, and multifocal Wilms tumor.

4. Persistent metanephric blastema (nephrogenic rests), which normally disappears by 36 weeks gestation.

Reference

Lonergan GJ: Nephrogenic rests, nephroblastomatosis, and associated lesion in the kidney, *Radiographics* 18(4):947–968, 1998.

Cross-Reference

Blickman JG, Parker BR, Barnes PD: *Pediatric radiology—the requisites*, ed 3, Philadelphia, 2009, Mosby, pp 140–141.

Comment

Nephroblastomatosis consists of diffuse or multifocal nephrogenic rests in the kidneys. The presenting ages range from birth to 7 years of age. Nephroblastomatosis is typically clinically occult and may incidentally be found as a palpable mass or in the work-up of children at risk for Wilms tumor. The imaging pearl is that nephroblastomatosis is homogeneous on all imaging modalities. Diffuse nephroblastomatosis is usually seen as renal enlargement with a thick peripheral rim of tissue that may show striated enhancement. Magnetic resonance imaging reveals nodules of low-signal intensity on both T1-weighted and T2-weighted images. Ultrasound may demonstrate hypoechoic nodules but is less sensitive than MRI and computed tomography. Contralateral involvement should be ruled out. The two pathologic subtypes are (1) perilobar rests (90%) and (2) intralobar rests (10%). Syndromes associated with these histologic subtypes are perilobar rests, which may have an association with Beckwith-Wiedemann syndrome and trisomy 18. Intralobar rests may be associated with Denys-Drash syndrome, sporadic aniridia, and WAGR (Wilms tumor, aniridia, genitourinary anomalies, and mental retardation) syndrome. Most cases regress spontaneously. Approximately 35% of diffuse hyperplastic perilobar nephrogenic rests will develop Wilms tumor.

No specific treatment method currently exists. Children with syndromes associated with Wilms tumor are typically screened regularly for the development of nephroblastomatosis and Wilms tumor. Nephroblastomatosis presents with nodules that are homogeneous, whereas Wilms tumor tends to be heterogeneous. However, differentiation between the two entities with imaging alone is not possible.

- diffuse multifocal Nephogenic Rests
- Birth - 7 years age
- homogenous on all modalities

- Diffuse — renal enlargment with thick peripheral Rim of tissue which may show striated enhancement

Perilobar 90%
Intralobar 10%

- MR - T₁/T₂ hypointense nodules

- Syndromes Associated (Perilobar)
  • Beckwith Wiedemann
  ◦ Trisomy 18

  Intralobar
  • Denys-Drash
  ◦ sporadic aniridia
  ◦ WAGR

- ~ 35% hyperplastic perilobar neph. rests will develop Wilms tumor

- Can't diff nephb. vs. Wilms tumor on imaging alone

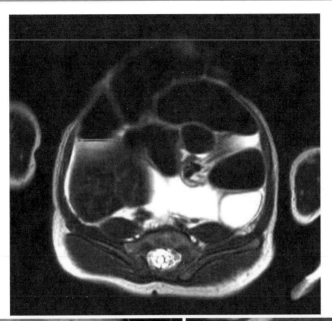

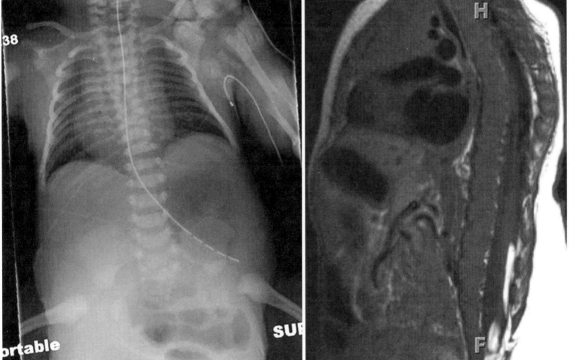

1. What are the imaging findings in this newborn infant with hypotonia and feeding intolerance?

2. What is the diagnosis?

3. Is this condition hereditary?

4. What are the synonyms for this entity?

Diagnosis: Omphalocele-Exstrophy-Imperforate Anus-Spinal Defects

1. Plain-film radiography of the abdomen shows a significant enlargement of the abdomen with air-filled bowel loops extending below the level of the pelvis. An apparent widening of the pubis and a superolateral displacement of the femoral heads are demonstrated. In addition, a segmentation anomaly of the thoracic vertebrae (T6 to T8) is revealed. An axial T2-weighted image through the pelvis shows a protrusion of significantly dilated bowel loops.
A sagittal T1-weighted image shows inferior displacement of the conus medullaris that terminates in an intradural lipoma. A normal bladder is not seen on the axial or sagittal images.

2. Omphalocele-exstrophy-imperforate anus-spinal defects (OEIS).

3. Yes. Sporadic recurrence has been reported in siblings.

4. Cloacal exstrophy, vesicointestinal fissure, splanchnica exstrophia, and exstrophy-epispadias sequence.

Reference

Soffer SZ, et al: Cloacal exstrophy: a unified management plan, *J Pediatr Surg* 35(6):932–937, 2000.

Cross-Reference

Blickman JG, Parker BR, Barnes PD: *Pediatric radiology—the requisites*, ed 3, Philadelphia, 2009, Mosby, pp 134–136.

Comment

OEIS is a rare complex and represents the most severe form of epispadias-exstrophy sequence, ranging from phallic separation with epispadias, pubic diastasis, exstrophy of the bladder (isolated), and cloacal exstrophy to complete spectrum of OEIS. OEIS occurs with an incidence of 1 in 250,000 live births. The occurrence of exstrophy of the bladder appears to be more common (1 in 30,000 to 40,000) than exstrophy of cloaca (1 in 200,000 to 250,000) or OEIS (1 in 200,000 to 400,000). The true incidence of OEIS is probably higher because many cases are incorrectly diagnosed as omphalocele, which is the most prominent component of this malformation complex. In humans, the cloaca is a phylogenetic embryonic structure where the genital, urinary, and digestive organs have a common outlet. The normal development gives origin to the lower abdominal wall with the bladder, intestine, anus, genital organs, part of the pelvis bones, and lumbosacral spine. OEIS is considered to be a defect in blastogenesis, beginning in the first 4 weeks of human development.

Differential diagnoses include omphalocele or gastroschisis (isolated), bladder exstrophy, and limb-body wall complex. Associated, cardiac, and renal anomalies can also be seen.

A multidisciplinary approach with collaboration among pediatric surgeons, urologists, orthopedic surgeons, neurosurgeons, gynecologists, and neonatologists is paramount in the management of children with cloacal exstrophy. Initial management first consists of identifying associated anomalies including renal anatomy, hydronephrosis, hydroureter, tethered cord, myelodysplasia, and a separated pubic symphysis. During the initial surgical management of the newborn, the omphalocele must be repaired, bladder exstrophy closed (either primarily or in stages) with or without osteotomies, and the fecal stream diverted.

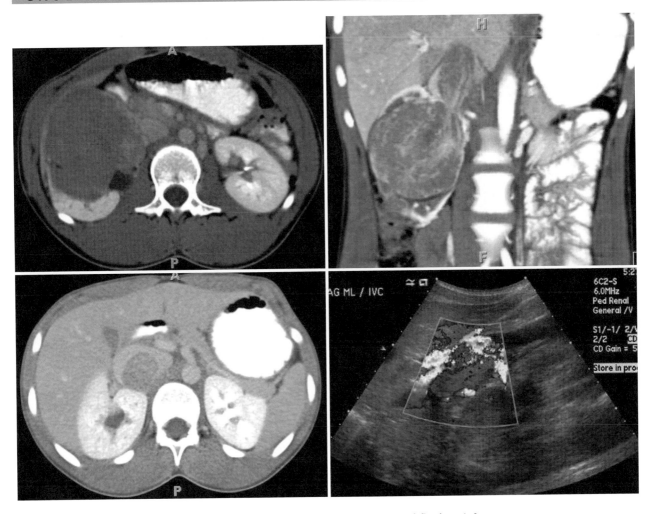

1. What are the imaging findings in this 12-year-old girl complaining of flank pain?

2. What is the diagnosis?

3. What is the differential diagnosis?

4. Does any association with a genetic disease exist?

Diagnosis: Renal Cell Carcinoma

1. A large, well-circumscribed, solid tumor with little enhancement extends into the inferior vena cava (IVC).

2. Renal cell carcinoma (RCC).

3. Wilms tumor.

4. Yes. RCC is associated with Hippel-Lindau disease.

References

Lowe LH, Isuani BH, Heller RM: Pediatric renal masses: Wilms tumor and beyond, *Radiographic* 20(6): 1585-1603, 2000.

Robson CJ: Staging of renal cell carcinoma, *Prog Clin Biol Res* 100:439-445, 1982.

Cross-Reference

Blickman JG, Parker BR, Barnes PD: *Pediatric radiology— the requisites*, ed 3, Philadelphia, 2009, Mosby, p 143.

Comment

RCC is rare in children, representing less than 0.1% of all malignant tumors and only 2% to 6% of all renal tumors. However, RCC shares an equal prevalence with Wilms tumor in the second decade of life. RCC presents a mean age of 9 to 11 years of age, with an equal male-to-female ratio.

Recent data have suggested that pediatric RCC may be a different entity from adult RCC, with different clinical presentations and behavioral characteristics, unique genetic abnormalities, and distinct pathologic characteristics. Children usually present with signs and symptoms related to their primary tumor (mass, pain, hematuria), whereas adults often present with signs and symptoms of metastatic disease or paraneoplastic symptoms. Pathologically, RCC in children differs from that in adults in that a great proportion of pediatric RCC exhibits a papillary histology (30% in children versus 15% in adults). In adults the majority (75%) of RCC has a clear-cell nonpapillary histology. The tumor forms an infiltrative solid mass with variable necrosis, hemorrhage, calcification, and cystic degeneration. The tumor invades locally with spread to adjacent retroperitoneal lymph nodes. Wilms tumor outnumbers RCC in childhood by a ratio of 30:1. Because RCC is usually significantly smaller than Wilms tumor at presentation, the mass may be subtle at intravenous urography and ultrasound and is most easily identified with computed tomography or magnetic resonance imaging as a nonspecific solid intrarenal mass with variable enhancement. Heterogeneous areas of hemorrhage and necrosis may be present. A higher frequency of calcification is demonstrated in RCC (25%) than in Wilms tumor (9%). Typically, RCC commonly invades the renal vein and may invade the IVC and extend into the right atrium. Identification of the tumor thrombus is extremely important for surgical planning because a combined abdominal and thoracic approach may be required. In addition, the contralateral kidney should be screened for additional RCC manifestations.

The Robson modification of Flocks and Kadesky classification correlates the stage at presentation with a prognosis. Tumor, nodes, metastasis (TNM) classification has been endorsed by the American Joint Committee on Cancer. The major advantage of the TNM system is that it clearly differentiates individuals with tumor thrombi from those with local nodal disease.

The prognosis is influenced by the stage at presentation, with an overall survival rate of approximately 64%. The best outcomes have resulted from radical nephrectomy and regional lymphadenectomy. The tumor is extremely resistant to chemotherapy, rendering metastatic disease difficult to treat.

RCC is a very rare pediatric disease and should be treated as an entity of its own because of the differences in symptoms, therapy, and prognosis from the adult form of the disease.

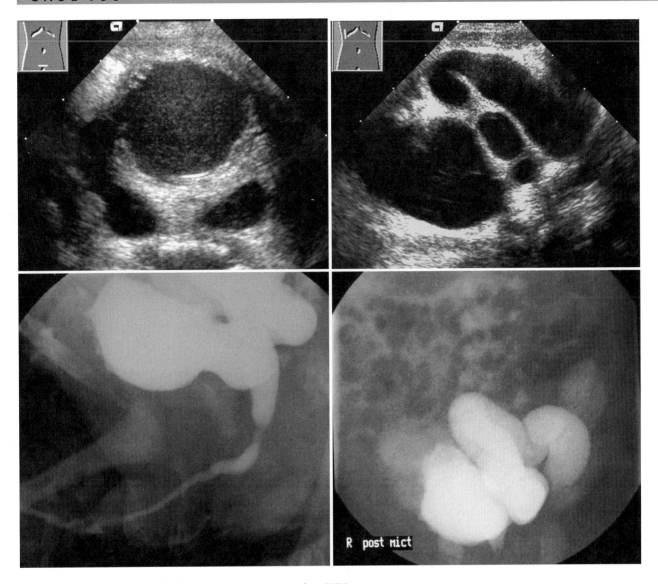

1. What are the imaging findings on ultrasonography (US)?

2. What does a voiding cystourethrogram (VCUG) reveal?

3. What could the imaging findings have been if the child had been imaged prenatally?

4. What is the value of renal nuclear medicine studies?

Diagnosis: Posterior Urethral Valves

1. Tortuous, elongated ureters.

2. A dilated posterior urethra, a thin valve distal to the verumontanum, and dilated, tortuous ureters.

3. Megacystis, oligohydramnios, bilateral hydroureteronephrosis, ascites, and pulmonary hypoplasia.

4. The ability to assess the degree of impaired renal function.

Reference

Bloom DA: Dilatation of the neonatal urinary tract. In Kuhn JP, Slovis TL, Haller JO, editors: *Caffey's pediatric diagnostic imaging*, ed 10, Philadelphia, 2004, Mosby, pp 204-223.

Cross-Reference

Blickman JG, Parker BR, Barnes PD: *Pediatric radiology— the requisites*, ed 3, Philadelphia, 2009, Mosby, pp 133-134.

Comment

Posterior urethral valves (PUVs) belong to the most frequent reasons for urethral obstruction in boys. PUVs result from the fusion and adhesions of mucosal folds in the urethra just below the verumontanum. The verumontanum is an elevation or crest in the wall of the urethra where the seminal ducts enter the urethra. These valves may result in a chronic outlet obstruction of the bladder. Depending on the degree and duration of intrauterine obstruction, significant morbidity may be seen as a result of renal dysfunction or failure and pulmonary hypoplasia. In the most severe cases, neonates die shortly after birth because of a Potter sequence. In less severe cases, the chronic obstruction results in a hypertrophic, thickened bladder wall with trabeculations, diverticula, and frequently additional hypertrophia of the interureteric ridge. Vesicoureteric reflux (VUR) and a ureterovesical junction obstruction are seen in 40% to 60% of patients. Chronic obstruction and VUR are believed to be the principal factors in the development of renal dysplasia. Occasionally, ascites, which may result from urine leaking into the peritoneal cavity after forniceal rupture, is seen on a prenatal US.

PUV can be diagnosed prenatally by US. Depending on the degree of obstruction, an enlarged urinary bladder and hydroureteronephrosis are seen. In addition, the more severe the obstruction and related renal failure, the more likely oligohydramnios with pulmonary hypoplasia is observed. In the postnatal period, US is the first-line imaging modality. US is highly sensitive in identifying the bladder wall thickening and hydroureteronephrosis. In addition, US allows the clinician to determine the degree of renal injury or dysplasia. Frequently, the kidneys are smaller in size, hyperechoic, and display a reduced corticomedullary differentiation. The gold standard for diagnosis is retrograde urethrography or VCUG. VCUG typically demonstrates a significant dilation of the posterior urethra up to the level of the posterior urethral valves. In addition, VCUG may reveal extensive VUR into dilated, tortuous ureters. Intrarenal reflux is occasionally noted. Catheterization of the urinary bladder may be difficult because the catheter may coil into the enlarged posterior urethra just superior to the valves. The use of a Coudé catheter may be helpful. Early diagnosis and prompt treatment are essential in limiting the degree of renal injury or failure.

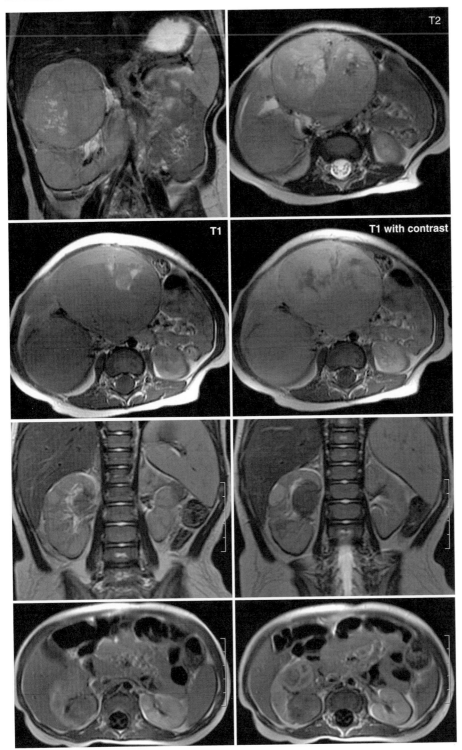

Follow up imaging after chemotherapy

1. What is the most likely diagnosis?

2. Which key anatomic structures can be invaded or involved?

3. Which syndromes and genetic abnormalities predispose a patient for this lesion?

4. What are the differential diagnoses?

Diagnosis: Wilms Tumor

1. Wilms tumor of the right kidney.

2. Tumor thrombus into the renal vein and the inferior vena cava possibly reaching the right atrium.

3. Nephroblastomatosis, Denys-Drash syndrome, hemihypertrophy, Beckwith-Wiedemann syndrome, and aniridia.

4. Clear-cell sarcoma, renal cell carcinoma, rhabdoid tumor, and mesoblastic nephroma.

Reference

Feinstein KA: Renal neoplasms. In Kuhn JP, Slovis TL, Haller JO, editors: *Caffey's pediatric diagnostic imaging*, ed 10, Philadelphia, 2004, Mosby, pp 1787–1795.

Cross-Reference

Blickman JG, Parker BR, Barnes PD: *Pediatric radiology— the requisites*, ed 3, Philadelphia, 2009, Mosby, pp 141–143.

Comment

Wilms tumor is the most common renal malignancy in children. The median age of presentation is 3½ years. Wilms tumors arise from a persisting primitive metanephric blastema. The presentation is most frequently unicentric; however, in 7% of children, Wilms tumors are multicentric, and in 5% of children, they are bilateral. Wilms tumors usually spontaneously occur; however, 1% of patients have a positive family history. An increased risk for developing Wilms tumors exist in nephroblastomatosis (multiple foci of nephrogenic rests within the kidney). In addition, Wilms tumors are more frequent in overgrowth syndromes such as hemihypertrophy or in Beckwith-Wiedemann syndrome and may occur in nonovergrowth syndromes like Denys-Drash syndrome (30% to 40% at risk). Finally, children without an iris (aniridia) have a 50% risk of developing a Wilms tumor. In these children, several studies recommend ultrasonographic (US) screening in 3-month intervals up to the age of 7 years.

Wilms tumors are usually large, asymptomatic abdominal masses. Occasionally, children report intermittent episodes of abdominal pain, which is probably related to traction to the renal capsula. Microscopic hematuria is seen in 30% of children, and hypertonia in found in 25% of children. Rarely a left varicocele is diagnosed, which may result from compression of the left renal vein by the tumor. Overall prognosis is favorable with survival in more than 90% of cases.

Plain-film radiographs of the abdomen may show indirect mass effects with displaced and compressed organs or bowel loops. Calcifications are rare. US is usually the first cross-sectional imaging modality. On US the tumor is easily identified. Because the tumor is frequently large on initial presentation, the small field of view of US may have difficulty identifying the exact architecture of the tumor and the degree of distortion of the involved kidney. Tumor staging requires additional studies, either contrast-enhanced computed tomography (CT) or, if available, multiplanar magnetic resonance imaging. Wilms tumors usually show a heterogeneous contrast enhancement. The renal architecture, especially the renal pelvis, may show a significant distortion. Extrarenal extension, retroperitoneal lymph node involvement and tumor thrombus extending into the ipsilateral renal vein may occur. The intravascular tumor thrombus can reach the right atrium. Metastases may involve the liver and lungs. CT of the lungs is recommended for tumor staging. If one Wilms tumor is diagnosed, the affected kidney and the contralateral kidney should be carefully studied to rule out additional tumor sites. Differential diagnoses include many other significantly less frequent primary renal malignancies. Because imaging does not always allow for reliable differentiation from Wilms tumor, tumor biopsy is frequently necessary. Wilms tumor usually responds well to chemotherapy with significant tumor size reduction facilitating surgical resection.

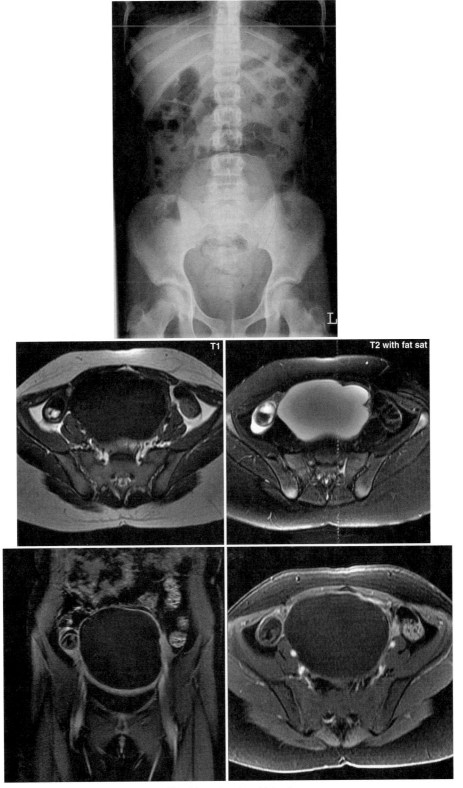

T1 with contrast and fat sat

1. What are the imaging findings on plain-film radiography in this 16-year-old girl with abdominal pain?

2. What are the imaging findings on magnetic resonance imaging (MRI)?

3. What is the most likely diagnosis, and what should be included in the differential diagnoses?

4. Which complications may occur?

Diagnosis: Bilateral Cystic Ovarian Teratomas

1. A large soft-tissue pelvic mass with peripheral calcification.

2. An MRI demonstrates bilateral, partially cystic, partially solid ovarian lesions left > right. Fat inclusions are confirmed on fat-saturated sequences. The urinary bladder is displaced downward.

3. Bilateral cystic teratoma is the most likely diagnosis. Differential diagnoses should include ovarian cyst, ovarian cystadenoma, malignant ovarian germ-cell tumor, and pregnancy.

4. Ovarian torsion with possible ovarian ischemia and rupture of the teratoma.

Reference

Siegel MJ, Coley BD: *Pediatric imaging*, Philadelphia, 2006, Lippincott Williams & Wilkins, pp 359–366.

Cross-Reference

Blickman JG, Parker BR, Barnes PD: *Pediatric radiology—the requisites*, ed 3, Philadelphia, 2009, Mosby, p 153.

Comment

Benign ovarian teratomas are the most frequent benign ovarian tumors in childhood (50% to 65%). The peak age of presentation is between 6 and 11 years of age. Clinically, teratomas may present as large, painless pelvic or abdominopelvic masses. If the child is suffering from an acute onset of pain, then ovarian torsion with resultant ovarian ischemia should be suspected. Most teratomas are predominantly cystic, usually with an excentric solid component that contains hair, fat, calcifications, and sebaceous material (dermoid plug). Occasionally, a dysplastic tooth may be encountered. If the solid component appears to be large or enlarging on follow-up imaging, a malignant transformation should be ruled out. In 25% of children, bilateral ovarian teratomas may be seen. Depending on the size of the cystic teratoma, determining, for certain, the ovary from which the lesion originates can be difficult. The affected ovary can be significantly displaced from its usual location. In addition, depending on the size of the teratoma, locating the contralateral ovary may also be difficult. Cystic ovarian teratomas can be suspected on plain-film radiography if a large pelvic or abdominal mass is identified with intralesional calcifications in a young girl. Ultrasound should be the second imaging modality to identify the lesion or to rule out pregnancy or both. If the lesion is large, ultrasound may be limited. On computed tomography (CT), the cystic component is hypodense. The calcium depositions, fat, and possibly teeth are easy to identify with CT. MRI is especially helpful for confirming the diagnosis. The selective signal suppression of the T1-hyperintense fatty components using selective fat saturation pulses facilitates diagnosis.

The most feared complications include ovarian torsion in which the teratoma acts as a fulcrum with ischemic injury of the ovary, spontaneous or traumatic rupture of the cystic teratoma, or malignant transformation. Cystic teratomas should be surgically resected while preserving the involved ovary if possible.

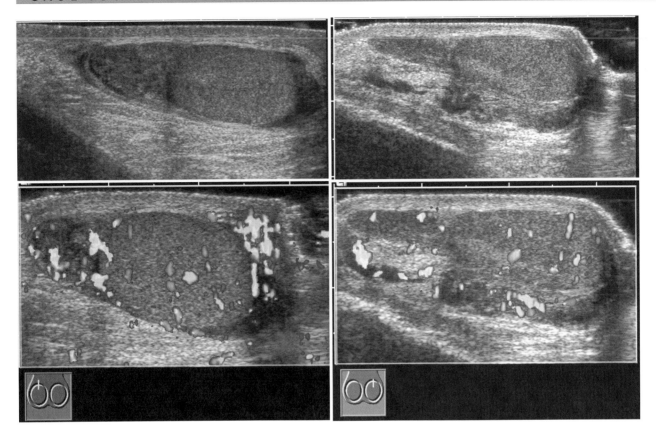

1. Describe the imaging findings.

2. What is the most likely diagnosis?

3. What should be included in the differential diagnoses?

4. Which ultrasound (US) protocol or technique is shown?

Diagnosis: Epididymitis

1. An enlarged, hypoechoic, hyperemic right epididymis, and mild scrotal wall thickening.

2. Right-sided epididymitis.

3. Epididymoorchitis, scrotal cellulitis, testicular torsion, and scrotal hernia.

4. High-frequency linear transducer and gray-scale and color-coded Doppler US using stand-off pad.

Reference

Donnelly LF: *Pediatrics, diagnostic imaging*, Salt Lake City, 2005, Amirsys Inc.

Cross-Reference

Blickman JG, Parker BR, Barnes PD: *Pediatric radiology—the requisites*, ed 3, Philadelphia, 2009, Mosby, p 154.

Comment

Epididymitis is an inflammation of the epididymis that can be acute or chronic. Children present with scrotal pain, edema, swelling, and erythema. Initially, pain may be centered to the flank and lower abdomen. With the progression of inflammation, the epicenter of the pain may migrate into the scrotum. In addition, the adjacent testicle may become involved, which is a condition known as *epididymoorchitis*. If untreated, epididymal abscess, testicular abscess, or sepsis may result.

Epididymitis is most frequently seen in adolescents who become sexually active; it may also, however, occur in infants and children. Acute epididymitis is bilateral in 5% to 10% of children. If epididymitis occurs in prepubertal children, a urologic evaluation should be initiated to rule out genitourinary anomalies (e.g., ectopic ureter, ectopic vas deferens, urethral duplication, posterior urethral valves, urethrorectal fistula). In genitourinary anomalies, epididymitis is most likely the result of a reflux of bacteria into the vas deferens. Hematogenous spread should be postulated if no anomaly is identified. Treatment includes antibiotic and antiinflammatory therapy to control inflammation, as well as supportive care that includes analgesics for pain control, bed rest, scrotal support with scrotal elevation, and ice packing for cooling. Aggressive treatment is especially indicated in bilateral inflammation because bilateral epididymitis may result in sterility. If treated adequately, the prognosis is excellent.

Next to a urine and blood work-up, US is especially helpful in diagnosing epididymitis. Gray-scale US will show an enlarged, usually hypoechoic epididymis with significant hyperemia on color-coded Doppler sonography. In addition, a scrotal wall thickening is frequently seen, as well as a mild degree of free fluid along the epididymis (reactive hydrocele). US is especially valuable to exclude abscess formation or coexisting or developing orchitis. In addition, US and color-coded Doppler sonography are extremely helpful to exclude testicular torsion that may present with a similar acute symptomatology. Finally, scrotal wall cellulitis and scrotal hernias can easily be differentiated from epididymitis by US.

In summary, a US examination in children with an *acute scrotum* is essential to (1) diagnose epididymitis, (2) exclude bilateral inflammation, (3) exclude testicular torsion, and (4) rule out complications similar to abscess formations. In addition, in young children, a urologic work-up should be considered to rule out genitourinary anomalies.

Computed tomography, magnetic resonance imaging, and vesicoureteral reflux examinations are rarely necessary but may be considered in complex cases.

US examinations should be performed with high-frequency linear transducers and should include gray-scale and color-coded Doppler imaging. The use of a stand-off pad may increase image quality and may also make the examination more comfortable for the child.

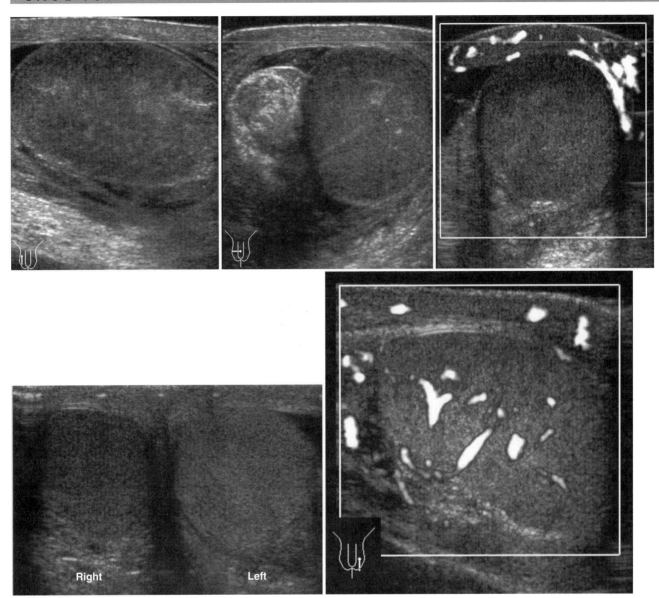

1. What are the imaging findings?

2. What is the diagnosis?

3. What should be excluded in the differential diagnoses?

4. Within how many hours should treatment be started after presentation?

Diagnosis: Testicular Torsion

1. An enlarged hypoechoic right testicle, an enlarged echogenic epididymis, no intratesticular blood flow, peripheral capsular blood flow, and a reactive hydrocele.

2. Acute right testicular torsion.

3. Epididymoorchitis, torsion of the testicular appendage, appendix epididymis, and testicular trauma.

4. Within 6 hours of presentation.

Reference

Cohen HL, Haller JA: Abnormalities of the male genital tract. In Kuhn JP, Slovis TL, Haller JO, editors: *Caffey's pediatric diagnostic imaging*, ed 10, Philadelphia, 2004, Mosby, pp 1917-1938.

Cross-Reference

Blickman JG, Parker BR, Barnes PD: *Pediatric radiology—the requisites*, ed 3, Philadelphia, 2009, Mosby, p 154.

Comment

Testicular torsion is a true urologic emergency. Testicular infarction is the result of venous and arterial occlusion caused by the twisting of the testicle along the spermatic cord–vascular pedicle. An early diagnosis is mandatory. Manual or surgical correction with detorsion within 6 hours of presentation saves a majority of testicles. If detorsion is performed later than 24 hours, irreversible testicular injury or ischemia has occurred in nearly 100% of cases.

Clinically, children present with a sudden onset of severe unilateral scrotal or inguinal pain or both. Frequently, patients report prior episodes of intermittent scrotal pain that spontaneously resolves. It is believed that these episodes represent intermittent torsions with spontaneous detorsions. In the acute phase, a swollen, tender, and erythematous hemiscrotum is observed. On physical examination, the affected testicle is swollen and painful to palpation. The testicle may be elevated in an oblique or horizontal position. The cremaster reflex is usually absent, and the Prehn sign is negative. Nausea and vomiting are common; fever occurs in only 10% to 15% of children.

Testicular torsion is seen in neonates and boys around 14 years of age. During development, the testicles are covered by and progressively attached to the tunica vaginalis and scrotal wall. Frequently in neonates the testicles have not yet descended into the scrotum, which prevents the appropriate attachment to the tunica vaginalis and increases the chance for torsion. In older children, the testicle can easily rotate along the long, free segment of the spermatic cord within the tunica vaginalis because of the high attachment of the tunica vaginalis. This predisposes the patient for an intravaginal testicular torsion. Testicular torsion is more frequently encountered in the colder times of the year, which may be related to the retraction of the testicle when exposed to colder temperatures.

Differential diagnoses include epididymoorchitis or orchitis, torsion of a testicular appendage, or appendix of the epididymis. In addition, testicular trauma, tumor, and incarcerated inguinal or scrotal hernias should be excluded. Occasionally, an acute appendicitis may clinically mimic acute testicular torsion.

Diagnosis is easily made with gray-scale ultrasound in combination with color-coded Doppler sonography. The involved testicle is usually enlarged and hypoechoic, and the ipsilateral epididymis is enlarged and either hypoechoic or hyperechoic. The scrotal wall is frequently thickened. On color-coded Doppler sonography, no flow is seen within the involved testicle. A rim of peripheral, capsular blood flow is often encountered. A reactive hydrocele may occur. Comparison with the contralateral testicle is helpful. Acute, bilateral torsion is very rare. Ultrasonography allows a differentiation from epididymoorchitis, tumor, or an incarcerated inguinal hernia, as well as appendicitis. Additional studies are rarely necessary.

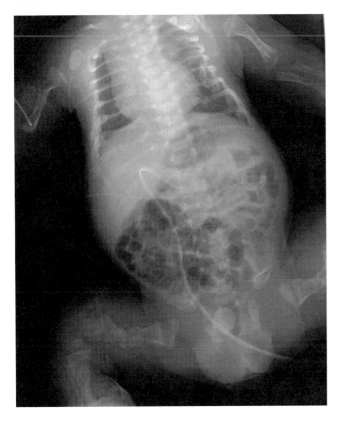

1. What key descriptive words help determine the radiographic classification of this entity?

2. What is the basic defect that causes these findings, and how is it usually inherited?

3. What classic physiognomic features aid in classification?

4. Which is the worst type to have?

Diagnosis: Osteogenesis Imperfecta

1. Fractures, osteopenia, bowing versus straight, and thin versus thick.

2. Defects in genes encoding type I collagen causes osteogenesis imperfecta (OI). Between 85% and 90% of new mutations are autosomal dominant.

3. Scleral color (blue versus white) and teeth (normal versus brittle).

4. Type II.

References

NIH Fact Sheet: Osteogenesis Imperfecta, Available at http://www.niams.nih.gov/Health_Info/Bone/Osteogenesis_Imperfecta/default.asp.

Sillence DO, Barlow KK, Garber AP, Hall JG, Rimoin DL: Osteogenesis imperfecta type II: Delineation of the phenotype with reference to genetic heterogeneity, *Am J Med Genet* 17:407-423, 1984.

Spranger JW, Brill PW, Poznanski AK: *Bone dysplasias: an atlas of genetic disorders of skeletal development*, ed 2, New York, 2002, Oxford University Press, pp 429-449.

Cross-Reference

Blickman JG, Parker BR, Barnes PD: *Pediatric radiology—the requisites*, ed 3, Philadelphia, 2009, Mosby, pp 165-167.

Comment

Similar to many syndromes with long histories, OI classification is in transition between the phenotype and the genotype. The traditional Sillence et al (1984) classification built on a still older, tripartite classification in a more systematic fashion. It enabled a rough clinical prognosis, using age at the first fracture, scleral color, dental fragility, and appearance of tubular bones to sort patients into four basic types with some inner subdivisions:

Type I: birth or later; blue sclerae; normal teeth (group A), fragile teeth (group B); straight or mildly bowed bones; has a good prognosis.

Type II ("OI congenita"): in utero or at birth; blue sclerae; broad crumpled long bones and ribs (group A), broad crumpled long bones and intact ribs (group B), thin fractured long bones and ribs (group C—a recessive type); is usually lethal.

Type III ("OI deformans progressiva"): in utero or later; white sclerae (though blue at birth); teeth variable; bones thick at birth then progressively thinning with bowing and "dumbbell" deformity; is a severe handicap and usually shortens lifespan.

Type IV: birth or later; white sclerae (blue at birth); normal teeth (group A), fragile teeth (group B); straight bones, occasional bowing; has a good prognosis, results in a short stature.

Note: Collagen names (e.g., type I, II, III, IV) are not related to the designation of OI types.

Genetic testing of patients with phenotypical type IV OI has found two groups that do *not* have type I collagen mutations:

Type V: Resembles type IV-group A, but with hyperplastic callus formation and calcification of interosseous membranes in the forearms and lower legs.

Type VI: Resembles type IV but may have recessive inheritance.

Further research has uncovered other genetic mutations that affect collagen formation and lead to OI type II-like recessive syndromes:

Type VII: Defect in CRTAP (cartilage-associated protein).

Type VIII: Is caused by a deficiency of Prolyl 3-hydroxylase 1 (P3H1) as a result of a mutation to the LEPRE1 gene.

One important differential diagnosis is child abuse. OI fractures are mainly diaphyseal, not the metaphyseal corner fractures that are classic in child abuse. However, it must be remembered that type I OI can have a tendency to easy bruising. A negative collagen-mutation test is not conclusive, and OI and child abuse can coexist.

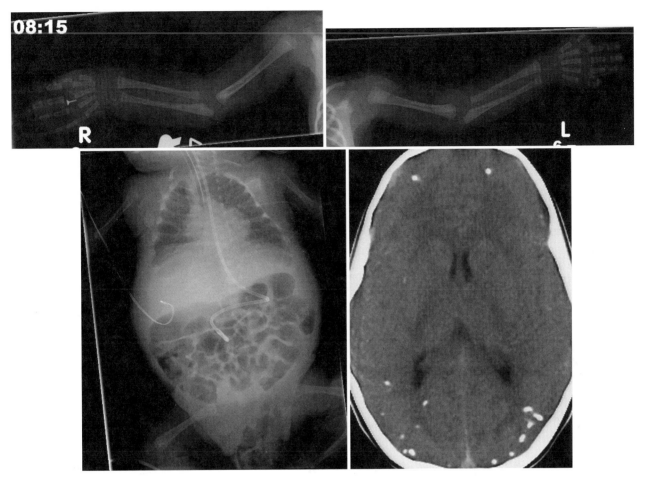

1. The mother of patient A tested positive for syphilis 1 month before delivery, did not get treated, and was rapid plasma reagin–positive (RPR+) 1:128 at delivery. The infant's serum was RPR reactive at 1:16 and had antitreponeme antibodies; cerebrospinal fluid (CSF) was Venereal Disease Research Laboratory (VDRL) negative (−). The first and second images were obtained. Should the infant be treated for congenital syphilis?

2. This premature infant (patient B, third image) was transferred to the neonatal intensive care unit (NICU) to confirm the suspicion of skeletal dysplasia. What are the long bone findings? What might be included in the differential diagnoses?

3. Patient C had seizures shortly after birth. What does a computed tomographic (CT) scan of the head (fourth image) show?

4. What other item might be in patient C's prenatal history?

Diagnosis: Congenital Infection

1. This infant should be treated for congenital syphilis. Even though the RPR reactivity was less than the mother's, the CSF was negative, and the source of the antibodies was likely maternal. The strong maternal history and the presence of characteristic bone lesions (metaphyseal fraying, submetaphyseal lucent bands) in all the infant's long bones (legs were not included here but were affected) were enough for treatment to be given in this case.

2. Long bone findings include widened, frayed metaphyses and poor mineralization. Rickets, scurvy, and congenital infection could be included in the differential diagnoses.

3. Diffuse cortical calcifications.

4. A pet cat in the house.

References

Barkovich AJ, editor: *Pediatric neuroradiology*, Salt Lake City, 2007, Amirsys Inc, pp I.1.198-202, 208-211.

Silverman FN, editor: *Caffey's pediatric x-ray diagnosis*, ed 8, Chicago, 1985, Yearbook-Medical Publishers, p 827, 835-840.

Cross-Reference

Blickman JG, Parker BR, Barnes PD: *Pediatric radiology—the requisites*, ed 3, Philadelphia, 2009, Mosby, pp 227-228.

Comment

Viruses, protozoa, and spirochetes cross the placenta and infect the fetus, interfering with developmental processes in all systems. The acronym TORCHS encompasses **to**xoplasmosis, **r**ubella (now very rare as a result of immunization), **c**ytomegalovirus (CMV), **her**pes, and **s**yphilis but has been expanded to include **h**uman immunodeficiency virus. The earlier in gestation the infection occurs, the greater the damage. Liver failure, chorioretinitis, hydrops, and seizures may all be present at birth.

In bones, the growing metaphysis is targeted, disrupting mineralization and destroying spongiosa. Metaphysitis is common to all of the infecting agents; frayed metaphyseal margins are seen acutely, then transverse bands of lucency migrate away from the recovering physis if the infection is contained. Periostitis can also be seen. In an acutely sick neonate with multisystem problems occupying the clinical staff in the first hours of life, the radiologist may be the first to raise the question of TORCHS infection when metaphysitis is seen in the proximal humerus on the chest radiograph. Prompt treatment may be instituted with antiviral drugs or with penicillin for syphilis.

Early transplacental infection corrupts the formation of neural tissue at its earliest stages; hydranencephaly can result. Later infection causes an inflammatory response, with meningoencephalitis leading to calcification, gliosis, and hydrocephalus. CMV infection, in particular, can result in cortical dysplasia and cerebellar hypoplasia; calcifications tend to be more periventricular. Herpes can be contracted acutely during passage through an infected birth canal with resulting multifocal encephalitis.

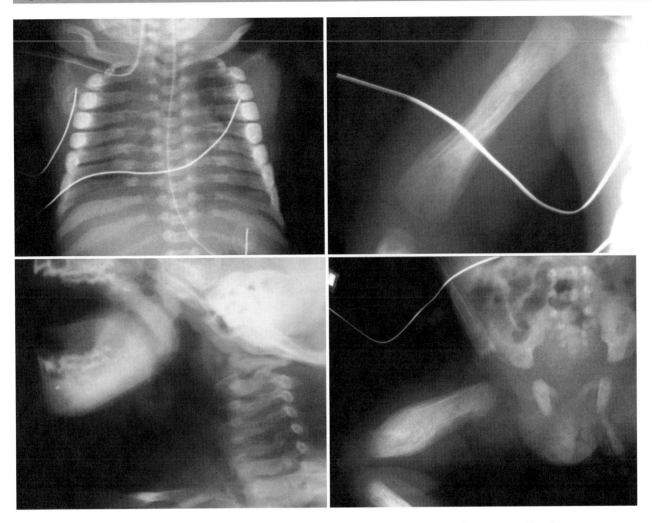

1. What are the differential diagnoses in this irritable 4-month-old child with soft-tissue swelling?

2. Which bones are most commonly involved?

3. What is the typical course of the disease?

4. List some possible long-term sequelae.

Diagnosis: Caffey Disease

1. Differential diagnoses of diffuse and significant periosteal new bone formation in an infant include infantile cortical hyperostosis (Caffey disease), scurvy, hypervitaminosis A, and trauma.

2. Multiple bones are typically involved in Caffey disease, most commonly flat bones, especially the mandible but also the clavicle, ribs, scapula, skull, and ilium. The diaphyseal region of the long bones may also be involved.

3. Typically, the signs and symptoms of Caffey disease regress spontaneously after many remissions and relapses.

4. Typically, Caffey disease is a self-limiting condition but rarely long-term sequelae such as facial asymmetry, exophthalmos, diaphragm paralysis, and bowing of the limbs result.

Reference

Azouz EM: Infections in bone. In Kuhn JP, Slovis TL, Haller JO, editors: *Caffey's pediatric diagnostic imaging*, ed 10, Philadelphia, 2004, Mosby, pp 2361–2368.

Cross-Reference

Blickman JG, Parker BR, Barnes PD: *Pediatric radiology—the requisites*, ed 3, Philadelphia, 2009, Mosby, pp 171–172.

Comments

Infantile cortical hyperostosis occurs in children under the age of 7 months and is characterized by hyper-irritability, soft-tissue swelling, and diffuse cortical thickening of the underlying bones. The mechanism is unclear, and no racial or sexual predominance exists. The disease is usually self-limited but typically has remissions and relapses over a period of 2 weeks and as long as 6 months. Plain-film radiographs may show soft-tissue swelling or cortical hyperostosis or both with significant widening of the bone. The periosteal reaction progresses to subperiosteal new bone formation. The bones most commonly affected are the flat bones—mandible (75% involvement), clavicle, rib (especially the lateral arches), scapula, skull, and ilium. The tubular bones most commonly affected are the ulnae, which usually show asymmetric involvement. Especially with a protracted course, a significant delay in musculoskeletal development and crippling deformities can occur in some cases, depending on the location of the lesion. Examples include facial asymmetry (mandibular lesion), exophthalmos (orbital lesion), ipsilateral diaphragmatic paralysis (scapular lesion), and bowing of the limbs. Possible residual radiographic changes include diaphyseal expansion or longitudinal overgrowth (leading to leg-length discrepancy), cortical thinning, bowing deformities, and osseous bridging with contiguous bones (e.g., ribs, radius, ulna). Differential diagnoses include hypervitaminosis A (typically older than 1 year of age with no mandibular involvement), healing scurvy (significant osteopenia, metaphyseal irregularity, decreased alkaline phosphatase), healing rickets (splaying, irregularity of the metaphysic with slower resolution of clinical and radiographic findings), trauma (fractures predominate), osteomyelitis (usually only one bone affected), leukemia (lytic bone lesions with metaphyseal bands), neuroblastoma, osteogenesis imperfecta, and neoplasm.

Caffey disease = infant cortical hyperostosis
- multiple bones usually are involved (flat bones especially)
- often self limiting disease

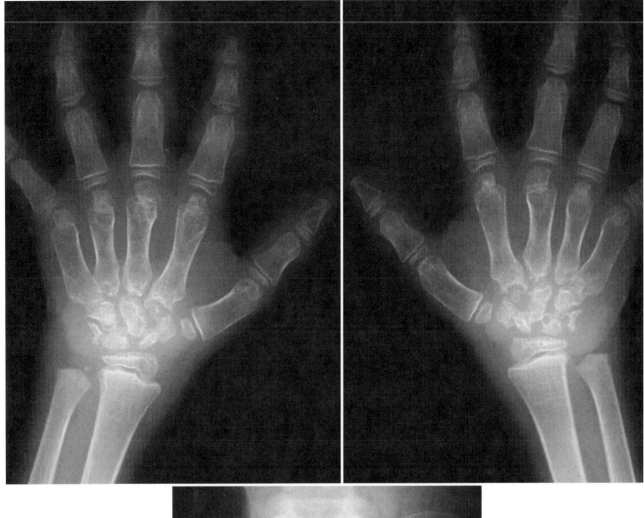

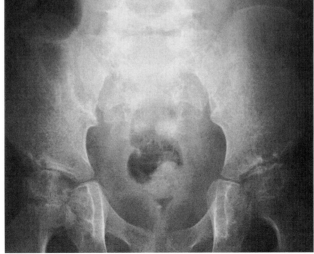

1. What is the diagnosis in this 7-year-old girl?

2. Name four imaging features or characteristics typically found with this disorder.

3. Which joints are most commonly affected?

4. What laboratory tests support the diagnosis?

Diagnosis: Juvenile Rheumatoid Arthritis

1. Juvenile rheumatoid arthritis (JRA).

2. Osteopenia, periarticular soft-tissue swelling, marginal erosions, and joint space narrowing.

3. Large joints are most commonly affected in monoarticular JRA; small joints of the hands and feet are most commonly involved in the polyarticular type.

4. An elevated level of C-reactive protein. In addition, antinuclear antibodies are positive in 25% of patients.

Reference

Babyn PS, Ranson MD: The joints. In Kuhn JP, Slovis TL, Haller JO, editors: *Caffey's pediatric diagnostic imaging*, ed 10, Philadelphia, 2004, Mosby, pp 2460–2469.

Cross-Reference:

Blickman JG, Parker BR, Barnes PD: *Pediatric radiology—the requisites*, ed 3, Philadelphia, 2009, Mosby, pp 182–183.

Comment

JRA is the most common cause of chronic arthritis in children and is classified as pauciarticular (up to four joints), polyarticular (at least five joints), or systemic (fever, rash, solid organ involvement). Onset is usually before the age of 16 years and, by definition, at least 6 weeks of symptoms including periarticular swelling, limited range of motion, stiffness, and tenderness and warmth overlying the involved joints must have occurred. Imaging findings include joint effusion, soft-tissue swelling, osteopenia, marginal erosions, narrowing of the joint space, subluxation, periosteal reaction, and growth disturbance. Differential diagnoses include psoriatic arthritis (large and small joints, spine, sacroiliac joint, nail changes); ankylosing spondylitis; Reiter syndrome; inflammatory bowel disease (sacroiliitis, enthesis); pigmented vilonodular synovitis (monoarticular with hemosiderin deposition); septic arthritis; and transient synovitis.

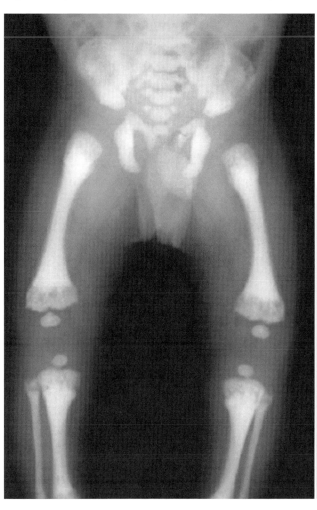

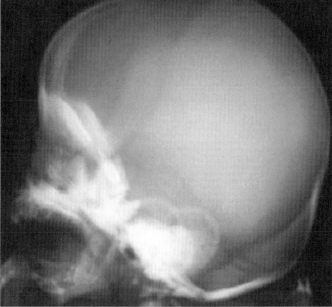

1. What is the diagnosis in this 4-month-old infant?

2. In what other disorders is the Erlenmeyer flask deformity seen?

3. Why do these patients present with anemia? With hepatomegaly?

4. Are cranial nerve palsies a feature? Why?

Diagnosis: Osteopetrosis

1. Osteopetrosis, also known as Albers-Schönberg or marble bone disease.

2. Chronic anemia (i.e., sickle cell disease), glycogen storage diseases (Gaucher, Niemann-Pick), and fibrous dysplasia. *Erlenmyer Flask Disease*

3. Bone marrow failure causes anemia, and extramedullary hematopoiesis results in hepatomegaly.

4. Yes, because of the narrowed neural foramina as a result of thickened bone.

Reference

Siegel MJ, Coley BD: *Pediatric imaging*, Philadelphia, 2006, Lippincott Williams & Wilkins, p 421.

Cross-Reference

Blickman JG, Parker BR, Barnes PD: *Pediatric radiology— the requisites*, ed 3, Philadelphia, 2009, Mosby, pp 170–171.

Comment

Osteopetrosis is a heterogeneous group of disorders characterized by dense, brittle bones caused by impaired bone resorption by osteoclasts. Autosomal dominant and recessive forms exist. Imaging characteristics include a bone-in-bone appearance of the vertebrae and pelvis, a metaphyseal widening or flaring (Erlenmeyer flask deformity), macrocranium with a thick skull base, absent or underdeveloped paranasal sinuses, a widening of the costochondral junctions, dense bones, bowing bones, and pathologic fractures.

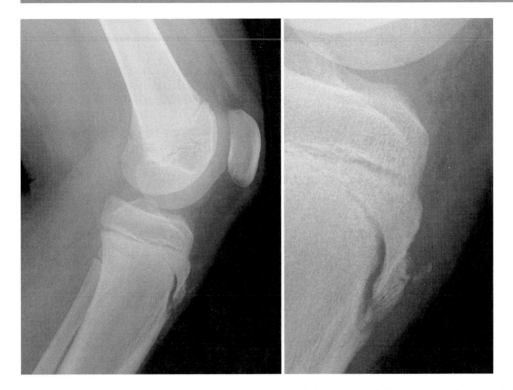

1. What is the diagnosis in this 12-year-old male adolescent with knee pain when participating in sports?

2. What is the classical clinical presentation?

3. How is the diagnosis made?

4. What are the characteristic findings on the lateral knee radiograph?

Diagnosis: Osgood-Schlatter Disease

1. Osgood-Schlatter (OS) disease.

2. Localized pain and soft-tissue swelling over the tibial tuberosity in an adolescent.

3. The diagnosis of OS disease is made clinically. Typically, a lateral radiograph of the symptomatic knee is obtained to rule out other pathologic conditions such as a neoplasm or infection.

4. Characteristic findings on the lateral radiograph of the knee include greater than 4-mm soft-tissue swelling over the anterior proximal surface of the tibial tuberosity, superficial ossicle in the patellar tendon (in 30% to 50% of patients), irregular ossification of the proximal tibial tuberosity, calcification within the patellar tendon, and thickening of the patellar tendon. Soft-tissue swelling is the key to this diagnosis because the other findings may be observed in normal patients.

Reference

Gholve PA, et al: Osgood-Schlatter syndrome, *Curr Opin Pediatr* 19(1):44–50, 2007.

Cross-Reference

Blickman JG, Parker BR, Barnes PD: *Pediatric radiology— the requisites*, ed 3, Philadelphia, 2009, Mosby, p 199.

Comment

OS disease, also known as tibial osteochondrosis or traction apophysitis of the patellar tendon insertion on the tibial tubercle, is one of the most common causes of knee pain in the adolescent. Most cases of OS disease are caused by chronic microtrauma in the deep fibers of the patellar tendon at its insertion on the tibial tuberosity, secondary to overuse of the quadriceps muscle. Typically, 8- to 13-year-old girls and 10- to 15-year-old boys present with pain and swelling over the tibial tubercle; the disease is bilateral in 20% to 30% of patients. Boys are affected more frequently than girls. The disease is generally benign and self limited. Approximately 50% of patients have a history of precipitating trauma. The diagnosis is primarily clinical but plain-film radiographs of the knee are often done to rule out other causes such as a neoplasm and infection. The lateral view visualizes the knee in slight internal rotation.

Visualizing the classic findings is most useful, and these findings include greater than 4 mm soft-tissue swelling over the anterior proximal surface of the tibial tuberosity, superficial ossicle in the patellar tendon (in 30% to 50% of patients), irregular ossification of the proximal tibial tuberosity, calcification within the patellar tendon, and thickening of the patellar tendon.

Soft-tissue swelling is the key to the diagnosis because the other findings may be found in normal patients. Computed tomography (CT) is not typically performed, but fragmentation of the tibial tuberosity, calcification within the patellar tendon, and thickening of the patellar tendon with adjacent soft-tissue edema would be characteristically demonstrated with CT. Magnetic resonance T2-weighted images would show increased signal intensity (edema) in the tibial tubercle, in the inferior patellar tendon, and within the surrounding soft tissues. Differential diagnoses include infrapatellar bursitis, patellar tendonitis, and Sinding-Larsen-Johansson disease. Analgesics and nonsteroidal antiinflammatory drugs may be given for pain relief and to reduce local inflammation. Rest from the offending activity is also recommended. Surgery is reserved for resistant cases.

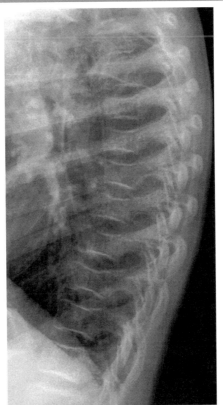

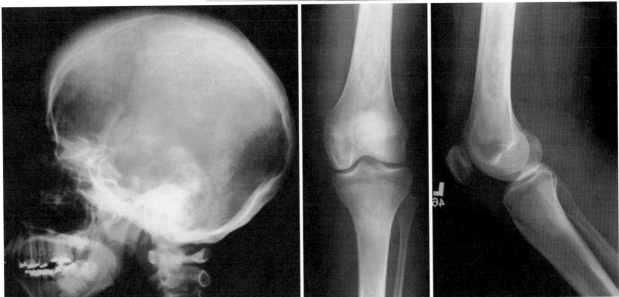

1. What are the imaging findings in this 17-year-old male adolescent, and what are the differential diagnoses?

2. What causes the skeletal changes in this disease?

3. What characteristic findings would be demonstrated on magnetic resonance imaging (MRI)?

4. What is the most common clinical presentation of bone involvement in this disease?

Diagnosis: Sickle Cell Anemia—Bone

1. On the lateral radiograph of the skull, evidence of a widening of the diploic space with the *hair-on-end* appearance is demonstrated. The frontal and lateral radiographs of the knee demonstrate mixed sclerosis and lucency in the distal femoral dia/metaphysis, which is consistent with a healed infarction. The lateral chest radiograph demonstrates central depression of multiple vertebral body endplates, resulting in the characteristic H-shaped vertebrae. The differential diagnosis includes sickle cell anemia and thalassemia.

2. Bone infarction and bone marrow hyperplasia.

3. On a T1-weighted MRI, a diffuse low signal of the marrow and hematopoietic marrow would be demonstrated, instead of the fatty marrow. With infarction, isointense or slightly hyperintense marrow is seen. With the injection of gadolinium, a lack of enhancement of areas of avascular necrosis and acute infarction is typical.

4. Pain.

Reference

Kottamasu SR: Bone changes associated with systemic disease. In Kuhn JP, Slovis TL, Haller JO, editors: *Caffey's pediatric diagnostic imaging*, ed 10, Philadelphia, 2004, Mosby, pp 2420-2422.

Cross-Reference

Blickman JG, Parker BR, Barnes PD: *Pediatric radiology—the requisites*, ed 3, Philadelphia, 2009, Mosby, pp 175-176.

Comment

Sickle cell disease is characterized by anemia associated with acute painful crises, usually beginning in the second or third year of life. The bone manifestations of sickle cell disease are the result of chronic tissue hypoxia, which causes changes in the bone marrow, as well as in the bone. Infarction, compensatory bone marrow hyperplasia, secondary osteomyelitis, and secondary growth defects all lead to bone and joint destruction in sickle cell disease. Bone changes seen on imaging reflect infarction with focal destruction and sclerosis of medullary and cortical bone and secondary periosteal new bone formation. Infarction of bone and marrow can lead to osteolysis (in acute infarction), osteonecrosis (avascular necrosis or aseptic necrosis), articular degeneration, vertebral endplate depression, dystrophic medullary calcification, and a *bone-within-bone* appearance. The shortened survival time of the erythrocytes in sickle cell anemia (10 to 20 days) leads to a compensatory marrow hyperplasia throughout the skeleton with resultant deossification that can bring about the characteristic changes in bone. These changes include decreased density of the skull, decreased thickness of the outer table of the skull caused by a widening of diploë, hair-on-end striations of the calvaria, osteoporosis that sometimes leads to biconcave vertebrae, coarsening of trabeculae in long and flat bones, and pathologic fractures.

Bone changes are very similar in both sickle cell anemia and thalassemia. In thalassemia, bone marrow expansion is typically more pronounced and paravertebral masses caused by extramedullary hematopoiesis are often seen. Avascular necrosis is less common in thalassemia than it is in sickle cell disease.

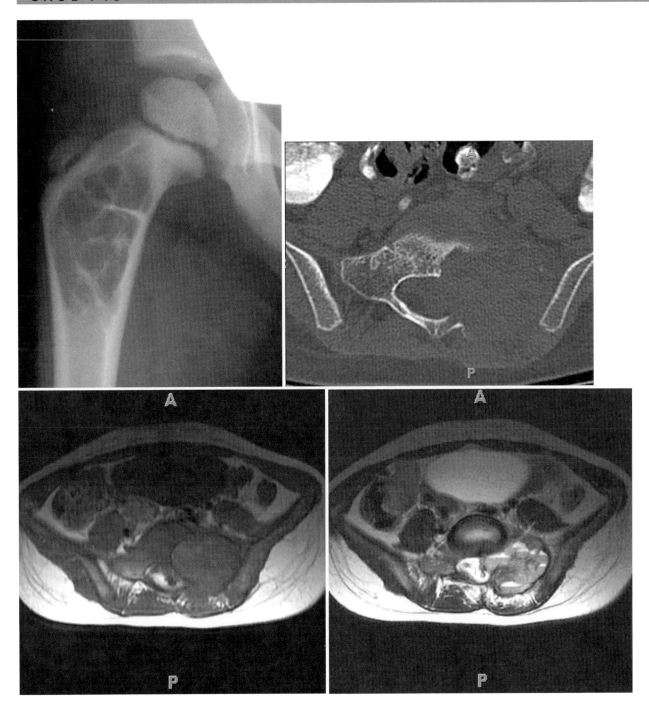

1. What are the imaging findings on the frontal radiograph of the right hip?

2. What are the imaging findings on the axial computed tomographic (CT) image of the pelvis and on the T1- and T2-weighted axial magnetic resonance images (MRIs) of the pelvis?

3. What is the diagnosis in these two patients?

4. What are the differential diagnoses of a bone lesion with a fluid-fluid level?

Diagnosis: Aneurysmal Bone Cyst

1. Imaging findings include an expansile lytic lesion that involves the metaphysis of the proximal right femur. The margins are well-defined, and multiple internal septations are demonstrated.

2. The CT demonstrates an expansile lytic lesion with well-defined margins in the left sacral ala. The MRIs demonstrate a well-defined, lobulated lesion with internal septations and multiple fluid-fluid levels.

3. An aneurysmal bone cyst (ABC).

4. ABC, fibrous dysplasia, chondroblastoma, giant cell tumors, myositis ossificans, nonossifying fibroma, simple bone cyst, and telangiectatic osteosarcomas.

Reference

Fletcher BD: Benign and malignant bone tumors. In Kuhn JP, Slovis TL, Haller JO, editors: *Caffey's pediatric diagnostic imaging*, ed 10, Philadelphia, 2004, Mosby, p 2381.

Cross-Reference

Blickman JG, Parker BR, Barnes PD: *Pediatric radiology—the requisites*, ed 3, Philadelphia, 2009, Mosby, p 192.

Comment

An ABC is an expansile osteolytic lesion with a thin wall containing blood-filled cystic cavities. It may be radiographically and histologically difficult to differentiate from telangiectatic osteosarcoma. ABCs occur in patients 10 to 30 years of age, with a peak incidence of 16 years; 75% of patients are younger than 20 years of age. Any bone may be affected, but the most common location is the metaphyseal region of the knee. The frequency in decreasing order is as follows: lower leg (24%), upper extremity (21%), spine with a predilection for the posterior elements (16%), femur (13%), pelvis and sacrum (12%), clavicle and ribs (5%), skull and mandible (4%), and foot (3%).

The common presentation includes the acute onset of pain that rapidly increases in severity over 6 to 12 weeks.

Trauma is considered an initiating factor. In approximately one third of patients, an ABC arises within a preexisting bone tumor (chondroblastoma, chondromyxoid fibroma, osteoblastoma, giant cell tumor, or fibrous dysplasia).

ABCs may be purely intraosseous, arising from the bone marrow cavity. In this case, they are primarily cystic and slowly expand into the cortex. They may be extraosseous, arising from the bone surface, eroding adjacent cortex, and extending into the marrow space. Four phases of pathogenesis are recognized: (1) initial osteolytic phase; (2) active growth phase, characterized by rapid destruction of bone and a subperiosteal blowout pattern; (3) mature phase, also known as the stage of stabilization in which the formation of a distinct peripheral bony shell and internal bony septae and trabeculae develop, producing the classic soap-bubble appearance; and (4) healing phase with progressive calcification and ossification of the cyst. On plain radiographs, ABCs are expansile lucencies with thin, smooth walls and possibly adjacent periosteal reaction. Radiographs are usually adequate for diagnosis. Cross-sectional imaging may be needed for better characterization of the lesion, especially in the axial skeleton.

CT demonstrates the intraosseous and extraosseous extents of the lesion. Fluid-fluid levels may be seen but are also present in malignant and other benign lesions such as fibrous dysplasia, chondroblastoma, giant cell tumors, myositis ossificans, nonossifying fibroma, simple bone cyst, and telangiectatic osteosarcomas.

MRI characterizes the lesion in greater detail than CT. On MRI, T1-weighted images show predominantly low-to-intermediate signal intensity with or without fluid levels. Acute hemorrhage into the cyst may have high-signal intensity. T2-weighted images show areas of low-to-intermediate signal intensity or some areas of heterogeneous high-signal intensity, depending on the content of the cyst. Septal enhancement is characteristic. A rim of low-signal intensity with internal septa may produce a multicystic appearance.

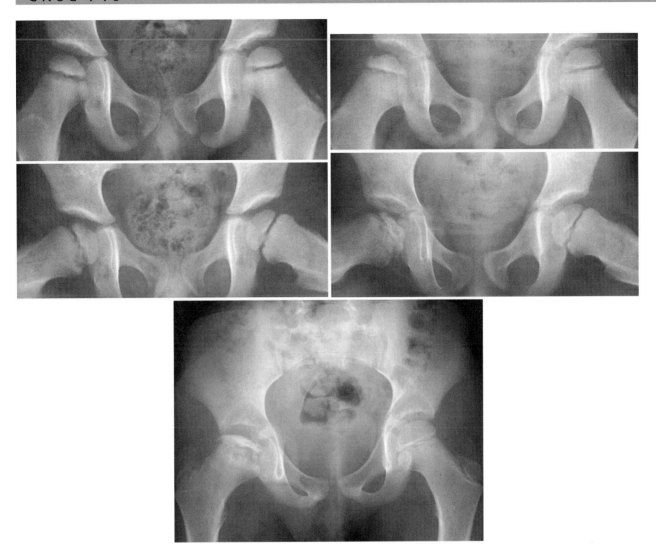

1. Explain the imaging findings on the frontal and frog-leg views of the hip in this 8-year-old boy.

2. What is the diagnosis?

3. What is visualized on early radiographic images?

4. What are the long-term complications?

Diagnosis: Legg-Calvé-Perthes Disease

1. Flattening, sclerosis, and irregularity of mineralization of the right capital femoral epiphysis.

2. Legg-Calvé-Perthes disease—the avascular necrosis of the capital femoral epiphysis.

3. Early radiographic images may be normal in Legg-Calvé-Perthes disease. The earliest appreciable change is mild, lateral displacement of the femoral head. *OR physeal widening*

4. Coxa vara deformity and painful osteoarthritis caused by the progressive destruction of the articular cartilage.

Reference

Harcke HT, Mandell GA: Osteochondroses and miscellaneous alignment disorders. In Kuhn JP, Slovis TL, Haller JO, editors: *Caffey's pediatric diagnostic imaging*, ed 10, Philadelphia, 2004, Mosby, pp 2319–2321.

Cross-Reference

Blickman JG, Parker BR, Barnes PD: *Pediatric radiology—the requisites*, ed 3, Philadelphia, 2009, Mosby, p 198.

Comment

Legg-Calvé-Perthes disease, or idiopathic avascular necrosis of the capital femoral epiphysis, affects male children four to five times more frequently than female children. It develops between 3 and 12 years of age with a peak incidence at 6 to 8 years of age. Findings are bilateral in approximately 10% of the cases, but typically both hips are not affected simultaneously. Patients typically present with hip pain, a limp, and limited range of motion.

Radiographs may be normal with the earliest findings being the mild, lateral displacement of the femoral head. With progression, subchondral lucencies may be seen, followed by flattening, sclerosis, and irregularity of mineralization. Further progression brings collapse and fragmentation of the sclerotic femoral head and a shortening and widening of the femoral neck with metaphyseal cystic changes and, ultimately, a coxa vara deformity. Painful osteoarthritis develops in the third and forth decades because of the progressive destruction of the articular cartilage. Four stages are recognized, according to the Catterall classification, which is based on radiographic findings. In stage I, no radiographic changes are demonstrated, and the diagnosis is based on clinical and histologic findings. In stage II, sclerosis of the femoral head is seen with the preservation of contour, with or without cystic change. A loss of structural integrity of the femoral head is seen in stage

III with additional changes occurring in the acetabulum in stage IV.

Hip ultrasound is helpful by demonstrating hip joint effusion, which causes capsular distention that is associated with Legg-Calvé-Perthes disease if it lasts longer than 6 weeks. Scintigraphy demonstrates early changes that are not appreciated on plain-film radiography. Initially, uptake is decreased in the femoral head as a result of the interruption of blood supply. Later, uptake is increased as a result of revascularization, bone repair, and degenerative osteoarthritis. Computed tomographic (CT) scans are helpful for early diagnosis of bone collapse and curvilinear zones of sclerosis and can also demonstrate subtle changes in the trabecular pattern of the bone.

Early on, magnetic resonance imaging (MRI) demonstrates appreciable thickening of the femoral head cartilage with a loss of the normally high-signal intensity from the epiphyseal marrow, which is replaced by irregular foci of low-signal intensity on T1- and T2-weighted images. Dynamic contrast-enhanced MRI demonstrates hypoperfusion.

Four phases of Legg-Calvé-Perthes disease are recognized. In the early destructive phase, blood supply is absent to the femoral head and the hip joint becomes inflamed, stiff, and painful. This phase may last from several months to 1 year. In the second phase, which may last 1 to several years, the femoral head begins to remodel into a round shape again. The joint is still irritated and painful. In the third stage, the femoral head continues to model itself back into a round shape with new bone. This phase lasts for 1 to 3 years. The fourth and last stage is the remineralization or healing phase, which can last up to a few years.

Idiopathic AVN

♂:♀ 5.1

peak incidence 6-8 years

Bilateral 10%, but not simultaneously

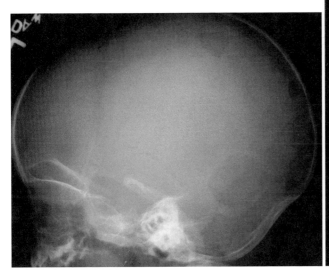
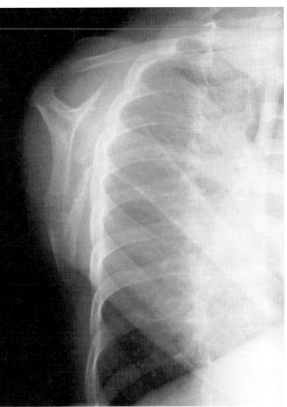

1. What are the imaging findings in the lateral skull and right shoulder radiographs of this 5-year-old boy? What is the diagnosis?

2. What bones are most commonly affected in this disorder?

3. What is the most common lesion seen in the spine?

4. What would be apparent on a radionuclide bone scanning with technetium-99m polyphosphate?

Diagnosis: Langerhans Cell Histiocytosis

1. Findings include well-defined lytic lesions with scalloped sclerotic borders. Langerhans cell histiocytosis (LCH) is the diagnosis.

2. In decreasing order, the skull, femur, mandible, pelvis, ribs, and spine.

3. Vertebra plana.

4. Localized increased uptake, which is characteristic of bone lesions in LCH.

Reference

Azouz EM, Saigal G, Rodriguez MM, Podda A: Langerhans cell histiocytosis: pathology, imaging and treatment of skeletal involvement, *Pediatr Radiol* 35 (2):103–115, 2005.

Cross-Reference

Blickman JG, Parker BR, Barnes PD: *Pediatric radiology—the requisites*, ed 3, Philadelphia, 2009, Mosby, p 179.

Comment

Eosinophilic granuloma refers to Langerhans cell histiocytosis localized to the skeleton. Boys in the first decade of life are most commonly affected, and painful swelling is the most common presenting sign. The skull is the bone most often affected, followed in frequency by the femur, mandible, pelvis, ribs, and spine. Adjacent soft-tissue swelling may occur. Multiple lesions develop in approximately 25% of cases. LCH localized to the skeleton carries a favorable prognosis, compared with multisystem involvement, which indicates a poorer prognosis, especially if present at the time of diagnosis.

Radiographically, a well-defined lytic lesion with scalloped sclerotic borders is characteristic. Vertebra plana is the most common spinal manifestation, but a lytic lesion involving the posterior elements is also recognized. Radionuclide bone scanning with technetium-99m polyphosphate may reveal a localized increased uptake. Magnetic resonance imaging is very sensitive but not specific with active lesions demonstrating low-signal intensity on T1-weighted images and high-signal intensity on T2-weighted images; it is specific with old lesions demonstrating low-signal intensity on both T1- and T2-weighted sequences. Extensive soft tissue and bone marrow edema are usually seen.

The cause of LCH is unknown. LCH may, in some instances, regress on its own without treatment. In other cases, very minimal treatment will result in the resolution of symptoms and a regression of the disease. For patients with more extensive disease, systemic chemotherapy will be beneficial.

LCH was formerly divided into three disease categories: (1) eosinophilic granuloma, (2) Hand-Schüller-Christian disease, and (3) Letterer-Siwe disease, depending on the severity and extent of involvement. This classification and its related risk groups are no longer used.

EG = LCH of the skeleton

♂ > ♀ 1st decade

skull
femur
mandible
pelvis
ribs
spine

25% Multiple

Rad – lytic lesion c̄ scalloped sclerotic borders

MR New: ↓T1, ↑T2 ++ Soft tissue & marrow edema
old ↓T1, ↓T2

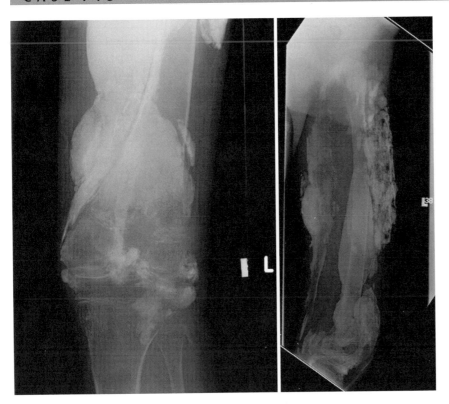

1. What are the findings on the frontal and lateral radiographs of the femur in this 15-year-old adolescent who is experiencing hand swelling and lower-extremity pain and swelling? No intravenous (IV) contrast was administered.

2. What typical abnormal laboratory values would radiographic studies be expected to find in this patient?

3. What are the characteristic clinical symptoms of this disorder?

4. What are the long-term complications?

Diagnosis: Mixed Connective Tissue Disorder

1. Extensive soft-tissue swelling with dense calcifications.

2. The diagnosis is based on clinical findings and significantly elevated antinuclear antibodies (ANAs) and antibodies to ribonucleoprotein (anti-RNP) in the patient's blood.

3. Raynaud phenomenon, swollen hands, arthritis or arthralgia, myositis, and esophageal dysmotility.

4. Pulmonary hypertension and infections.

Reference

Ostendorf B, Cohnen M, Scherer A: Diagnostic imaging for connective tissue diseases, *Z Rheumatol* 65: 553–562, 2006.

Comment

Mixed connective tissue disorder (MCTD) was first described in 1972 as an *overlap* of three diseases: (1) systemic lupus erythematosus, (2) scleroderma, and (3) polymyositis. Patients present with clinical features of all three of these diseases and typically have very high quantities of ANAs and anti-RNP detectable in their blood. MCTD affects people from ages 5 to 80 years of age with the onset typically in those 15 to 25 years of age. Its cause is unknown, but it seems to be an autoimmune disorder. The female-to-male ratio of MCTD is approximately 10:1.

MCTD has been more completely characterized in recent years and is now recognized to consist of the following core clinical and laboratory features: Raynaud phenomenon (96%), swollen hands (66%), arthritis or arthralgia (96%), acrosclerosis or esophageal dysmotility (66%), myositis (51%), pulmonary hypertension (23%), high level of anti–U1-RNP antibodies, and antibodies against U1-70 kd small nuclear ribonucleoprotein (snRNP).

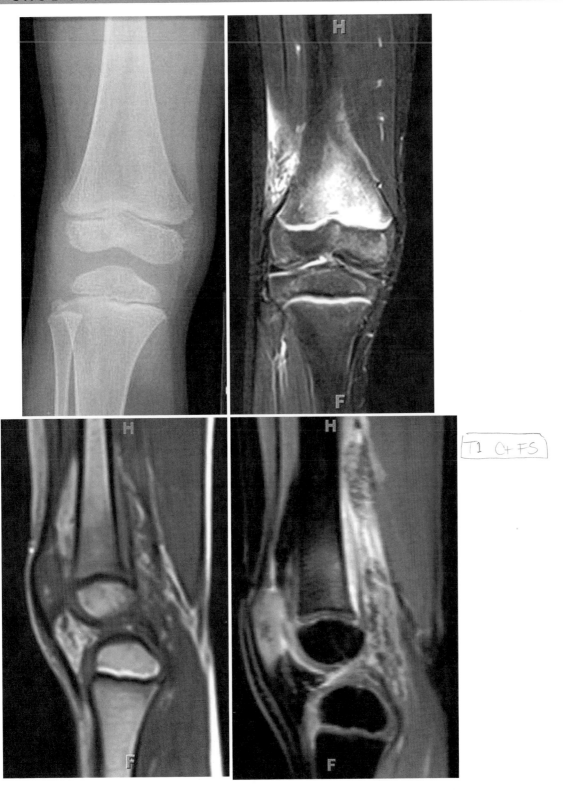

T1 C+ FS

1. What are the imaging findings in this 4-year-old male child refusing to bear weight?

2. What is your diagnosis?

3. Can ultrasound (US) be helpful in cases with this entity?

4. What is the differential diagnosis?

C A S E   1 4 9

Diagnosis: Acute Osteomyelitis

1. A plain-film reveals focal osteopenia in the medial inferior aspect of femoral metaphysic and minimal loss of fat planes with no evidence of destruction in the cortex or periosteal reaction. Magnetic resonance imaging (MRI) reveals an increased T2-weighted signal in the metaphysis of the femur with increased T2-weighted signal in the adjacent soft tissue. A T1-weighted sagittal image shows periosteal elevation, and minimal subperiosteal fluid. Postcontrast, fat-suppressed images show abnormal contrast enhancement in the bone marrow and surrounding soft tissue, indicating edema and inflammation in these areas.

2. Acute osteomyelitis.

3. US changes may be demonstrated within 48 hours of the onset of infection. The US appearance of osteomyelitis includes loss of normal soft-tissue architecture and periosteal elevation, which may appear as single or multiple echogenic lines surrounding the cortical bone. US may also help demonstrate some irregularity and interruption of the cortical bone, although these findings would be better demonstrated with plain-film radiographs or computed tomography (CT). US helps not only in making an accurate diagnosis but also aids in image-guided aspiration of the effusions.

4. Imaging findings may not be specific and may be simulated by other diseases. Osteomyelitis is primarily a disease of the infants and young children but can be seen in any age group. A permeative bone lesion in a child younger than 5 years old should raise the suspicion for Langerhans cell histiocytosis (LCH) and neuroblastoma metastasis. If the child is older than 5 years of age, Ewing sarcoma, lymphoma, leukemia, or LCH should be considered.

Reference

Saigal G, Azouz EM, Abdenour G: Imaging of osteomyelitis with special reference to children, *Semin Musculoskelet Radiol* 8:255–265, 2004.

Cross-Reference

Blickman JG, Parker BR, Barnes PD: *Pediatric radiology— the requisites*, ed 3, Philadelphia, 2009, Mosby, p 181.

Comment

Osteomyelitis implies bone and bone marrow inflammation, secondary to an infectious cause. Acute osteomyelitis is primarily the disease of infants and younger children, approximately 50% of the cases presenting before 5 years of age. Osteomyelitis is most commonly caused by bacterial organisms, most commonly by *Staphylococcus aureus,* followed by β-hemolytic streptococcus, although it can also be caused by fungi, parasites, and viruses. In cases with direct penetrating trauma, *Pseudomonas aeruginosa* is the most common organism. *Salmonella* is the most common cause in children with sickle cell disease.

The route of infection is hematogeneous in the great majority of cases, followed by contiguous involvement and direct inoculation.

Acute osteomyelitis commonly presents in the metaphysis of the long bones (femur, tibia, humerus, fibula), followed by short bones, pelvis, spine, and calvarium. The metaphysis have rich blood supply and relatively slow circulation, making it more susceptible for infectious involvement.

Neonates are at higher risk for osteomyelitis, given the weaker developing immune system. In addition, the transphyseal sinusoids connect metaphyseal and epiphyseal blood vessels, allowing metaphyseal and epiphyseal infection spread, which results in increased epiphyseal damage.

Radiographic changes in acute hematogenous osteomyelitis lag 7 to 10 days behind the evolution of infection. The earliest finding is soft tissue swelling and displacement or obliteration of fat planes. Bony destruction may become visible after 7 to 14 days or even later. Periosteal reaction can be seen at 7 to 10 days. In MRI, acute osteomyelitis shows loss of the high marrow signal on the T1-weighted images, with increased corresponding signal intensity on the T2-weighted and short T1-weighted inversion recovery (STIR) images. T1-weighted fat-suppressed postcontrast images are better because suppression of intrinsic fat results in better evaluation of the enhancing soft tissues and fatty marrow. The high intramedullary T2-weighted signal is secondary to edema, hyperemia, and exudate. Cortical bone initially appears normal, which explains the initially normal-appearing radiographs. The muscular and fascial planes adjacent to the infected bone may demonstrate localized or diffuse increased signal intensity on the T2-weighted and STIR images. Well-established intraosseous, subperiosteal, and soft tissue abscess collections are marked by peripheral enhancement with central hypointensity on T1-weighted postgadolinium images. Anatomical detail of MRI is better than in Tc-bone scintigraphy, and the absence of ionizing radiation is an advantage, especially in the pediatric age group. Three phasic bone scans, although highly sensitive in the early detection (may be positive in 24 to 72 hours of onset) of infection, can sometimes be ineffective in separating a bone marrow process from soft tissue disease, given the lack of anatomical detail in bone scans. Tc-bone scintigraphy, or whole body MRI, is superior to other imaging modalities in detecting multifocal involvement.

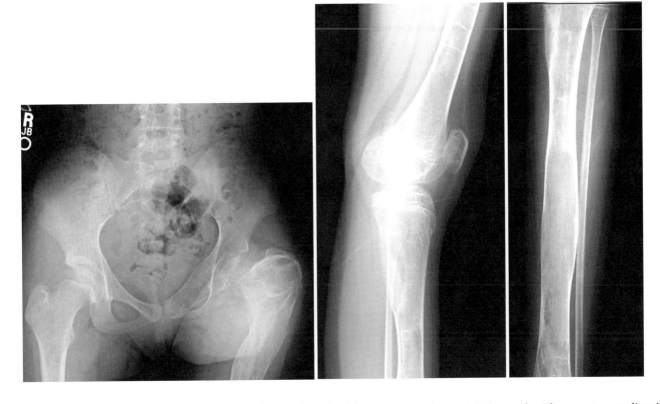

1. What are the imaging findings in this 14-year-old girl with asymmetry in the left leg and with an apparent limp?

2. What is the diagnosis, and what are the differential diagnoses?

3. What is McCune-Albright syndrome?

4. What is the cause?

Diagnosis: Polyostotic Fibrous Dysplasia

1. The plain-film radiograph shows a loss of the normal trabecular pattern with a ground-glass appearance of the bony matrix in the proximal left femur, distal left femur, and proximal and middiaphyses of the left tibia. The curvature of the femoral neck and proximal shaft of the femur is significantly increased because the proximal femoral lesion causes a severe coxa vara abnormality (shepherd's crook deformity), which is a characteristic sign of the disease.

2. The diagnosis is polyostotic fibrous dysplasia. Differential diagnoses include enchondroma, eosinophilic granuloma, giant cell tumor, chronic osteomyelitis, and postradiation changes.

3. McCune-Albright syndrome involves precocious puberty in girls, with polyostotic fibrous dysplasia and cutaneous hyperpigmentation.

4. Polyostotic fibrous dysplasia is a nonhereditary disorder of unknown cause.

Reference

Smith SE, Kransdorf MJ: Primary musculoskeletal tumors of fibrous origin, *Semin Musculoskelet Radiol* 4 (1):73–88, 2000.

Cross-Reference

Blickman JG, Parker BR, Barnes PD: *Pediatric radiology—the requisites*, ed 3, Philadelphia, 2009, Mosby, pp 178–179.

Comment

Fibrous dysplasia is a skeletal developmental abnormality of the bone-forming mesenchyme that manifests as a defect in osteoblastic differentiation and maturation. Virtually any bone in the body can be affected. Histologically, the medullary bone is replaced by fibrous tissue, which appears radiolucent on radiographs with the classically described ground-glass appearance. The initial manifestations of fibrous dysplasia are most commonly found in children 3 to 15 years of age. Approximately 70% to 80% of patients with fibrous dysplasias are monostotic. This form most frequently occurs in the rib (28%), femur (23%), tibia or craniofacial bones (10% to 25%), humerus, and vertebrae in decreasing order of frequency. Approximately 20% to 30% of fibrous dysplasias are polyostotic. Polyostotic fibrous dysplasia more frequently involves the skull and facial bones, pelvis, spine, and shoulder girdle. The sites of involvement are the femur (91%), tibia (81%), pelvis (78%), ribs, skull and facial bones (50%), upper extremities, lumbar spine, clavicle, and cervical spine, in decreasing order of frequency.

Fibrous dysplasia may be associated with endocrinopathies in 2% to 3% of cases; these include precocious puberty in girls, hyperthyroidism, hyperparathyroidism, acromegaly, diabetes mellitus, and Cushing syndrome. Radiologically, a lucent lesion is seen in the diaphysis or metaphysis with endosteal scalloping and with or without bone expansion and the absence of periosteal reaction. Usually, the matrix of the lucency is smooth and relatively homogeneous; classically, this finding is described as a ground-glass appearance. Irregular areas of sclerosis may be present with or without calcification. The lucent lesion has a thick sclerotic border and is called the *rind sign*. Plain-film radiographs are highly specific when characteristic features are present in a lesion. However, the specificity decreases when the lesion occurs at more complex sites such as the spine, skull, and, sometimes, pelvis. Computed tomographic findings complement plain-film radiographic findings. Magnetic resonance imaging (MRI) shows decreased signal in both T1- and T2-weighted images. Typically, no contrast enhancement is used. Cartilaginous islands may reveal increased T2-weighted signal. MRI is helpful after surgery in demonstrating fibrocellular tissue proliferation. Malignant degeneration is rare.

Two thirds of patients with polyostotic fibrous dysplasia are symptomatic before they are 10 years old. The initial symptom is often pain in the involved limb, associated with a limp, spontaneous fracture, or both. In one series, a pathologic fracture was present in 85% of patients with polyostotic fibrous dysplasias. Leg-length discrepancy of varying degrees occurs in approximately 70% of patients with limb involvement. No cure for fibrous dysplasia exists, and treatment focuses on relieving the signs and symptoms.

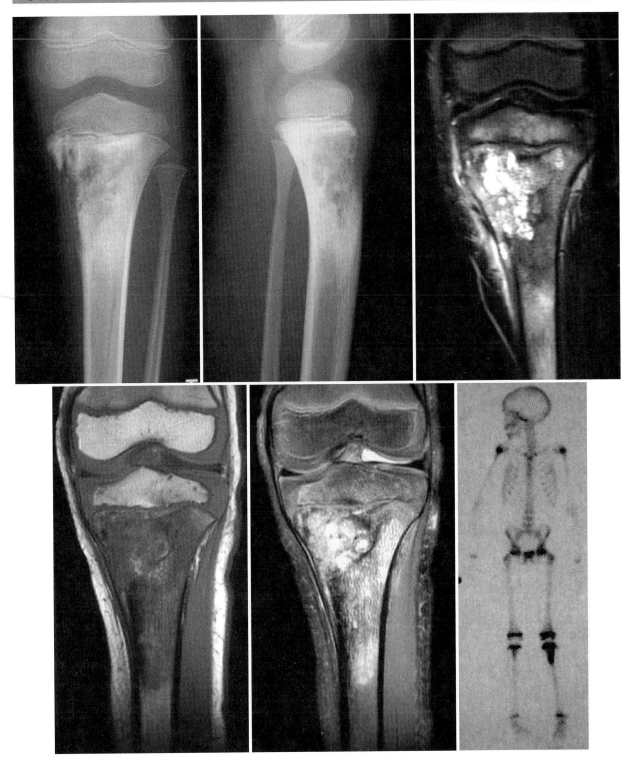

1. List the three most likely diagnoses.

2. List at least five plain-film imaging findings indicating malignancy.

3. Describe how to differentiate bone tumors based on location and the patient's age.

4. What is the value of nuclear medicine studies?

Diagnosis: Osteosarcoma

1. Osteosarcoma, Ewing sarcoma, and osteomyelitis.

2. Findings include (1) ill-defined destruction of trabecular bone, (2) permeative or moth-eaten appearance of the lesion, (3) wide zone of transition, (4) pathologic fracture, (5) irregular cortical destruction, (6) aggressive periosteal reaction, (7) Codman triangle, (8) sun burst appearance with spiculae, (9) lamellated onion skin, and (10) associated soft-tissue mass.

3. Osteosarcomas frequently involve the metaphysis of long tubular bones, especially around the knee, with a peak age of 10 to 15 years. Ewing sarcomas involve flat bones and diaphysis of tubular bones and are extremely rare in patients younger than 5 years of age. The tumor may arise in bone or soft tissues.

4. Nuclear medicine studies facilitate differentiation between malignant and benign bone lesions. These studies help identify undetected tumor sites, bone and bone marrow metastases, and may give information concerning tumor viability.

Reference

Stoller DW: *Magnetic resonance imaging in orthopedics and sports medicine*, ed 3, Philadelphia, 2006, Lippincott Williams & Wilkins, pp 2095-2104.

Cross-Reference

Blickman JG, Parker BR, Barnes PD: *Pediatric radiology—the requisites*, ed 3, Philadelphia, 2009, Mosby, p 186.

Comment

Osteosarcomas are the most frequent primary malignant bone tumors in children. The overall incidence of primary bone tumors is, however, low. Osteosarcomas are diagnosed in 5.6 million children per year. Osteosarcomas are most frequently diagnosed between 10 and 15 years of age during the adolescent growth spurt. Children most frequently present with pain, spontaneous pathologic fractures, or a focal swelling. An increased risk for the development of osteosarcomas has been reported in certain genetic disorders such as hereditary retinoblastoma, or it may occur in the setting of preexisting bone diseases such as Paget disease or fibrous dysplasia. In addition, an increased risk for osteosarcoma exists in children who have been exposed to radiation. Osteosarcomas may metastasize into the lungs, lymph nodes, liver, brain, and bones. Metastases may show central calcifications. Plain films are usually the first-line imaging modality, providing a good overview of the findings. Additional diagnostic work-up is, however, essential and should provide information on

the exact location, extension, and biologic characteristics of the primary tumor. For limb-saving surgical procedures, the orthopedic surgeons and oncologists are especially interested to know which anatomic compartments are involved, the possible extension into the adjacent growth plate or infiltration of the adjacent joint capsule (or both), and the degree of subperiosteal tumor extension. Magnetic resonance imaging (MRI) is the best imaging modality for local tumor staging. Imaging both adjacent joints is essential. Distant metastases can be identified using nuclear medicine studies (bone scintigraphy, positron emission tomography, computed tomography [CT]). CT should be used to exclude pulmonary, liver, and lymph node metastases. Brain MRI is used to rule out brain metastases. Differentiation from osteomyelitis can be challenging, and nuclear medicine studies may be helpful. Biopsies may be considered but should be carefully planned together with the orthopedic surgeon. If biopsy confirms a malignancy, the orthopedic surgeon may have to resect the biopsy canal because of possible tumor contamination.

Osteosarcoma - metaphysis of tubular long bones
- 10-15 yrs peak (during growth spurt)
- Knee
- most frequent 1° malignancy of childhood
- ↑ in hereditary retinoblastoma, Paget, FD, prior radiation
- metx to lung, liver, nodes, brain bones
  ↳ may have central Ca2+
- MR for tumor staging
- Bone scan for metx bone
- CT for metx liver, lung, nodes
- MR Brain for metx

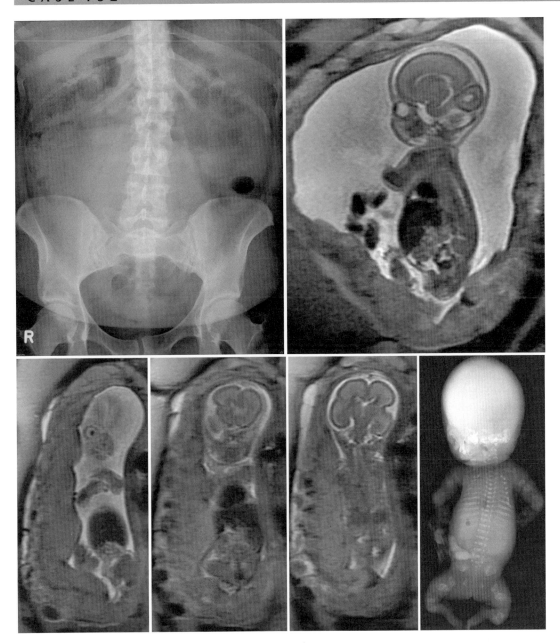

1. What is the striking finding on this abdominal radiograph of a 24-week pregnant woman?

2. What are the imaging findings on this fetal magnetic resonance image (MRI)?

3. What are the imaging findings on this postmortem radiograph?

4. What is the final diagnosis?

Diagnosis: Osteogenesis Imperfecta Type II

1. The abdominal radiograph does not show the osseous skeleton of the fetus (invisible fetus).

2. Short, deformed limbs, and an abnormally sized heart (which appears large because the chest cage is small with hypoplastic lungs).

3. Short, deformed, osteopenic bones, multiple insufficiency fractures with excessive callus formation, and a small chest cage.

4. Osteogenesis imperfecta (OI) type II.

Reference

Solopova A, Wisser J, Huisman TA: Osteogenesis imperfecta type II: fetal magnetic resonance imaging findings, *Fetal Diagn Ther* 24(4):361–367, 2008.

Cross-Reference

Blickman JG, Parker BR, Barnes PD: *Pediatric radiology— the requisites*, ed 3, Philadelphia, 2009, Mosby, pp 165–167.

Comment

OI or brittle bone disease is a heterogeneous group of inherited disorders characterized by increased bone fragility. OI is the result of either a reduction of the normal type I collagen production or from an abnormal collagen synthesis. Typically, four different types of OI are distinguished. Type I is the most frequent form. Clinical symptoms are usually mild. Type II is the most severe form. All children die within the perinatal period. Children with type III and IV survive the neonatal period but suffer from significant complications. OI is classified by clinical and molecular analysis.

Skeletal manifestations result from a generalized deficiency of the membranous and endochondral bone development and include significantly thinned calvarium with a delayed closure of the fontanelles, sutures, and excessive wormian bone formation. The classical clinical stigmata include fragile bones, blue sclerae, and ligamental laxity.

Bone changes may be identified as early as the twelfth week gestation by prenatal ultrasound examination. Imaging findings include shortened, deformed extremities. In addition, a reduced acoustic shadowing of the long bones is observed, as well as an increased nuchal translucency. Intrauterine growth retardation is often present. Death usually occurs in the neonatal period as a result of complications from infection, respiratory distress (narrowed thorax as a result of multiple rib fractures with pulmonary hypoplasia), cardiac insufficiency, or cerebral injury.

Newborns present with soft calvarian bones, a peculiar triangular-shaped face with a beaked nose and blue sclerae. Clinically, the extremities are usually short and deformed as a result of the multiple fractures and are typically in a froglike position. The radiologic hallmarks are short, deformed, or angulated long bones with multiple fractures in varied stages of healing with excess callus formation, wormian bones, and poor skeletal mineralization.

Typically, abdominal radiography of the mother will not show the fetal skeleton (invisible fetus) because of the poor mineralization of the fetal skeleton. Abdominal radiography is rarely performed but may, however, be considered in rare, potentially lethal skeletal malformations of the fetus.

Fetal magnetic resonance imaging (MRI) is helpful because an MRI simultaneously displays the skeletal malformation and the hypoplastic chest and lungs. This image may render valuable information about the immediate postnatal time.

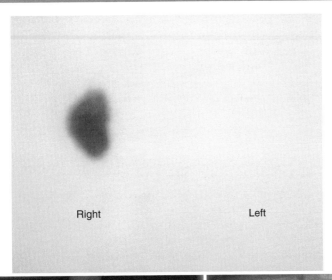

Right   Left

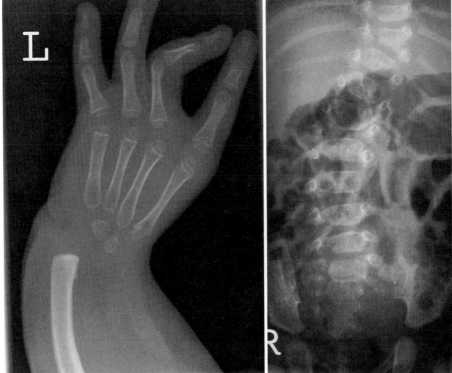

1. What are the combined imaging findings?

2. Is this disorder an association or syndrome, and what is the name?

3. What are the additional possible findings that should be excluded?

4. This is a genetic disorder. Is this statement *true* or *false*?

C A S E 1 5 3

Diagnosis: VACTERL Association

1. Findings include a vertebral segmentation anomaly, left renal agenesis, and radial aplasia.

2. The disorder is an association with the name VATER or VACTERL.

3. Imperforate anus, cardiovascular anomalies, tracheoesophageal malformation, esophageal atresia, single umbilical artery, or limb anomalies.

4. False. This disorder is not genetic in origin.

Cross-Reference

Blickman JG, Parker BR, Barnes PD: *Pediatric radiology— the requisites*, ed 3, Philadelphia, 2009, Mosby, pp 76-77.

Comment

VATER or VACTERL is an acronym that refers to a constellation of associated anomalies. The acronym relates to the following findings: vertebral segmentation anomalies, anal atresia, cardiovascular anomalies, tracheoesophageal fistula, esophageal atresia, renal or radial anomalies or both, and limb anomalies. Duodenal atresia and a single umbilical artery have also been described. This disorder is called an association rather than a syndrome because the findings are linked, but no specific genetic or chromosomal defect has been identified. The VACTERL association has an estimated incidence of 16 in 100,000 live births. The diagnosis is made if at least three of the seven defects are present. Children with a VACTERL association have normal development and intelligence. Vertebral anomalies, tracheoesophageal fistula, and limb defects are seen in approximately 70% of children. Renal or radial defects (or both) or anal atresia are less frequent (50% to 55% of patients). Cardiac defects are even less frequent. Treatment is usually directly related to the present birth defects.

[Handwritten annotations:]

3/7

Anomalies of:

Vertebral Segmentation
Anal atresia
Cardiovascular
Tracheoesophageal fistula
Esophageal atresia
Renal / Radial
Limb

+ Duodenal atresia
+ Single uterine artery

- Not a genetic disorder

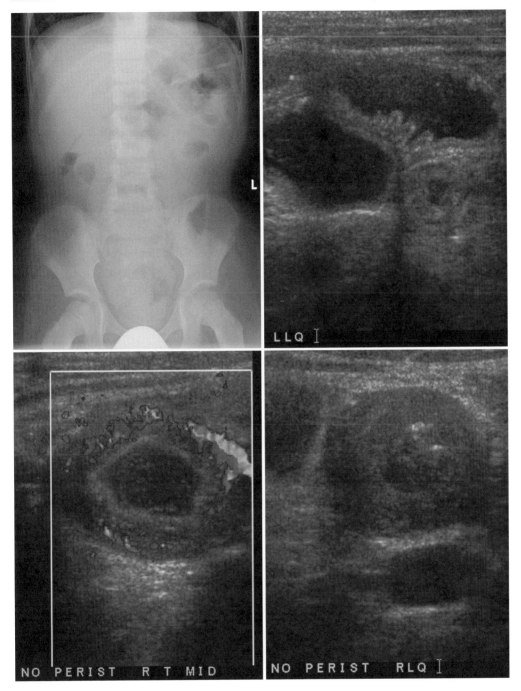

1. This 5-year-old developmentally delayed boy had crampy abdominal pain for several days. His pediatrician was treating him for constipation. What can be seen on his abdominal radiograph (first image)?

2. The emergency department clinician sent the child for an ultrasound to rule out intussusception. What should be the focus as he is examined?

3. What is important to note about the ultrasound images (second, third, and fourth images)?

4. As his abdomen is being observed during the scan, a purplish flat rash is seen in the groin. His mother explains that the boy has complained about pain in his legs for the last few days. What additional question should be asked of the emergency department clinician?

Diagnosis: Henoch-Schönlein Purpura Syndrome

1. Very little bowel gas, no sign of a large mass, and stool impaction or obstruction.

2. The child is at the upper end of the age range for uncomplicated, postinfectious intussusception. In his age group, a lead point (polyp, hematoma, lymphoma, lipoma, duplication cyst) becomes more likely.

3. The ultrasound reveals a fluid-filled small bowel that has thickened with clubbed, mucosal folds (second image). One area of the small bowel in the midabdomen has a very thick, hyperemic wall (third image). No *target* sign of intussusception is demonstrated. Low echogenicity is seen in the submucosal region, consistent with nonacute hematoma (fourth image).

4. If hematuria is present.

Reference

Stringer DA, Babyn PS, editors: *Pediatric gastrointestinal imaging and intervention*, ed 2, Hamilton, Ontario, 2000, BC Decker, pp 406–407.

Cross-Reference

Blickman JG, Parker BR, Barnes PD: *Pediatric radiology—the requisites*, ed 3, Philadelphia, 2009, Mosby, p 149.

Comment

Henoch-Schönlein purpura syndrome is an acute but self-limiting diffuse vasculitis of uncertain causes that affects the gut, skin, joints, kidneys, and (occasionally) the central nervous system. The skin shows a purpuric rash that spreads centrifugally. No signs of thrombocytopenia are presented. The bowel wall, usually in the jejunum, can be affected at multiple points. The hematoma can act as a lead point and cause intussusception that may have to be surgically relieved.

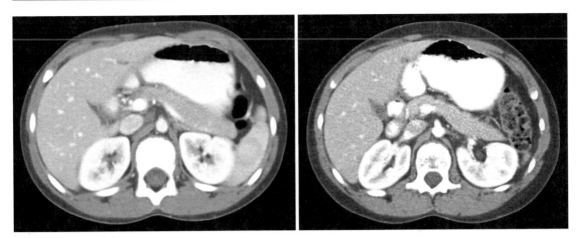

1. This 9-year-old patient had two computed tomographic (CT) scans 8 months apart. What is the difference between them?

2. What portion of the total radiation burden in the U.S. population is now attributed to CT scanning?

3. Why is the concept of radiation dose especially important in pediatric radiology?

4. What four machine factors have the greatest effect on dose delivery?

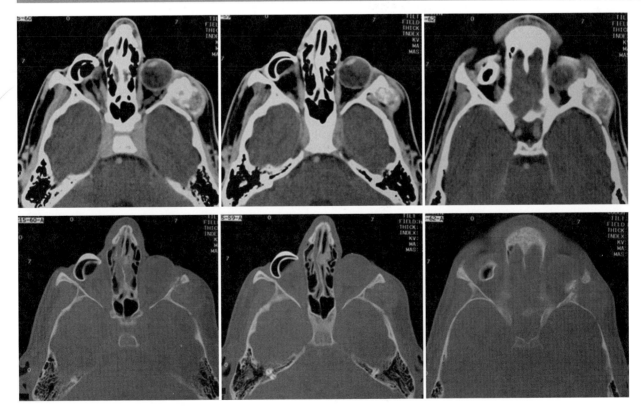

1. What are the imaging findings?

2. What is the most likely history?

3. How frequently does this complication occur?

4. Which anatomic area related to the primary lesion should be checked for additional lesions?

Diagnosis: Radiation Exposure in Children from Computed Tomography

1. The second scan has less than one half of the radiation dose of the first scan.

2. 25%.

3. Young tissues are more susceptible to radiation damage. Children live longer, which allows expression of the damaged DNA as cancer. In addition, a greater dose deposition is given to small bodies because the same scan parameters are used for adults as used for children.

4. Tube mA (direct, linear), kVp (direct; linear at lower levels, nonlinear [greater effect] at higher levels), gantry cycle time (direct, linear), and pitch (indirect, linear).

References

Coursey CA, Frush DP: CT and radiation: what radiologists should know, *Applied Radiology* 37(3):22–29, 2008.

Alliance for radiation safety in pediatric imaging: image gently. (Web site) www.pedrad.org/.

Comment

Multidetector CT is a powerful tool for diagnosing disease, but it comes at a price—an ever-increasing radiation dose. No visual penalty is paid for the higher doses as it is with plain films; rather, the images become incrementally more crisp and clear. The newer scanners have wider effective beams for better overlap of slices, which means more detailed three-dimensional reconstructions. However, because the dose recorders are built into the scanners, calculating the dose only by overall volume scanned can lead to an underestimation of the actual dose by up to 35%.

Turning down the mA and kVp, rotating the gantry faster, and passing the patient through the scanner faster will all decrease the deposited radiation. Add bismuth breast shields or eye patches for a head scan, and the dose decreases further. However, the tradeoff is increased noise in the image. Depending on the reason for the scan, more or less noise might be tolerable. Persuading the clinician to select an ultrasound or magnetic resonance imaging is the surest form of dose reduction. After all, the CT scan that is not used has a dose of 0.

Diagnosis: Posttreatment for Hereditary Bilateral Retinoblastoma and Sphenoid Wing Osteosarcoma

1. Enucleation of the right eye ball and a partially calcified tumor of the left sphenoid wing (osteosarcoma).

2. Posttreatment of bilateral retinoblastomas, enucleation on the right, and radiotherapy on the left.

3. Osteosarcomas may result from radiotherapy. Osteosarcomas are also seen associated with hereditary bilateral retinoblastoma.

4. The pineal gland.

Cross-Reference

Blickman JG, Parker BR, Barnes PD: *Pediatric radiology— the requisites*, ed 3, Philadelphia, 2009, Mosby, p 331.

Comment

Retinoblastoma is the most common malignant ocular tumor in childhood. The typical age of presentation for unilateral cases is between 1 and 3 years. Bilateral cases typically present during the first year. Trilateral retinoblastomas are rare and are usually hereditary. In 2% to 5% of children with hereditary bilateral retinoblastoma, a third tumor may be found in the pineal gland. In hereditary bilateral neuroblastoma, children are at risk for secondary nonocular tumors later in life. The mean latency of second tumors is 9 years. Osteosarcomas are the most frequently encountered second malignancies. Development of osteosarcoma may be accelerated by focal radiotherapy. Osteosarcomas typically develop in the field of radiation. Other tumors that may occur are pinealomas, brain tumors, soft-tissue sarcomas, and melanomas. The prognosis of children who develop a second tumor is poor. In children with a unilateral (sporadic) retinoblastoma, a 20% chance exists for developing a retinoblastoma in the contralateral eye. Close monitoring using magnetic resonance imaging is mandatory. If diagnosed early and treated adequately (a combination of surgery, chemotherapy, and radiotherapy), the prognosis today is favorable. The main factor that determines the prognosis is direct tumor extension via the optic nerve or adjacent sclera.

Secondary osteosarcomas are treated as primary osteosarcomas.

Challenge

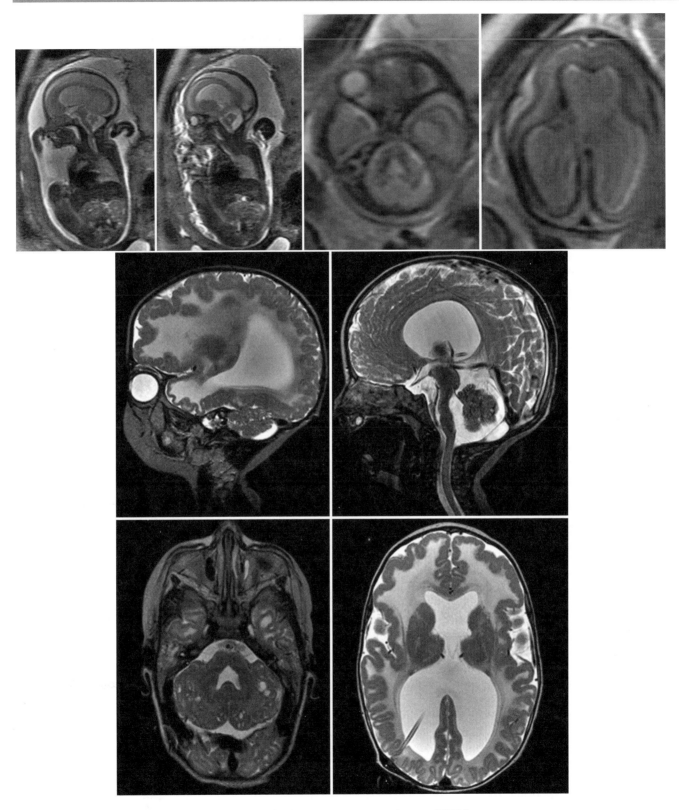

1. What are the imaging findings on a prenatal magnetic resonance image (MRI)?

2. What are the imaging findings on a postnatal MRI at 5 months?

3. What is the most likely diagnosis?

4. To which group does this diagnosis belong?

Diagnosis: Muscle-Eye-Brain Disease

1. Ventriculomegaly and a small, hypoplastic, kinked brainstem.

2. Ventriculomegaly; diffuse cerebral polymicrogyria; multiple subcortical cerebellar cysts; swollen, T2-hyperintense cerebral white matter; hypoplastic pons; malformed tectal plate; and elongated mesencephalon.

3. Muscle-eye-brain disease (MEB).

4. Congenital muscular dystrophies (CMDs).

Reference

Van der Knaap MS, Valk J: Congenital muscular dystrophies. In *Magnetic resonance of myelination and myelin disorders*, ed 3, New York, 2005, Springer Berlin Heidelberg, pp 451-468.

Cross-Reference

Blickman JG, Parker BR, Barnes PD: *Pediatric radiology—the requisites*, ed 3, Philadelphia, 2009, Mosby, p 215.

Comment

MEB belongs to the group of CMDs, which is a heterogeneous group of congenital, hereditary myopathies that are often progressive. Frequently, the name of the diagnosis is based on the combined abnormalities of the eyes and brain. MEB is inherited autosomal recessive. Early clinical symptoms include muscular hypotonia and poor visual contact. A hydrocephalus is seen in the majority of patients. Motor development is generally severely delayed. In addition, severe mental retardation is usually present in combination with seizures. Ocular signs include severe myopia, glaucoma, retinal degeneration, choroidal hypoplasia, and optic nerve hypoplasia. MEB is caused by a defect in the O-mannosyl glycan synthesis. No curative treatment is available.

MRI findings are extensive and prominent. Ventriculomegaly frequently ranges from mild-to-significantly dilated. Additional striking features include a hypoplastic pons and brainstem, multiple subcortical cerebellar cysts, and variable degrees of cerebral polymicrogyria. The cortex is characteristically thickened, and the inner contour of the cortex reveals the polymicrogyria most prominently. In addition, the cerebral white matter is edematous and swollen with a significantly increased T2-weighted signal. The mesencephalon is frequently elongated with a malformation of the tectal plate. The superior and inferior colliculi may be fused. In addition, neuronal heterotopias may be seen within the cerebral hemispheres, as well as a thinned, hypoplastic corpus callosum and a partial absence of the septum pellucidum.

The characteristic features, especially the combination of a ventriculomegaly and a hypoplastic, elongated, and kinked brainstem may already be observed on prenatal, fetal MRI. The cerebellar cysts may, however, be too small to be detected intrauterine or may progress after birth.

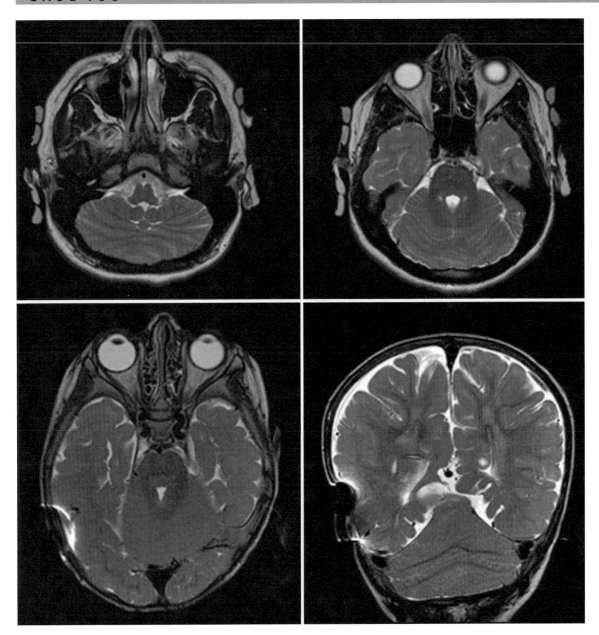

1. What are the imaging findings?

2. What is your diagnosis?

3. What is the underlying pathologic condition?

4. Which associated lesions may be observed?

Diagnosis: Rhombencephalosynapsis

1. A single-lobed cerebellum, no vermis, a keyhole fourth ventricle, and fused dentate nuclei.

2. Rhombencephalosynapsis.

3. A disruption of failed dorsal induction.

4. Hydrocephalus (the current patient is shunted), corpus callosum anomalies, and midline anomalies.

Reference

Patel S, Barkovich AJ: Analysis and classification of cerebellar malformations, *AJNR Am J Neuroradiol* 23: 1074–1087, 2002.

Cross-Reference

Blickman JG, Parker BR, Barnes PD: *Pediatric radiology—the requisites*, ed 3, Philadelphia, 2009, Mosby, p 212.

Comment

Rhombencephalosynapsis is a complex congenital malformation of the posterior fossa, characterized by a fusion of the cerebellar hemispheres, dentate nuclei, and hypoplastic or fused superior cerebellar peduncles (single-lobed cerebellum). In addition, the cerebellar vermis is absent or hypoplastic. This malformation is believed to be the result of a defective dorsal induction or a differentiation of the cerebellar midline structures or both. Rhombencephalosynapsis has been linked to several gene defects, but it is also observed in conditions such as Gomez-Lopez-Hernandez syndrome. Rhombencephalosynapsis is extremely rare; the clinical presentation is usually nonspecific with ataxia, gait abnormalities, and developmental delays. Associated findings, such as corpus callosum agenesis or dysgenesis, septo-optic dysplasia, and hydrocephalus as a result of aqueductal stenosis, are frequently observed. Migrational abnormalities with cerebral polymicrogyria have also been described. Rhombencephalosynapsis may be diagnosed intrauterine by fetal magnetic resonance imaging (MRI) or by postnatal MRI. Imaging findings are usually obvious with the identification of a single-lobed cerebellum with folia and cerebellar fissures crossing the midline (transverse folia). In addition, the dentate nuclei are fused and usually in a more midline position dorsally to a narrowed or keyhole-shaped fourth ventricle. Midsagittal images may be misleading; however, the pattern of the midline fissures do not match the normal anatomy of the vermis (i.e., the primary fissure is missing). Coronal and axial images are most useful. The prognosis is variable; most children do not survive until adulthood. Additional lesions or complications such as hydrocephalus or both shorten survival.

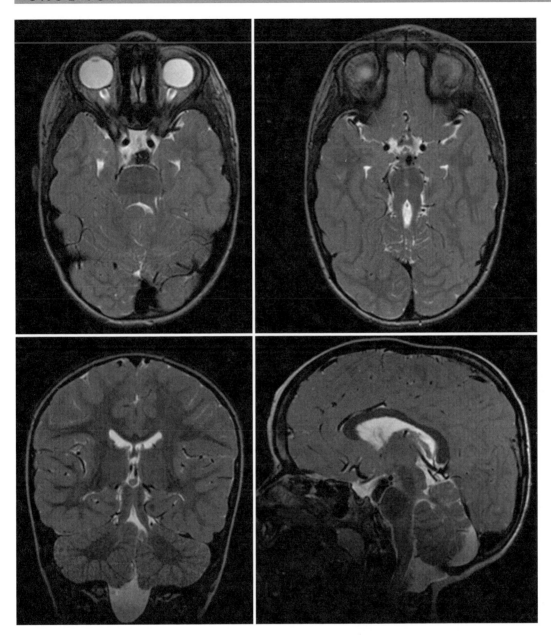

1. What are the imaging findings on magnetic resonance imaging (MRI)?

2. What is the diagnosis?

3. What characteristic is special on the corticospinal tracts in this syndrome?

4. Which other organs may show a pathologic condition?

Diagnosis: Joubert Syndrome

1. Aplasia of the vermis, molar tooth appearance of the brainstem, superior cerebellar peduncles that are thickened and run horizontally, and a bat wing– or umbrella-shaped fourth ventricle.

2. Joubert syndrome.

3. The absence of the pyramidal decussation.

4. The kidneys.

Reference

Poretti A, Boltshauser E, Loenneker T, et al: Diffusion tensor imaging in Joubert syndrome, *AJNR Am J Neuroradiol* 28:1929-1933, 2007.

Cross-Reference

Blickman JG, Parker BR, Barnes PD: *Pediatric radiology—the requisites*, ed 3, Philadelphia, 2009, Mosby, p 212.

Comment

Joubert syndrome was originally reported by Dr. Marie Joubert who described several children with a similar clinical presentation that included episodic hyperpnea, abnormal eye movement, rhythmic tongue protrusions, ataxia, and mental retardation. Anatomically, the cerebellar vermis is lacking. On MRI, the axial images show a characteristic molar tooth appearance of the brainstem, resulting from a horizontal course of the thickened superior cerebellar peduncles. The fourth ventricle is deformed and resembles an umbrella or bat wing on axial planes. Because the vermis is lacking, both cerebellar hemispheres reach each other in the midline; consequently, the midline slices reveal cerebellar fissures on sagittal imaging instead of vermian sulci. In addition, dentate nuclei are lateralized. Tractography studies have shown that the corticospinal tracts do not cross at the pyramidal decussation, which may, in part, explain the clinical presentation. Multiple gene loci that are linked to Joubert syndrome have been identified. The expression may vary; children with Joubert syndrome may show different degrees of mental retardation and gait disturbance. Currently, no prenatal test is available for early diagnosis. Rarely associated supratentorial anomalies occur, and cortical dysplasia and gray-matter heterotopia have been reported. In children with Joubert syndrome, the kidneys may be affected (cerebelloocculorenal syndrome). Renal ultrasound should be considered during the diagnostic work-up of these children. Experienced pediatric neurologists may suspect a diagnosis, based on the facial characteristics that are not specific but indicative. With ongoing research, many more malformations of the brainstem and cerebellum that share a *molar tooth* appearance of the brainstem are described. Perhaps, Joubert syndrome is simply one of a spectrum of brainstem malformations.

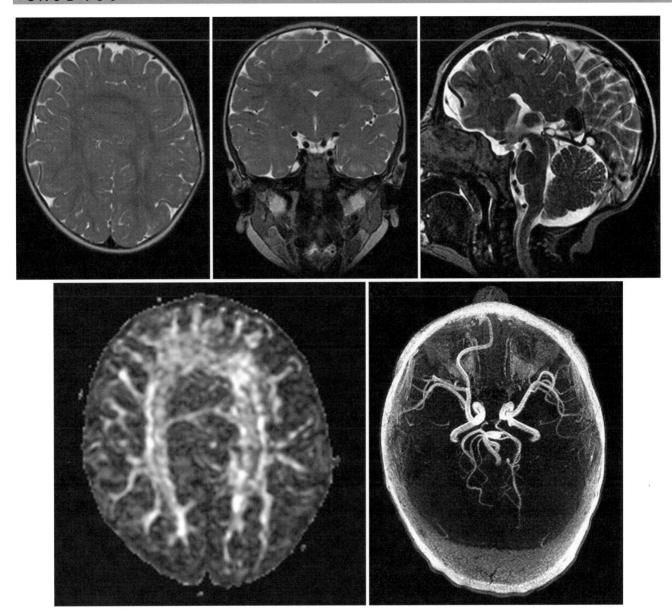

1. What are the imaging findings on magnetic resonance imaging (MRI) and magnetic resonance angiography?

2. What is seen on the fractional anisotropy map?

3. What is the diagnosis?

4. To which group of anomalies does this malformation belong?

Diagnosis: Semilobar Holoprosencephaly

1. Fused frontal lobes, small lateral ventricles, lack of the anterior corpus callosum, unpaired anterior cerebral artery (azygos artery), hypoplastic falx cerebri, rudimentary temporal horns, and partial separation of the thalami.

2. Continuous fiber tracts between the fused frontal lobes and a horseshoe appearance.

3. Semilobar holoprosencephaly.

4. The ventral induction group of anomalies or the diverticulation or cleavage group of disorders.

Cross-Reference
Blickman JG, Parker BR, Barnes PD: *Pediatric radiology—the requisites*, ed 3, Philadelphia, 2009, Mosby, pp 212–213.

Comment
A group of holoprosencephalies results from a disorder of diverticulation or cleavage. Holoprosencephalies are also known as disorders of ventral induction. Holoprosencephalies encompass an entire spectrum of malformations; the mildest form is septo-optic dysplasia; the most severe form is alobar holoprosencephaly. They both result from a failure of cleavage of the prosencephalic vesicle during organogenesis. Frequently, associated anomalies of the face are seen—"*The face predicts the brain.*" Cyclopia has been described in cases of alobar holoprosencephaly. Clinically, depending on the severity of the malformation, different symptoms may occur and include seizures, mental retardation, dystonia, microcephaly, hypothalamic-pituitary dysfunction, cyclopia, and fused metopic suture. Symptoms may be mild in lobar holoprosencephaly and severe in alobar holoprosencephaly. In septo-optic dysplasia, the anterior horns of the ventricles have a boxlike configuration on coronal MRI. In addition, an optic nerve pathologic abnormality is seen on fundoscopy. Various degrees of hypothalamic-pituitary dysfunction are observed. In the lobar holoprosencephaly, a lobar brain is seen with hypoplastic frontal lobes, some frontal horn formation, and the falx cerebri extends frontally. In semilobar holoprosencephaly, a partially formed fax cerebri and a partially formed interhemispheric fissure are seen in the posterior part. The anterior brain is fused, the thalami are partially separated, and a small third ventricle and rudimentary temporal horns are demonstrated. The septum pellucidum is absent, the splenium of the corpus callosum is present, whereas the truncus of the corpus callosum is lacking. Hypoplastic olfactory bulbs and optic nerves may exist. In alobar holoprosencephaly, a small holosphere and monoventricle are seen, as well as fused thalami. However, no third ventricle, falx cerebri or corpus callosum, or interhemispheric fissure is seen. In addition, no temporal horns are demonstrated, and malformations of the Willis circle are observed with an azygos or unpaired anterior cerebral artery. The prognosis is frequently poor, especially in the most severe forms of holoprosencephalies. Diagnosis is usually made prenatally by either ultrasound or fetal MRI. In septo-optic dysplasia, the prognosis will be determined by the associated malformations. In up to 50% of cases, additional lesions are identified by MRI. Postnatally, MRI is indicated to identify all details of the malformation.

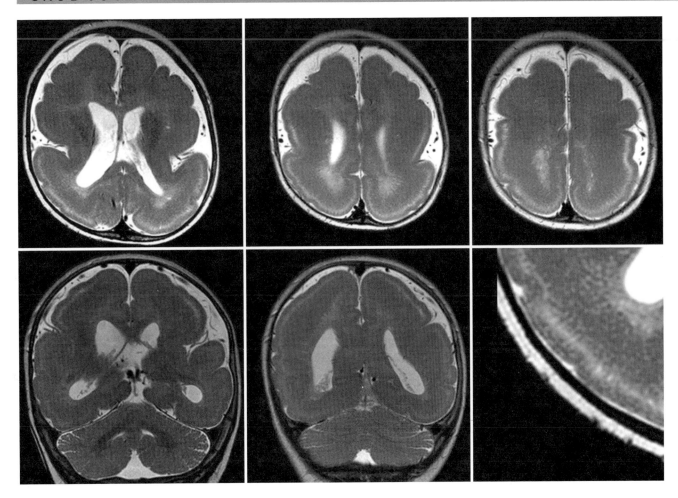

1. What are the findings on magnetic resonance imaging (MRI)?

2. What is the diagnosis?

3. To which group of lesions does this malformation belong?

4. How many layers does the normal cortex have, and how many do you expect to find in this child?

Diagnosis: Lissencephaly Type I

1. Symmetric T2-hypointense bands within the cerebral white matter, lissencephalic cortex, and mild ventriculomegaly.

2. Lissencephaly (type I) with extensive and arrested neuronal migration.

3. Neuronal migration anomalies.

4. The normal cortex has six layers; this child has four layers.

Cross-Reference

Blickman JG, Parker BR, Barnes PD: *Pediatric radiology— the requisites*, ed 3, Philadelphia, 2009, Mosby, pp 219–222.

Comment

Neuronal migration anomalies and malformations of cortical development occur between the second and fourth months gestation. In neuronal migration anomalies, cells that should migrate from the periventricular germinal matrix to the cortical surface of the brain are arrested somewhere along their paths. These cells may rest at multiple locations, either focal or as bands. Heterotopic gray matter may be recognized on imaging focally as subependymal heteroptopic cell masses or as bands within the periventricular, central, or subcortical white matter of the cerebral hemispheres. Disorders of cortical organization may result in agyria, pachygyria, polymicrogyria, or focal cortical dysplasia. Frequently, combined malformations of neuronal migration and cortical organization are seen. In lissencephaly (type I), an extensive arrest of the neuronal migration results in a wide, T2-hypointense band of neurons within the white matter of both hemispheres separated from the overlying cortex by a thin band of T2-hyperintense white matter. The overlying cortex is typically lissencephalic and has a four-layer architecture combined with a smooth brain surface. The anomaly is usually symmetric. Ventriculomegaly may be associated. The cerebellum is usually unremarkable. Children may present with intractable seizures and a developmental delay. The cause is not yet fully determined but is at least known to be mediated genetically but is also believed to be the result of intrauterine infections. MRI is the imaging modality of choice to identify the exact anatomy of the anomaly. High-resolution imaging will also display that the subcortical white matter has multiple linear bands of T2-hypointensity, which most likely represents streaks of neurons that *almost* reached the lissencephalic cortex. Prenatal diagnosis on ultrasound may be difficult because the overlying fetal skull prevents a detailed study of the cortex; the arrested neurons within the white matter are also difficult to detect. Lissencephaly (type I) should be differentiated from the neuronal migration anomalies and malformations of cortical development because differentiation will help determine prognosis.

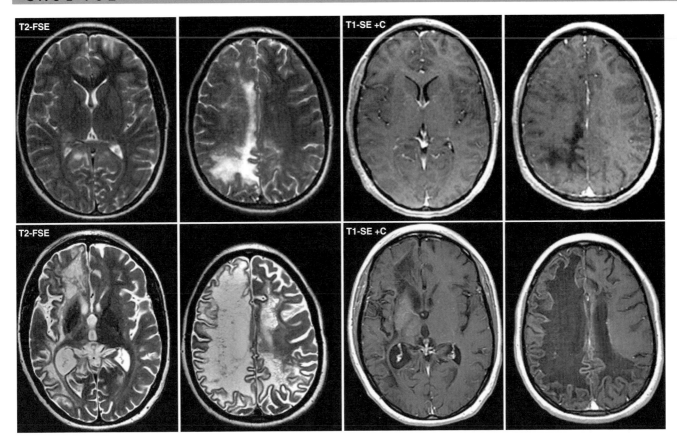

1. What are the imaging findings on an initial magnetic resonance image (MRI) in this 15-year-old girl?

2. Does the follow-up imaging, performed 13 months later, narrow the differential diagnoses?

3. What is the most likely diagnosis?

4. What is the prognosis?

Diagnosis: Progressive Multifocal Leukoencephalopathy

1. Areas of T2-hyperintensity and nonenhancing T1-hypointensity within the white matter of both hemispheres (right is greater than left), minimal mass effect, preserved superficial layers of the cortex, and asymmetric distribution.

2. Rapid progression of the lesions, cortical thinning, a strikingly asymmetric presentation, a metabolic disease, or acute disseminated encephalomyelitis is less likely.

3. Progressive multifocal leukoencephalopathy (PML) in the immunocompromised child.

4. The prognosis of PML in a child with human immunodeficiency virus (HIV) is poor, in general; rapid increase makes the prognosis even worse.

Cross-Reference
Blickman JG, Parker BR, Barnes PD: *Pediatric radiology—the requisites*, ed 3, Philadelphia, 2009, Mosby, p 231.

Discussion
PML is a severe, demyelinating disease of the central nervous system as a result of JC papovavirus infection of the myelin-producing oligodendrocytes. The name *JC virus* is derived from the initials of the index patient. PML typically occurs in immunocompromised individuals, such as children with congenital HIV infection or other conditions associated with impaired T-cell function. In the course of the infection, extensive myelin breakdown results in white matter destruction. Neurologic symptoms are unspecific and include focal neurologic deficits and dementia. Without treatment, patients have a relentless downhill course. The disease is usually fatal within 1 year of diagnosis in 90% of patients. The diagnosis can be established by the detection of the JC virus deoxyribonucleic acid (DNA) in cerebrospinal fluid by polymerase chain reaction testing. Many reports have described MRI findings in patients with PML, but only few MRI abnormalities correlate with patient survival. Conventional MRI reveals patchy areas of T2-hyperintense and T1-hypointense demyelination within the white matter. These lesions do not usually show any contrast enhancement and have minimal or no mass effect. Typically, these lesions are asymmetric. On diffusion tensor imaging, the lesions have a reduced fractional anisotropy, confirming the injury to the white matter by the infection. On follow-up imaging, lesions may show a rapid increase without treatment. The overlying cortex may be thinned. Any child with a rapidly expanding, focal white matter lesion with a compromised immune system should be suspected for PML until proved otherwise. The differential diagnoses may include acute disseminated encephalomyelitis and radiation necrosis or metabolic white matter diseases. The rapid progression and the clinical history are usually helpful in differentiating the cause of the observed lesions.

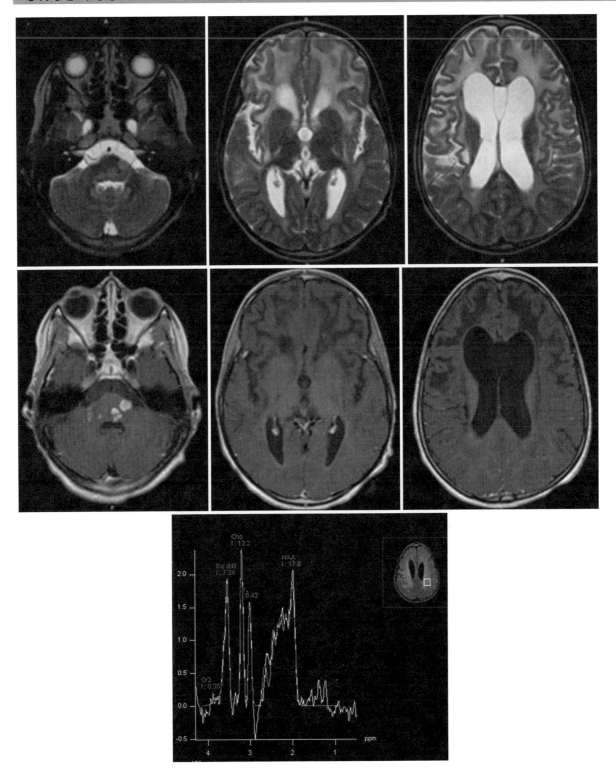

1. What are the findings in a magnetic resonance image (MRI) of a 10-year-old girl with a history of progressive loss of developmental milestones?

2. What does the 1H–magnetic resonance spectroscopy (1H-MRS) of the hemispheric white matter show?

3. What is the most likely diagnosis?

4. How can this diagnosis be confirmed?

C A S E   1 6 3

Diagnosis: Alexander Disease

1. Symmetric T2-hyperintense, T1-hypointense signal of predominantly the frontal white matter and posterior limb of internal capsule; multifocal contrast-enhancing brainstem lesions; periventricular T1-hyperintensity; subcortical cysts; mild ventriculomegaly; and cavum septi pellucid.

2. Increased levels of myoinositol and choline, decreased N-acetyl aspartate, and mild lactate within the white matter.

3. Alexander disease, a form of leukodystrophy.

4. Brain biopsy will confirm the diagnosis and reveal an accumulation of Rosenthal fibers in hypertrophic, fibrillary astrocytes and a mutation in the glial fibrillary acidic protein (GFAP) gene located on the long arm (q) of chromosome 17 at position 21 (17q21).

Reference

Van der Knaap MS, Valk J: Congenital muscular dystrophies. In *Magnetic resonance of myelination and myelin disorders*, ed 3, New York, 2005, Springer Berlin Heidelberg, pp 416–441.

Cross-Reference

Blickman JG, Parker BR, Barnes PD: *Pediatric radiology—the requisites*, ed 3, Philadelphia, 2009, Mosby, pp 267–268.

Comment

Alexander disease is a leukodystrophy first described by W. Stewart Alexander in 1949 as progressive fibrinoid degeneration of fibrillary astrocytes associated with mental retardation in a hydrocephalic infant. Three subgroups have been identified: infantile, juvenile, and adult. In the juvenile subgroup, the patients become symptomatic between 4 and 14 years of age, typically with a progressive loss of previously mastered developmental milestones. In addition, patients may present with progressive bulbar and pseudobulbar symptoms, an increase in swallowing problems and apneic attacks, impaired speech or loss of speech, dysarthria, hoarseness, spasticity, cerebellar ataxia, seizures, and progressive behavioral and cognitive deterioration. Average duration of the illness is 8 years. Most cases are sporadic, but familial cases have been described. Imaging features are rather characteristic with predominant frontal lobe involvement that may progress over the course of the disease into the parietal regions. Five characteristic MRI criteria have been defined, and four of the five have to be fulfilled for diagnosis: (1) symmetric cerebral white matter abnormalities with predominant frontal involvement, (2) T2-hypointense, T1-hyperintense rim of tissue along the ventricles, (3) focal lesions in the basal ganglia and thalami, (4) brainstem abnormalities (midbrain and medulla), and (5) contrast enhancement of the described lesions including optic chiasm. In addition, 1H-MRS will show increased myoinositol and choline levels within the affected white matter, as well as a reduced N-acetyl aspartate peak. Lactate may also be observed. On microscopic examination, countless Rosenthal fibers are seen throughout the brain within hypertrophic fibrillary astrocytes. Macrocephaly results from the combination of astrocytic hyperplasia and massive deposition of Rosenthal fibers.

Alexander Disease

- predominant frontal lobe involvement, may progress to parietal regions

MRI Criteria 4/5

(1) Symmetric cerebral WM abn with predominal frontal involvement

(2) T₂ hypointense > Rim tissue around ventricles T₁ hyperintense

(3) focal lesions in thalamus & basal ganglia

(4) brainstem abn

(5) Contrast enhancement of such lesions

- Microscopy ⇒ Rosenthal fibers c̄ hypertrophic fibrillary astrocytes

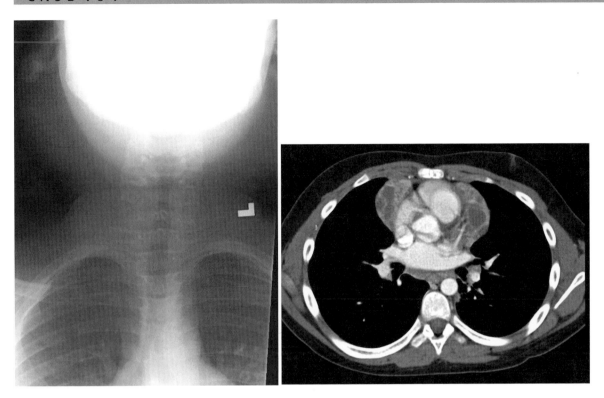

1. At 7 years of age, this boy presented with parotitis (first image). What are the differential possibilities?

2. At 12 years old, the patient developed a cough. What were the findings on a computed tomographic (CT) scan of the chest (second image)?

3. What does this combination of findings suggest?

4. What are the vectors for this condition in children?

HIV – parotitis and thymic cysts

Diagnosis: Positive Human Immunodeficiency Virus: Parotitis and Thymic Cysts

1. All of the following differential possibilities are very rare: acute bacterial parotitis, recurrent parotitis with sialectasia, viral parotitis (mumps, Ebstein-Barr virus [EBV], human immunodeficiency virus [HIV]), and Sjögren's syndrome, this patient's first diagnosis.

2. CT findings included thymic cysts.

3. This combination of findings suggests HIV and acquired immunodeficiency syndrome (AIDS).

4. The vectors for this condition in children are congenital infection acquired through transfusion.

Reference

Kuhn JP, Slovis TL, Haller JO: *Caffey's pediatric diagnostic imaging*, ed 10, Philadelphia, 2004, Mosby, pp 1184–1189.

Cross-Reference

Blickman JG, Parker BR, Barnes PD: *Pediatric radiology—the requisites*, ed 3, Philadelphia, 2009, Mosby, pp 324–325.

Comment

All parotitis is rare in children; consequently, all of the unusual entities in the differential list have a good chance of being correct. EBV, HIV, recurrent parotitis, and Sjögren syndrome all have similar clinical presentations and relapsing and remitting courses. This patient was not tested for HIV until the thymic cysts were discovered.

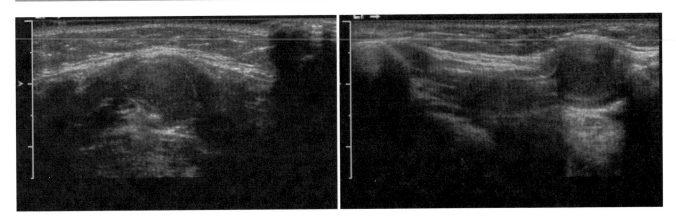

1. What is the finding in these transverse and midline sagittal plane images of the anterior upper neck of a 4-year-old patient?

2. What are the differential diagnoses?

3. The lesion is located in the midline of the anterior neck. If it were found in the lateral aspect, what would be a likely diagnosis?

4. Why is localizing the thyroid gland important in this situation?

Diagnosis: Thyroglossal Duct Cysts

1. A 1 to 2 cm round cystic structure with a high level of echoes suggests a complicated cyst.

2. A thyroglossal duct cyst and lymphadenitis with abscess are the most likely differential diagnoses. Sebaceous cyst, lymphatic malformation, thymic cyst, dermoid cyst, teratoma, lipomas, and sarcoma are less likely because of the size or ultrasound characteristics.

3. Branchial cleft cyst.

4. If the thyroid tissue is not seen in the normal location, then the gland may be ectopic and possibly incorporated in the thyroglossal duct cyst.

Reference

Tunkel DE, Domenech EE: Radioisotope scanning of the thyroid gland prior to thyroglossal duct cyst excision, *Arch Otolaryngol Head Neck Surg* 124:597-599, 1998.

Cross-Reference

Blickman JG, Parker BR, Barnes PD: *Pediatric radiology—the requisites*, ed 3, Philadelphia, 2009, Mosby, pp 309-311.

Comment

Thyroglossal duct cysts are the most common congenital cysts in the neck representing 75% of midline masses and resulting from cystic dilation of epithelial remnants of the thyroglossal duct tract, which is present during the embryologic inferior migration of the thyroid from the base of the tongue to its normal final location. These cysts present as midline neck masses at the level of the thyrohyoid membrane and are closely associated with the hyoid bone. Most patients present as children, although presentation at any age is possible. Males and females are equally affected, and the cysts are usually asymptomatic, but they may become infected and form abscesses and draining fistulas.

In this example, the cyst is small; if larger, both an elevation of the tongue and a swallowing dysfunction would have developed. Ultrasound is the imaging modality of choice because it is ideal for determination of the nature of the mass and the localization of thyroid tissue. In this case, the lesion appears as a complex cyst, which is likely because of prior infection or hemorrhage. Computed tomography (CT) and magnetic resonance imaging (MRI) is also diagnostic but radiation (CT), length of study (MRI), and expense make both modalities impractical and unnecessary. Scintigraphy may be helpful to localize ectopic location of the thyroid gland.

Surgical resection is considered the treatment of choice. If the patient is euthyroid and thyroid tissue is seen in the normal location, no further imaging of the thyroid gland is necessary. In cases of abnormal thyroid function, nuclear thyroid scans are indicated to search for ectopic thyroid. Ectopic thyroid tissue may be located in the sublingual space in 10% of patients and at the base of the tongue in 90% of patients. In 75% of patients, the ectopic tissue is the only functioning thyroid tissue. However, these patients are usually hypothyroid anyway because the ectopic tissue is dysplastic. A careful histologic study of the specimen is important; a small incidence of carcinoma arising in thyroglossal duct remnants exists.

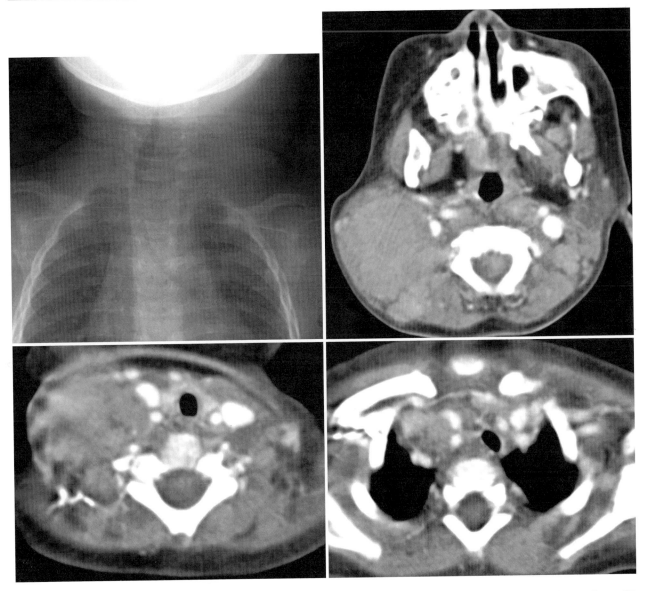

1. What are the imaging findings in this 3-year-old African-American child that presented with right neck swelling? What are the differential diagnoses?

2. What is Rosai-Dorfman disease?

3. What is Castleman disease?

4. What are the characteristic pathologic findings?

Diagnosis: Rosai-Dorfman Disease

1. A frontal chest radiograph and intravenous contrast-enhanced computed tomographic scans through the neck and upper chest demonstrate massive cervical and mediastinal lymphadenopathy. The differential diagnoses include lymphoma, infection, Castleman disease, and Rosai-Dorfman disease.

2. Painless bilateral cervical lymph node enlargement with the possible involvement of various extranodal sites.

Rosai Dorfman Disease

3. A benign process of angiofollicular hyperplasia of the lymph nodes and typically does not affect children.

4. In Rosai-Dorfman disease, extensive reactive process within the lymph node is typically seen, including significant dilated sinuses containing sheets of histiocytes with eosinophilic cytoplasm and small nuclei with no evidence of malignancy.

References

Rosai J, Dorfman RF: Sinus histiocytosis with massive lymphadenopathy: a pseudolymphomatous benign disorder, *Cancer* 30:1174–1188, 1972.

La Barge DV 3rd, Salzman KL, Harnsberger HR, et al: Sinus histiocytosis with massive lymphadenopathy (Rosai-Dorfman disease): imaging manifestations in the head and neck, *AJR Am J Roentgenol* 191(6): W299–W306, 2008.

Comments

Rosai-Dorfman disease is a rare sinus histiocytosis and a benign source of massive lymphadenopathy, which may mimic a neoplastic process. This disease commonly presents in children and young adults and in blacks more commonly than in whites. It is characterized by painless bilateral cervical lymph node enlargement and, less commonly, other groups of lymph nodes. Up to 43% of patients have involvement of extranodal sites, especially the soft tissues of the head and neck, paranasal sinuses, and nasal cavity. Other sites that may be involved include the upper respiratory tract, skin, salivary glands, orbit, bones, and testis. These extranodal lesions may appear before lymphadenopathy is apparent.

Pathologic examination of the biopsied lymph nodes demonstrates exaggerated reactive process with no evidence of malignancy. Characteristic features include significantly dilated sinuses containing sheets of histiocytes with eosinophilic cytoplasm and small nuclei.

Differential diagnoses include Castleman disease, dermopathic lymphadenitis, mucocutaneous lymph node syndrome (Kawasaki disease), histiocytic necrotizing lymphadenopathy (Kikuchi disease), vascular transformation of the lymph nodes, and inflammatory pseudotumor of the lymph nodes.

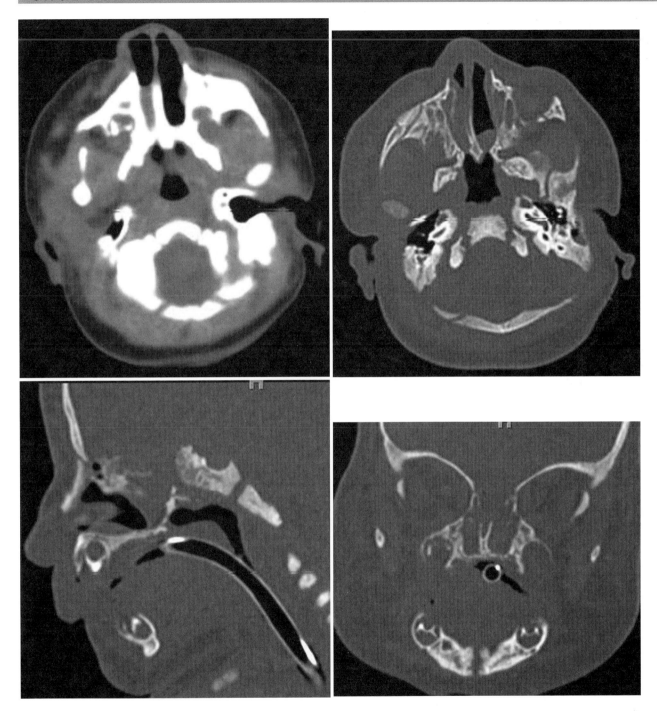

1. What are the imaging findings in this newborn with respiratory distress?

2. What is the diagnosis?

3. Does this condition have any association with other congenital anomalies?

4. What is the cause?

Diagnosis: Choanal Atresia

1. A thickening and medial bowing of the lateral walls of the nasal cavity, an enlargement of the vomer, and fusion of these elements. These findings are nicely depicted in axial soft-tissue windows and reformatted coronal and sagittal images.

2. Bilateral choanal atresia.

3. Choanal atresia is associated with Down, Treacher Collins, and Apert syndromes, as well as Crouzon disease. In addition, cardiac malformations; cleft palate; malformations of the hands, fingers, and ears; stunted growth; tracheoesophageal fistula; and musculoskeletal abnormalities are all part of the condition. In 30% of patients, choanal atresia is associated with the CHARGE syndrome (the acronym means Coloboma, Heart anomalies, choanal Atresia, Retardation of growth and development, and Genital and Ear anomalies).

4. Causes include a lack of reabsorption of the buccopharyngeal membrane, the permanence of the Hochstetter nasobuccal membrane, and the theory in which an alteration exists in the orientation of the mesodermal cells that make up the nasal cavities.

Reference

Valencia MP, Castillo M: Congenital and acquired lesions of the nasal septum: a practical guide for differential diagnosis, *Radiographics* 28:205–223, 2008.

Cross-Reference

Blickman JG, Parker BR, Barnes PD: *Pediatric radiology— the requisites*, ed 3, Philadelphia, 2009, Mosby, p 302.

Comment

Newborns are obligatory nasal breathers; therefore nasal obstruction is an airway emergency in this population. Choanal atresia is the result of an occluded nasal airway and typically presents with respiratory distress during feeding, which may be alleviated by crying. Theories proposed to explain the embryogenesis of choanal atresia include persistence of the buccopharyngeal membrane and the oronasal membrane, as well as the mesodermal flow theory, in which a misdirection of neural crest cell migration, secondary to local factors, is implicated. Bilateral congenital choanal atresia should be suspected when the infant presents signs of asphyxia and cyanosis that improves with crying. Choanal atresia will only present as an airway emergency if it is bilateral. Choanal atresia occurs in 1 of 8000 live births and is commonly (>75%) associated with syndromes and systemic anomalies. Approximately two thirds of patients are bilateral. In the most severe form of this condition,

the hard palate and vomer are fused with the ventral clivus, and the nasopharynx is very small (nasopharyngeal atresia). In another form, membranous choanal atresia is a result of the failure of the buccopharyngeal membrane to perforate. In more than 90% of patients with choanal atresia, the abnormality is partly or completely osseous; pure membranous atresia is rare. Female infants are affected twice as often as male newborns. Computed tomography is the imaging modality of choice to diagnose and help determine whether the obstruction is bony or membranous. Multiplanar reconstructions should be performed to better evaluate the anatomy. Normal choanal orifices measure more than 0.37 cm in children younger than 2 years of age. The width of the posterior and inferior parts of the vomer is normally less than 0.34 cm in patients younger than 8 years. Additional congenital anomalies are present in approximately 50% of the patients and should be actively searched for in the presence of choanal atresia.

Choanal Atresia

- >75% associated c̄ syndromes or systemic anomalies

- 2/3 bilateral

- osseous vs. membranous
  90% ↳ pure is rare

- ♀ : ♂   2:1

- CT modality of choice

- Actively search for other anomalies

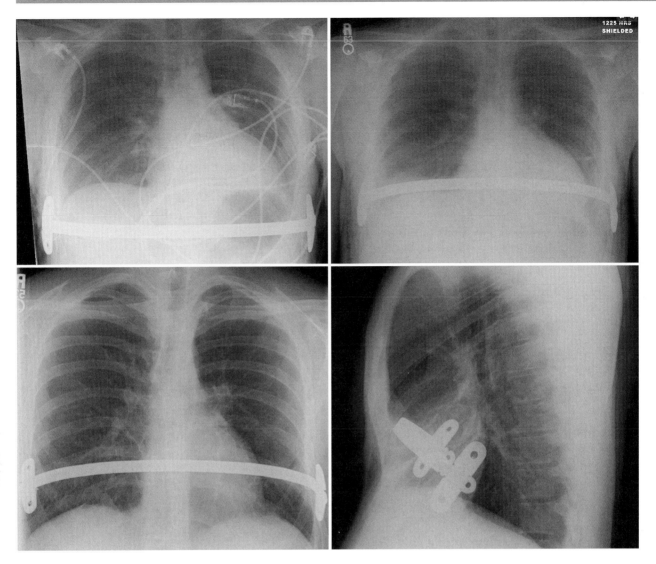

1. This series of films shows a complication of the Nuss procedure to repair the pectus excavatum in a teenage boy. The first film was on the first day after surgery, the next film was 2 days later, and the posteroanterior (AP) and lateral films were taken 1 month after surgery. What is visualized?

2. What is the Haller index?

3. Why is pectus excavatum repaired?

4. At what age is the repair usually performed?

CASE 168

Diagnosis: Pectus Excavatum Repair Complication

1. The Nuss bar became displaced as shown on the film 3 days and 1 month after surgery. It has rotated superiorly 45 degrees. The pneumothorax and left lower lobe atelectasis are also present on the early postoperative films.

2. The ratio of the width of the chest (inside the rib cage) to the narrowest AP diameter of the chest (between the sternum and the anterior aspect of the thoracic spine) as shown on a computed tomographic scan. Haller Index

3. In addition to the cosmetic deformity, pectus excavatum may result in cardiac compromise and restrictive lung disease.

4. During the mid-to-late teenage years, although the timing is controversial.

Reference

Vegunta RK, Pacheco PE, Wallace LJ, et al: Complications associated with the Nuss procedure: continued evolution of the learning curve, *Am J Surg* 195 (3):313-316, 2008.

Cross-Reference

Blickman JG, Parker BR, Barnes PD: *Pediatric radiology—the requisites*, ed 3, Philadelphia, 2009, Mosby, pp 15-17.

Comment

Pectus excavatum is the most common congenital abnormality of the chest wall and occurs in 1 out of 1000 children and more often in boys than in girls. The Nuss procedure is relatively new; it was first described in 1998 and uses a minimally invasive approach. The Nuss bar is left in place for approximately 36 months and then removed. The repair of the deformity is generally recommended when the Haller index is greater than 3.25.

Minor complications of the Nuss procedure are common and include pneumothorax, pleural fluid, atelectasis, breakage of wires used to secure the lateral stabilizer plate, intraoperative rupture of the intercostal muscles, and pericardial tears without clinical significance. Major complications are rare and include organ perforation (heart and liver), laceration of the internal mammary artery, pericardial effusion, ossification around the Nuss bar, bar infections, and significant bar displacement. Careful study of the postoperative films will allow recognition of bar displacement. Although not routinely obtained, a lateral film may be helpful as it was in this example.

Haller Index
- on CT

$$\frac{\text{Width of chest (inside rib)}}{\text{Narrowest AP diameter}}$$

> 3.25   repair suggested

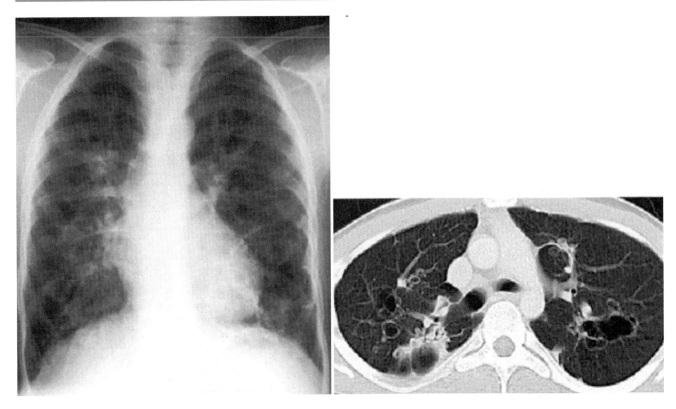

1. What are the imaging findings in this 6-year-old boy who presented with stridor? What is the diagnosis?

2. What is the most frequent location of the lesions in this disease?

3. How do the lungs get involved?

4. Describe the typical presentation of these patients.

Diagnosis: Respiratory Papillomatosis

1. A chest radiograph and intravenous contrast-enhanced computerized axial tomographic scan of the chest demonstrate hyperinflation with multiple lung nodules and cavitations. These findings are consistent with the diagnosis of respiratory papillomatosis.

2. In the larynx.

3. The lungs become involved due to endobronchial spread of laryngeal lesions.

4. Most commonly with hoarseness, but may also have a weak cry, stridor, and a failure to thrive in infancy.

References

Kuhn J: Larynx and cervical trachea. In Kuhn JP, Slovis TL, Haller JO, editors: *Caffey's pediatric diagnostic imaging*, ed 10, Philadelphia, 2004, Mosby, pp 812–813.

Effman E: Pulmonary neoplasms, tumor-like conditions and miscellaneous diseases. In Kuhn JP, Slovis TL, Haller JO, editors: *Caffey's pediatric diagnostic imaging*, ed 10, Philadelphia, 2004, Mosby, pp 1129–1130.

Cross-Reference

Blickman JG, Parker BR, Barnes PD: *Pediatric radiology—the requisites*, ed 3, Philadelphia, 2009, Mosby, pp 37–38.

Comment

Recurrent respiratory papillomatosis (RRP) is relatively rare in children. However, papillomas are the most common tumor found in the larynx in childhood.

Benign tumors of the aerodigestive tract from the human papilloma viral infection result in papillomatosis. Lesions may be 1 mm to several centimeters in size. The most frequent location is the larynx (95%) with the tracheobronchial tree, lung parenchyma, nasopharynx, and oropharynx and esophagus less common. Endobronchial spread leads to lung nodules that may cavitate. Complications include airway obstruction, hemorrhage, and rarely malignant degeneration.

Hoarseness is the most common clinical presentation, but it may also include a weak cry, stridor, and failure to thrive. Most patients present between the ages of 2 and 5 years. At least one half of affected children have mothers with condyloma acuminata, but most infants of mothers with genital papilloma viral infection do not develop RRP.

Diagnosis is made with laryngoscopy. Most cases can be treated with laser therapy, but lesions frequently recur.

Laryngeal tracheopapillomatosis spreads to the lungs in less than 1% of patients and is associated with a poor prognosis. Radiographic findings include thin-walled cystic lesions, as well as solid pulmonary lesions that tend to grow peripherally and lead to lung destruction. Lesions are distributed predominantly in the posterior lower lobes and are frequently associated with atelectasis, bronchiectasis, and associated infections. Differential diagnoses include granulomatous disease (Wegener disease), metastatic disease, and septic emboli.

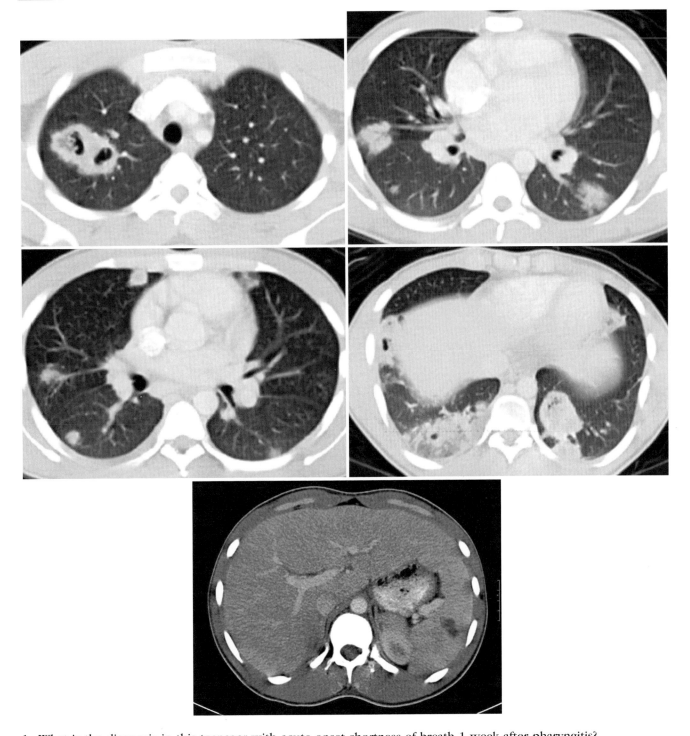

1. What is the diagnosis in this teenager with acute onset shortness of breath 1 week after pharyngitis?

2. What is the most common causative agent?

3. What are the features of this syndrome?

4. What are the possible complications?

Diagnosis: Lemierre Syndrome

1. Lemierre syndrome–pharyngitis with septic thrombosis of the internal jugular veins.

2. *Fusobacterium necrophorum*.

3. Septic thrombosis of the internal jugular vein develops after pharyngitis.

4. The direct spread from the internal jugular vein into the mediastinum or cranial vault.

References

DeSena S, Rosenfeld DL, Santos S, et al: Jugular thrombophlebitis complicating bacterial pharyngitis (Lemierre's syndrome), *Pediatr Radiol* 26:141-144, 1996.

Lustig LR, Cusick BC, Cheung SW, et al: Lemierre's syndrome: two cases of postanginal sepsis, *Otolaryngol Head Neck Surg* 112:767-772, 1995.

Cross-Reference

Blickman JG, Parker BR, Barnes PD: *Pediatric radiology—the requisites*, ed 3, Philadelphia, 2009, Mosby, pp 8-9.

Comment

Lemierre syndrome is pharyngitis with septic thrombosis of the internal jugular veins and is usually caused by the bacterium *Fusobacterium necrophorum*. It typically affects young, previously healthy patients. Lemierre syndrome develops most often after oropharyngeal infection; the pathogens spread to the internal jugular vein by several anatomic routes including local draining veins, lymphatic tissue, or direct extension through the soft tissue of the neck. The bacteria penetrate the jugular vein, causing an infected clot, from which bacteria are seeded throughout the body. Pieces of the infected clot break off and travel to the lungs as emboli, blocking branches of the pulmonary artery. If untreated, supportive infection can spread directly into the ear, mediastinum, and cranial vault. Findings on clinical examination of patients with Lemierre syndrome are quite variable. Signs of exudative tonsillitis, pharyngitis, and thick gray pseudomembranes, as well as oral ulcers, have been reported. However, oropharyngeal examination may be normal because sepsis typically occurs 1 week after primary infection, allowing time for physical findings to resolve. Neck pain, swelling, and trismus along the anterior border of the sternocleidomastoid muscle and at the angle of the mandible are the clinical manifestations of a septic thrombophlebitis of the ipsilateral internal jugular vein. Signs and symptoms of pulmonary embolism may be the presenting clinical finding, especially in patients in whom oropharyngeal manifestations have resolved. Persistent fever and rigors despite antibiotics, followed by the complaint of pleuritic chest pain, hemoptysis, or dyspnea, may be all that is required for a presumptive diagnosis.

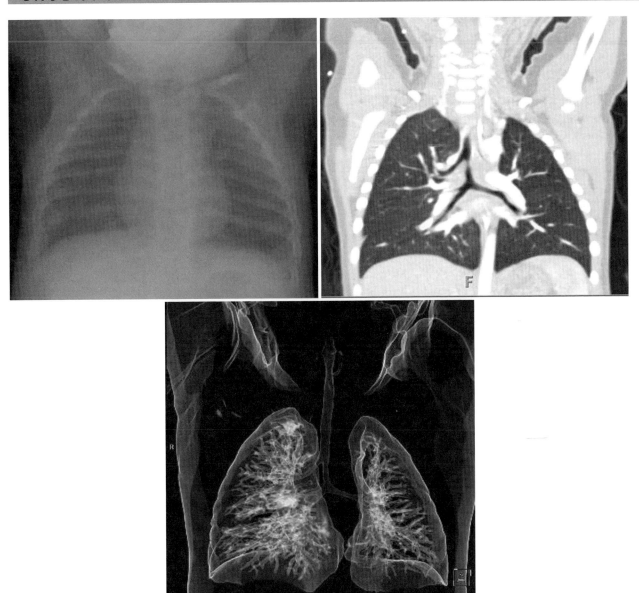

1. What are the imaging findings in this 6-month-old girl with chronic cough, wheezing, and noisy breathing?

2. What is the diagnosis?

3. What is the differential diagnosis?

4. Are any associated congenital anomalies identified?

Diagnosis: Tracheobronchial Anomaly (Pig Bronchus)

1. Imaging findings include an extra bronchus branching from the upper right lateral wall of the trachea, nicely displayed as a supernumerary bronchus; otherwise, the lung parenchyma and interstitium are normal. The extra bronchus branching was an incidental finding, and the plain-film radiography was negative.

2. The diagnosis is true right tracheal bronchus. This type of tracheobronchial anomaly is called *pig bronchus* because this morphologic condition is normal in pigs.

3. In the light of computed tomographic findings, no other differential diagnosis is evident.

4. Bronchiectasis, focal emphysema, and cystic lung malformations may coexist. The prevalence of tracheal bronchus in association with infantile lobar emphysema is unknown, but the association is more frequent with a left tracheal bronchus.

Reference

Berrocal T, Madrid C, Novo S, et al: Congenital anomalies of the tracheobronchial tree, lung, and mediastinum: embryology, radiology, and pathology, *Radiographics* 24(1):e17, 2004.

Comment

Between 1% and 12% of patients who undergo bronchography or bronchoscopy demonstrate some form of congenital tracheobronchial variant or anomaly. Contrary to the numerous variations of lobar or segmental bronchial subdivisions, abnormal bronchi originating from the trachea or main bronchi are rare.

Tracheal bronchus was first described in 1785 as an airway malformation in which the right upper lobe bronchus originates in the trachea. The term *tracheal bronchus* includes a variety of bronchial anomalies that affect the trachea or main bronchus and are directed toward the upper lobe territory. This anomalous bronchus usually exits the right lateral wall of the trachea less than 2 cm above the major carina and can supply the entire upper lobe or its apical segment. The two types are (1) displaced and (2) supernumerary bronchi. If the anatomic upper lobe bronchus is missing a single branch, then the tracheal bronchus is defined as *displaced*; if the right upper lobe bronchus has a normal trifurcation into apical, posterior, and anterior segmental bronchi, then the tracheal bronchus is defined as *supernumerary*. The supernumerary bronchi may end blindly; in that case, they are also called *tracheal diverticula*. If they end in aerated or bronchiectatic lung tissue, they are termed *apical accessory lungs* or *tracheal lobes*. Right tracheal bronchus has a prevalence of 0.1% to 2% and left tracheal bronchus a prevalence of 0.3% to 1% in bronchographic and bronchoscopic studies. The displaced type of tracheal bronchus occurs more frequent than the supernumerary type.

Multidetector computed tomography (MDCT) is a reliable, noninvasive imaging technique for the diagnosis of tracheal bronchus. Diagnostic sensitivity of MDCT has been shown to be 100%. Three-dimensional reconstruction of the airways makes the diagnosis easier. The angle between the tracheal bronchus and trachea varies from 22 to 108 degrees. During endotracheal intubation, an endotracheal tube can occlude the lumen of the tracheal bronchus, resulting in atelectasis of the involved lobe or segment. Recognition of the distance between the tracheal bronchus and carina, the size of tracheal bronchus and angle between the tracheal bronchus and trachea are important for the anesthesiologist and helps avoid complications of intubation.

Patients are usually asymptomatic, but the diagnosis of tracheal bronchus should be considered in cases of persistent or recurrent upper lobe pneumonia, atelectasis or air trapping, and chronic bronchitis. Identification of this anatomic variant would allow appropriate changes in airway management.

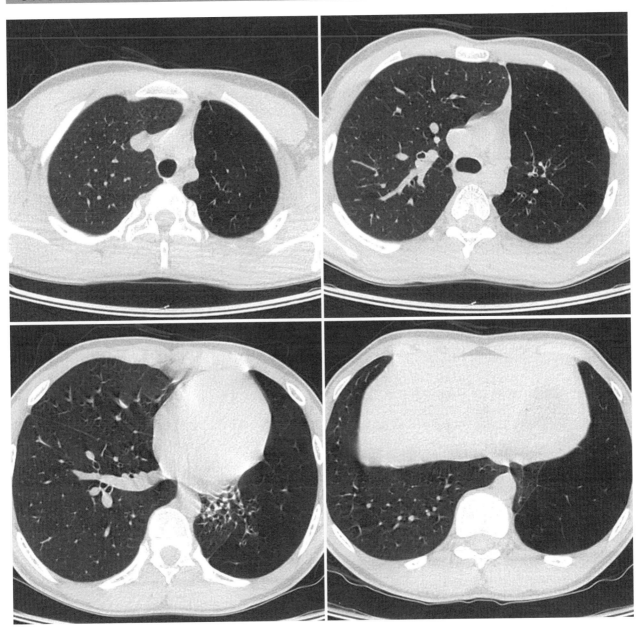

1. What are the imaging findings?

2. What is your diagnosis?

3. What are the differential diagnoses?

4. What is the cause?

Diagnosis: Swyer-James Syndrome

1. A hyperlucent, hypoperfused small left lung with bronchiectasis.

2. Swyer-James syndrome (SJS).

3. Hypoplastic pulmonary artery and primary or secondary lung hypoplasia.

4. Severe bronchiolitis obliterans early during life (<8 years of age).

Reference

Fraser RG, Paré PD, Fraser RS, Genereux GP: *Diagnosis of disease of the chest*, ed 3, Philadelphia, 1996, Saunders, pp 2177–2186.

Cross-Reference

Blickman JG, Parker BR, Barnes PD: *Pediatric radiology—the requisites*, ed 3, Philadelphia, 2009, Mosby, pp 22–23.

Comment

SJS refers to a small, hyperlucent lung with overdistended alveoli and diminished pulmonary perfusion. SJS is the result of an obliterative bronchiolitis early in life; that is, before pulmonary alveolarization is completed (<8 years of age). Early obliterative bronchiolitis results in concentric fibrosis of the submucosal and peribronchial tissues of the terminal bronchi. As a consequence, progressive peripheral air trapping and diminished pulmonary vascularization will result in pulmonary hypoplasia. SJS is seen after *Mycoplasmal*, streptococcal, or staphylococcal infection. SJS has also been described after severe respiratory syncytial virus or influenza virus bronchiolitis.

The clinical findings are nonspecific. Most children present with wheezing, episodes of hypoxemia, pneumonia, or atelectasis. Occasionally, SJS is clinically asymptomatic and is discovered accidentally on chest films. Pulmonary function tests show abnormal time-attenuation curves during inspiration and a prolonged forced expiration. Air trapping is frequently confirmed. On physical examination a unilateral small chest may be observed. Typically, children with SJS have a history of severe pneumonia, bronchitis, or bronchiolitis before 8 years of age. SJS may become apparent on imaging within a few months of infection but may, however, take several years to become apparent.

Diagnosis of SJS is suggested on plain-film imaging, especially if supported by a history of severe pneumonia in early childhood. Plain-films of the chest will reveal a hyperlucent small lung with small vessels. The mediastinal structures may be shifted to the affected side as a result of hyperinflation of the contralateral lung. An expiration film shows little change in the lung volume, compared with inspiration views. Follow-up chest films may be helpful because the affected lung will not show a significant growth.

Findings on high-resolution computer tomography (CT) include a mosaic pattern of hyperlucency, a paucity of pulmonary vessels, and irregularly dilated and deformed segmental bronchi (cylindrical or saccular bronchiectasis). The contralateral lung is usually hyperexpanded. High-resolution CT should be performed in inspiration and deep expiration if possible. Especially, the forced expiration images will show focal air trapping and the mosaic perfusion pattern.

Differential diagnoses include primary congenital lung hypoplasia, secondary lung hypoplasia after repair of a congenital diaphragmatic hernia, or pulmonary hypoplasia caused by a hypoplastic pulmonary artery. The clinical history usually limits the differential diagnoses. Biopsy is rarely necessary.

SJS
- hyperluscent lung overdistended alveolis, ↓ pulmonary perfusion

- results from obliterative bronchiolitis early in life (<8) before alveolarization is completed.

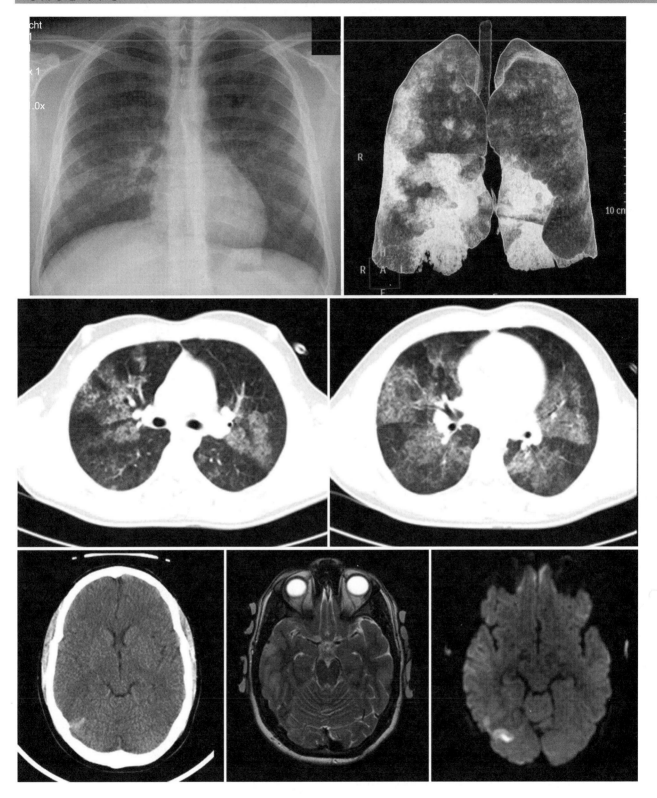

1. What are the imaging findings in this 15-year-old patient with acute hemoptysis, dyspnea, and cough?

2. How would the imaging findings on chest computed tomography (CT) be described?

3. What is the differential diagnosis?

4. Which complication is visualized on CT and magnetic resonance imaging (MRI) (axial T2-weighted and diffusion tensor images)?

Diagnosis: Systemic Lupus Erythematosus

1. Bilateral, ill-defined airspace consolidation without pleural effusion.

2. Patchy, bilateral, predominantly central, ground-glass opacities.

3. Systemic lupus erythematosus (SLE) with acute lupus pneumonitis versus Goodpasture syndrome.

4. Acute right-sided venous thrombosis with temporooccipital venous ischemia.

Reference

Swigris JJ, Fischer A, Gillis J, et al: Pulmonary and thrombotic manifestations of systemic lupus erythematosus, *Chest* 133:271–280, 2008.

Comment

Acute lupus pneumonitis may present with an acute onset of dyspnea, cough, fever, pleuritic chest pain, and, occasionally, hemoptysis. Chest radiographic findings are usually extensive. CT findings are nonspecific with multiple areas of ground-glass opacities that may mimic diffuse alveolar hemorrhage. The distribution is similar to the "crazy paving" pattern as can be observed in Goodpasture disease.

SLE is a systemic autoimmune disease with multisystem involvement. The entire pulmonary system may be affected including the airways, lung parenchyma, vasculature, and pleura or respiratory musculature.

One feared complication of pulmonary involvement is diffuse alveolar hemorrhage. The sudden onset of dyspnea, acute ground-glass opacities, and declining hematocrit with or without hemoptysis should raise the suspicion of diffuse alveolar hemorrhage. Patients with SLE are at increased risk for developing pneumonia as a result of the treatment with glucocorticoids or an immunomodulatory drug. Respiratory distress syndrome may occur in 5% to 15% of patients. Pulmonary arterial hypertension results from the involvement of the pulmonary arteries.

Antiphospholipid antibodies may be present in a significant number of patients and are associated with an increased risk of thrombosis including dural venous thrombosis, as seen in this patient.

Diagnosis can be difficult and relies on the combination of imaging findings and immunologic studies. SLE may have its onset in childhood and is significantly more common in girls than in boys. Pleural and pericardial effusions may be seen in addition to the pulmonary manifestations. Imaging findings are nonspecific, and the initial differential diagnoses include Goodpasture syndrome, extrinsic allergic alveolitis, and various other collagen-vascular diseases.

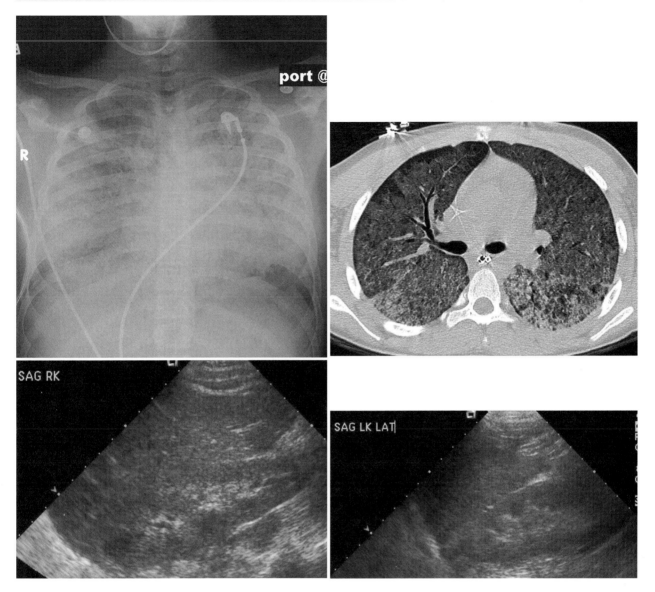

1. This 13-year-old girl presented to the emergency department with hemoptysis. A chest x-ray film (first image) and then a chest computed tomographic (CT) scan (second image) were obtained. What were the findings?

2. What were some differential possibilities for this finding?

3. Her urinalysis showed hyaline casts and red cells; consequently, a renal ultrasound (US) was obtained (third and fourth images). What were the findings?

4. How does this change the differential diagnoses?

Diagnosis: Microscopic Polyangiitis

1. Diffuse alveolar infiltrate consistent with pulmonary hemorrhage.

2. Vasculitis, idiopathic pulmonary hemosiderosis, capillary hemangiomatosis, lymphangioleiomyomatosis, and tuberous sclerosis.

3. Enlarged kidneys (11.5 cm in length) with echogenic parenchyma.

4. Narrowed to include abnormalities that affect both the lungs and the kidneys and include Goodpasture syndrome, Wegener granulomatosis, and microscopic polyangiitis.

References

Bansal PJ, Tobin MC: Neonatal microscopic polyangiitis secondary to transfer of maternal myeloperoxidase-antineutrophil antibody resulting in neonatal pulmonary hemorrhage and renal involvement, *Ann Allergy Asthma Immunol* 93(4):398–401, 2004.

Fotter R, editor: *Pediatric uroradiology*, ed 2, Berlin Heidelberg New York, 2008, Springer, pp 366–367.

Kuhn JP, Slovis TL, Haller JO, editors: *Caffey's pediatric diagnostic imaging*, ed 10, Philadelphia, 2004, Mosby, pp 1057–1059.

Comment

Autoimmune disease has different manifestations, depending on the tissue-specific antibodies involved. One of the antibody markers in vasculitis is myeloperoxidase-antineutrophil cytoplasmic antibody (MPO-ANCA), which was positive in this case. Capillary inflammation and fragility leads to pulmonary hemorrhage in 12% of these patients.

The renal enlargement and echogenicity on US reflected edema and inflammation. A renal biopsy found focal necrotizing and crescentic glomerulonephritis, characteristic of MPO-ANCA positive vasculitis and found in approximately 80% of patients. Goodpasture syndrome also affects kidneys and lungs but through antibasement membrane (ABM) antibodies; these patients are ABM positive but MPO-ANCA negative.

Wegener granulomatosis is also MPO-ANCA positive but has a preponderance of granulomatous inflammation, especially in the upper respiratory tract, which is not a feature of microscopic polyangiitis.

MPO-ANCA is a very potent antibody and crosses the placenta, where it can result in pneumonitis and neonatal pulmonary hemorrhage, as well as renal disease. Exchange transfusion decreases the antibody burden, and steroid administration blunts the effect of the antibodies already in action. Symptoms will abate as long as the infant is not making new antibodies.

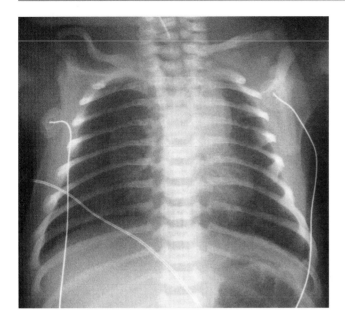

1. Is this newborn infant blue or pink?

2. Why must the ductus arteriosus remain open?

3. This patient had a successful correction but then suffered myocardial infarction. Why?

Diagnosis: Pulmonary Atresia with Intact Ventricular Septum

1. This infant is blue.

2. The ductus arteriosus is the largest supplier of blood flow to the disconnected pulmonary arteries and must be kept open. Prostaglandins must be given to prevent closure of the ductus arteriosus.

3. The small, high-pressure right ventricle (RV) decompresses through the sinusoids to the coronary arteries, which can be otherwise obstructed. When the outflow tract is opened and the RV is no longer high pressure, the sinusoids close and the coronaries and myocardium are without blood supply.

Reference

Park MK: *Pediatric cardiology for practitioners*, ed 4, St Louis, 2002, Mosby, pp 214–218.

Cross-Reference

Blickman JG, Parker BR, Barnes PD: *Pediatric radiology—the requisites*, ed 3, Philadelphia, 2009, Mosby, pp 47–56.

Comment

Pulmonary atresia with an intact ventricular septum is a rare defect, accounting for less than 1% of congenital heart disease. In some ways it represents a step beyond the classic Fallot tetralogy and the tetralogy variant with atresia of the pulmonic valve. In these two abnormalities a ventriculoseptal defect (VSD) exists, and the RV experiences at least a modicum of blood flow and is less severely hypoplastic than where the septum is intact. With pulmonic atresia, the lack of a VSD completely isolates the RV. Moreover, because much of the shaping of the fetal vascular system depends on blood flow passing through it, this defect also results in small, inadequate central pulmonary arteries. Meanwhile, the fetal systemic collateral vessels (including the ductus arteriosus) that connect the aorta to the pulmonary arterial bed persist. An atrial septal defect must also exist to allow right-to-left passage of deoxygenated blood.

The infant who is born with this defect is profoundly hypoxemic. Surgery must first improve pulmonary blood flow, which is usually performed with a Glenn shunt (superior vena cava to the pulmonary artery), if adequate central arteries exist. If not, but enough large aortic collateral vessels exist, these can be *unifocalized* to construct central, shuntable pulmonary arteries. If the RV is adequate in size, it can then be connected to the reconstructed arteries; if not, then it is bypassed with a conduit that brings the inferior vena cava blood back to the pulmonary circulation.

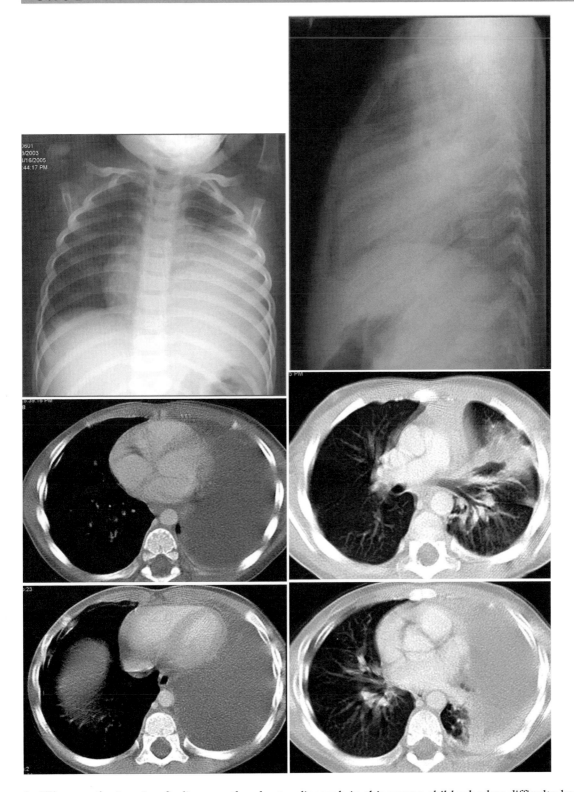

1. What are the imaging findings on the chest radiograph in this young child who has difficulty breathing?

2. A computed tomographic (CT) scan was obtained 2 weeks after symptoms resolved, but the findings on the chest radiograph were essentially unchanged. What were the CT findings?

3. What were the differential diagnoses?

4. What is the most common congenital intrathoracic cyst?

Diagnosis: Pericardial Cyst

1. Opacification of the middle and lower left hemithorax with no significant mediastinal shift, making atelectasis unlikely. The differential diagnosis includes infiltrate with large pleural effusion of space occupying the lesion.

2. A large pericardial cyst, which was described as a nondependent fluid density occupying much of the left hemithorax and originating from the middle mediastinum.

3. Pericardial cyst, bronchogenic cyst, and thymic cyst.

4. The most common intrathoracic cystic lesion is a bronchogenic cyst. Most are found in the middle mediastinum, but they can occur in the posterior mediastinum or, less commonly, between the intrapulmonary arteries.

Cross-Reference
Blickman JG, Parker BR, Barnes PD: *Pediatric radiology—the requisites*, ed 3, Philadelphia, 2009, Mosby, p 59.

Comment
Pericardial cysts are an uncommon benign congenital anomaly in the middle mediastinum. They represent 6% of mediastinal masses and 33% of mediastinal cysts. Other cysts in the mediastinum are bronchogenic (34%), enteric (12%), and thymic and others (21%). Of the middle mediastinum masses, 61% are cysts. Pericardial and bronchogenic cysts share the second most common cause after lymphomas.

The incidence of a pericardial cyst is approximately 1 in 100,000. They are thought to result from a failure of fusion of one of the mesenchymal lacunae that form the pericardial sac; 75% have no associated symptoms and are usually found incidentally during routine chest x-ray or echocardiographic studies.

On a CT scan, pericardial cysts are thin-walled, sharply defined, oval homogeneous masses. Their attenuation is slightly higher than water density—30 to 40 Hounsfield units (HU). They fail to enhance with intravenous contrast.

The indications for resection of pericardial cysts include size, symptoms, patient concern, and an uncertainty of malignant potential, as well as to prevent life-threatening emergencies. Before the development of thoracoscopy, thoracotomy was the approach of choice. Currently, however, video-assisted thoracoscopic surgery (VATS) is the approach most commonly used. The VATS approach has many accepted advantages over open procedures, including cosmetic, improved intraoperative visualization, shorter postoperative recovery, reduced pain, and patient preference.

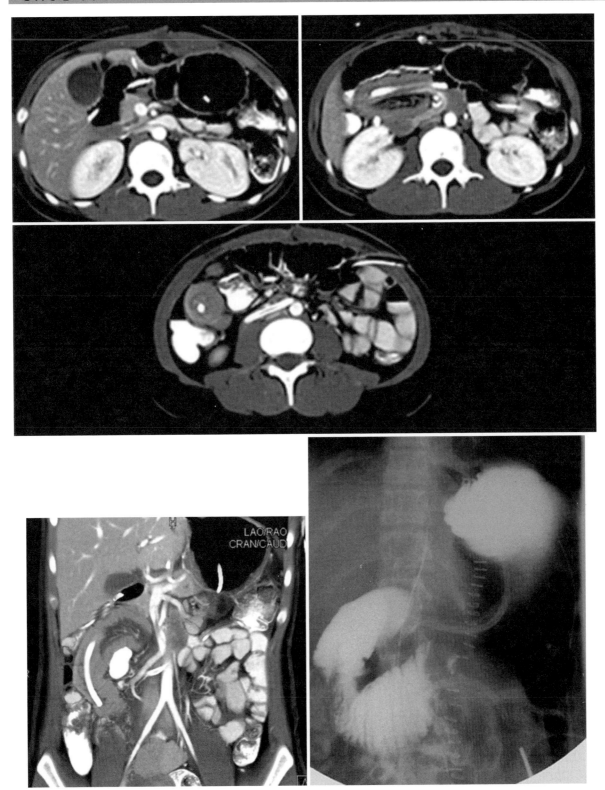

1. What are the most significant findings on computed tomography (CT) and an upper gastrointestinal (UGI) study in this teenager recovering from a stab wound to the right upper quadrant and chest?

2. What symptoms would the patient have?

3. What is the likely cause of this problem?

4. What other causes should be considered?

Diagnosis: Duodenojejunal Intussusception around the Feeding Tube

1. Nearly complete obstruction of the duodenum by duodenojejunal intussusception. A metal-tipped intestinal tube courses through the bowel involved in the intussusception.

2. Bilious vomiting and pain.

3. The feeding tube is likely acting as a lead point for the intussusception.

4. Other lead points should be considered. In this patient, bowel wall hematoma or other bowel wall injury may have been present. A preexisting bowel wall mass may also act as a lead point.

Reference

Redmond P, Ambos M, Berliner L, Pachter HL, et al: Iatrogenic intussusception: a complication of long intestinal tubes, *Am J of Gastroenterol* 77:39-42, 1982.

Cross-Reference

Blickman JG, Parker BR, Barnes PD: *Pediatric radiology—the requisites*, ed 3, Philadelphia, 2009, Mosby, pp 73-75.

Comment

Upper small bowel intussusception is a well-known but uncommon complication of gastrostomy tube placement and intubation of the upper stomach and small bowel. It may be transient; however, it usually results in partial or complete upper intestinal obstruction. A gastrostomy tube may migrate into the duodenum or into even the jejunum and, when pulled back, may result in retrograde duodenogastric or jejunoduodenogastric intussusception, or an antegrade intussusception may occur around a long intestinal tube.

The intussusception may be diagnosed by UGI, CT, or ultrasound examination. UGI examination in this patient shows the nearly complete obstruction of the duodenum with a luminal mass effect at the level of obstruction. CT shows a rounded or sausage-shaped mass that contains multiple layers representing the intussuscepted bowel loops. In this patient, the enteric tube is seen within the intussusception. Ultrasound findings are characteristic with a targetlike mass seen when the intussusception is visualized in a cross-sectional image.

Careful withdrawal of the enteric or gastric tube usually results in the resolution of the intussusception. However, in this patient, removal of the feeding tube and two endoscopic procedures were unsuccessful. The intussusception was easily reduced with laparotomy; however, a small mass was palpated in the proximal jejunum and a short segment was removed. The pathologic examination revealed ulceration and granuloma formation likely to be the result of irritation from the indwelling feeding tube.

The ileocolic type of intussusception is most common in the distal small bowel extending into the colon. This type is most often seen in the young child from 6 months to 3 years of age. It is usually idiopathic, although, perhaps caused by the lymphatic tissue in the bowel wall, which becomes more prominent after a viral illness. In ages below and above the idiopathic range, lead points such as lymphoma, Meckel diverticulum, duplication cyst, or bowel wall hematoma should be considered.

Enteroenteric intussusceptions fall into two general categories: (1) tumor related and (2) postoperative. Both are less likely idiopathic. Tumor- or mass-related intussusceptions are the result of a lead point within the bowel wall that promotes abnormal peristalsis. In addition to those previously listed, other intussusceptions are leiomyomas, polyps, lipomas, metastatic lesions, and rarer entities. Postoperative intussusceptions may be the result of adhesions, abnormal motility, or presence of intestinal tubes as in this patient. With the now-widespread usage of CT imaging, intussusception is more commonly encountered and, in many cases, an insignificant finding.

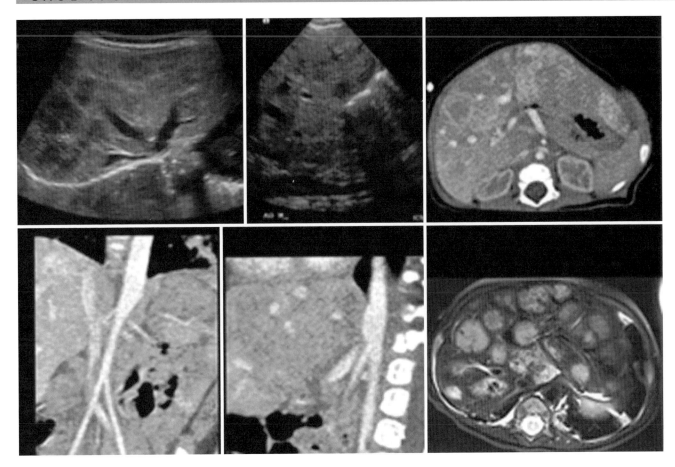

1. What are the findings?

2. What is the likely diagnosis in this 3-month-old infant? Are there any other considerations?

3. What causes the aortic findings?

4. Does the patient need treatment?

Diagnosis: Infantile Hemangioma of the Liver

1. Multiple discrete lesions are visualized in the liver—hypoechoic on ultrasound and low-density on computed tomographic (CT) studies (portovenous phase). Magnetic resonance (MR) imaging shows that the lesions are T2-hyperintense and discrete. As shown on ultrasound and CT, the aorta is wide above the origin of the celiac trunk and smaller below.

2. The diagnosis is multifocal infantile hemangioma of the liver. A significantly less likely diagnosis is a multifocal hepatoblastoma or metastatic neuroblastoma. Imaging findings in these entities would be atypical for hemangioma, and biopsy would be necessary.

3. The significantly increased blood flow and shunting in the liver results in the dramatic caliber change.

4. If the patient is symptomatic, treatment is indicated. With the significant shunting in the liver, this patient presented with heart failure.

Reference

Kassarjian A, Zurakowski D, Dubois J, et al: Infantile hepatic hemangiomas: clinical and imaging findings and their correlation with therapy, *AJR Am J Roentgenol* 182:785–795, 2004.

Cross-Reference

Blickman JG, Parker BR, Barnes PD: *Pediatric radiology—the requisites*, ed 3, Philadelphia, 2009, Mosby, pp 108–109.

Comment

Infantile hemangioma of the liver is a proliferative endothelial cell neoplasm that is characterized by initial rapid growth in the first few months of life and spontaneous involution. In this way, infantile hemangioma of the liver is quite similar to hemangiomas affecting the skin and other organs in infants. It must be differentiated, however, from an epithelioid hemangioendothelioma, which is a tumor that has malignant potential and does not involute.

The infantile hemangioma of the liver may be solitary and large, multifocal or diffuse. Imaging findings are nearly pathognomonic and, in combination with the clinical presentation, may allow determination of follow-up and treatment without biopsy. With ultrasound, the lesions are typically hypoechoic and discrete. Considerable blood often flows in them, hepatic arteries and veins are large, and portal and hepatic venous flow may be more arterial in nature with Doppler interrogation. The aorta tapers just after its take off of the celiac trunk. CT shows low-density lesions with gradual enhancement after intravenous contrast with the lesion filling in from the periphery and eventually becoming isodense with the adjacent normal liver. MR T1-weighted images show slight hypointensity of the lesions, which are bright on T2-weighted sequences. After contrast administration, the enhancement pattern is similar to that seen in CT. The aortic finding is seen in both CT and MR imaging. A calcification associated with this lesion may exist.

Patients with infantile hemangioma of the liver may present with high output heart failure. If the lesion is large or the liver is diffusely involved, abdominal compartment syndrome may occur. Especially in the diffuse type, an association with hypothyroidism exists, probably because the tumor produces high levels of type 3 iodothyronine deiodinase. Often cutaneous hemangiomas are revealed in these patients. Infantile hemangioma of the liver is more common in girls than it is in boys (3-2:1) and greater than one half of patients with these lesions are asymptomatic.

Treatment may be medical, embolization by noninvasive techniques, or surgical. The mainstay of medical management is steroid administration. The use of interferon alfa-2a has been curtailed since the side effect of spastic diplegia has been reported. Recent reports of the addition of Propranolol to the steroid regimen in the treatment of cutaneous lesions, large enough to have associated heart failure, have been encouraging. This treatment was successful in the patient discussed here. Catheter-based intervention, surgical resection, or liver transplant is reserved for patients who are refractory to medical management.

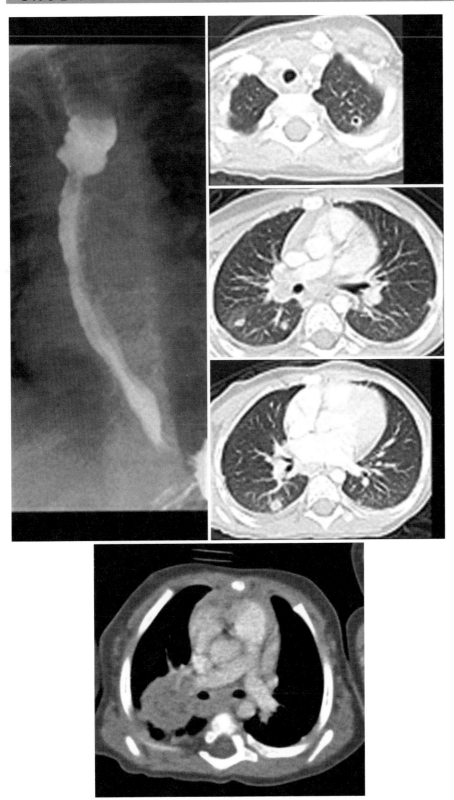

1. What are the findings in these studies of three patients under 10 years of age?

2. All of these patients have had unexplained fevers. What category of disease is most likely?

3. If a biopsy of the lung lesions in two of these patients shows granulomas, what disease should be considered?

4. What causes the esophageal lesions?

Diagnosis: Chronic Granulomatous Disease

1. Findings include nodularity and diffuse narrowing of the distal two thirds of the esophagus; multiple small-lung nodules, one of which is cavitary; and a large, rounded infiltrate or mass with subcarinal fullness.

2. Immunodeficiency is the most likely category.

3. Chronic granulomatous disease (CGD) should be considered.

4. In this patient with CGD and dysphagia, the causes may include granuloma formation, causing obstructive symptoms or dysmotility or both.

Reference

Marciano BE, Rosenzweig SD, Kleiner DE, et al: Gastrointestinal involvement in chronic granulomatous disease, *Pediatrics* 114(2):462–468, 2004.

Cross-Reference

Blickman JG, Parker BR, Barnes PD: *Pediatric radiology—the requisites*, ed 3, Philadelphia, 2009, Mosby, pp 38–39.

Comments

CGD is a genetic immunodeficiency caused by the inability of the phagocyte to kill certain bacteria and fungi because of the reduced production of superoxide anions. This results in recurrent infection and, in addition, the formation of granulomas as a result of an abnormal response to inflammation. Infection is usually caused by catalase-producing organisms. Granulomas are most frequently found in the gastrointestinal tract but may be present in almost any organ of the body.

CGD is an inherited X-linked disorder in 65% of the patients and autosomal recessive in the others. This disease was first described in the 1950s as a constellation of recurrent infection—hypergammaglobulinema, hepatosplenomegaly, and lymphadenopathy—mostly in boys and usually fatal in the first 10 years of life. CGD is now known to be caused by deficiency of nicotinamide adenine dinucleotide phosphate (NADPH) oxidase enzyme of phagocytes. The most common molecular defect in CGD is a mutation in the cytochrome b, b subunit (CYBB) gene. It is located on the X chromosome and encodes for gp91, which is the b subunit of cytochrome b558.

Differential diagnoses include other immunodeficiency syndromes, some of which are leukocyte-adhesion deficiency, human immunodeficiency viral infection, severe combined immunodeficiency, and Wiscott-Aldrich syndrome.

The standard assay for phagocytic oxidase activity is the nitroblue tetrazolium (NBT) test. The colorless compound NBT is reduced to blue formazan by the activity of the NADPH or phagocyte oxidase (phox) enzyme system.

Treatment for CGD includes infection prophylaxis, improvement of neutrophil function, treatment of actual infection, and eradication of the disease. Interferon gamma has proved useful in the long term and reduces infection by improving phagocytosis. Hematopoietic stem cell transplant may be curative; however, it has potentially high morbidity.

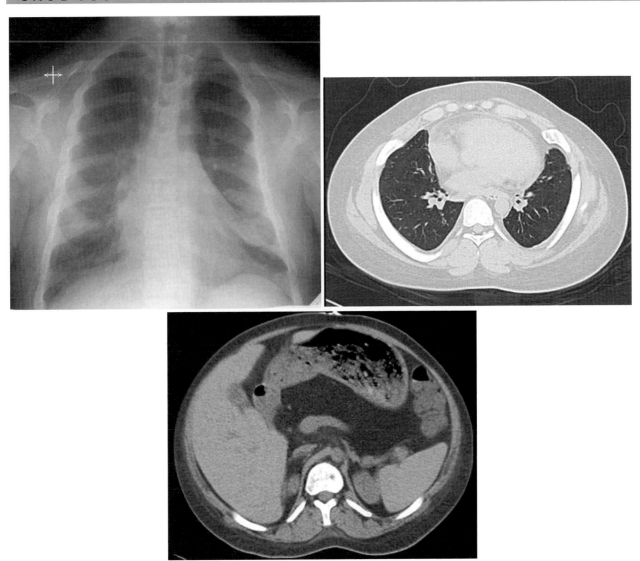

1. What are the imaging findings in a 16-year-old adolescent with short stature and dry skin?

2. What is the diagnosis?

3. What are the differential diagnoses?

4. What is the cause of this condition?

Diagnosis: Shwachman-Diamond Syndrome

1. Narrow thoracic cage, costochondral thickening, short-flaring lower ribs, and fatty replacement of the pancreas.

2. Shwachman-Diamond syndrome (SDS).

3. Cystic fibrosis, Pearson syndrome, severe combined immunodeficiency disease, and thrombocytopenia-absent radius syndrome. *of fatty replacement of pancreas*

4. In most patients, SDS is associated with mutations in the Shwachman-Bodian-Diamond syndrome gene located on chromosome 7. SDS is inherited in an autosomal recessive fashion.

Reference

Robberecht E, Nachtegaele P, Van Rattinghe R, et al: Pancreatic lipomatosis in the Shwachman-Diamond syndrome. Identification by sonography and CT-scan, *Pediatr Radiol* 15(5):348–349, 1985.

Comment

SDS is a rare congenital disorder characterized by exocrine pancreatic insufficiency, bone marrow dysfunction, and skeletal abnormalities. SDS is the second most common cause of inherited pancreatic insufficiency after cystic fibrosis and the third most common inherited bone marrow failure syndrome after Fanconi anemia and Blackfan-Diamond anemia. More than 200 cases of SDS have been reported in the literature.

The patients present with diarrhea, short stature, weight loss, and dry skin. Recurrent bacterial infections of the upper respiratory tract, otitis media, sinusitis, pneumonia, osteomyelitis, bacteremia, skin infections, aphthous stomatitis, fungal dermatitis, and paronychia are common because of a neutropenia-neutrophil migration defect. These patients may appear emaciated with abdominal distension accentuated by hypotonia and hepatomegaly.

Ultrasonographic findings of the pancreas reveal increased echogenicity of the pancreas as a result of fatty infiltration, whereas the same findings reveal as decreased density on computed tomographic studies. The size of the pancreas may be normal or atrophic.

Radiographic findings include delayed bone age and thoracic dysostosis, consisting of costochondral thickening, short-flaring lower ribs, and a narrow thoracic cage that is most obvious when the individual with SDS is younger than 2 years of age. Metaphyseal chondrodysplasia, shortening of the extremities, metaphyseal widening, and "cup" deformity of the ribs (40% to 80%), as well as valgus deformities of the elbows and knees, can be seen.

Imperforate anus and Hirschsprung disease have been associated with SDS. These associations may delay the diagnosis of SDS because the presenting symptom is constipation and not diarrhea. The sweat test helps differentiate SDS from cystic fibrosis. In SDS, no increase in chloride occurs. Pathologically, in contrast to cystic fibrosis, the pancreatic ductal architecture is spared; thus an intact anion secretion and fluid flow occurs.

No therapy has been successful in completely reversing neutropenia, anemia, or thrombocytopenia. Death usually occurs from overwhelming sepsis or malignancy. Median survival age is 35 years for all patients with SDS. For patients whose course is complicated by aplastic anemia, the median survival age is 24 years, whereas patients whose course is complicated by leukemia have a median survival age of 10 years.

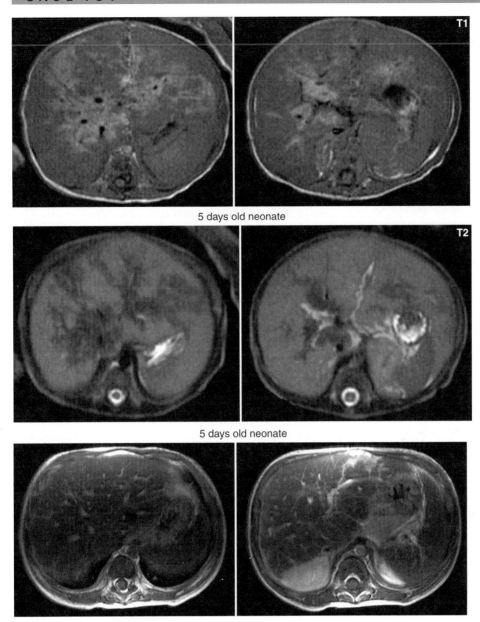

5 days old neonate

5 days old neonate

Follow up at 10 months

1. What is the most likely diagnosis in this neonate?

2. If no additional lesions are present, in what stage would this child be categorized?

3. What finding appeared on follow-up imaging?

4. What is the prognosis?

Diagnosis: Neuroblastoma—Stage 4S

1. Neuroblastoma of the left adrenal gland with extensive liver metastases.

2. Stage 4S, using the International Neuroblastoma Staging System (INSS).

3. Spontaneous regression.

4. The prognosis is favorable.

Reference

Daneman A: Adrenal gland. In Kuhn JP, Slovis TL, Haller JO, editors: *Caffey's pediatric diagnostic imaging*, ed 10, Philadelphia, 2004, Mosby, pp 1894–1908.

Cross-Reference

Blickman JG, Parker BR, Barnes PD: *Pediatric radiology— the requisites*, ed 3, Philadelphia, 2009, Mosby, pp 143–145.

Comment

Neuroblastoma is the most frequent solid neoplasm in childhood (8% to 10%) and the most frequent malignancy in the first year of life. Median age of diagnosis is 22 months. Neuroblastomas arise from neural crest cells either within the adrenal medulla or along the course of the sympathetic nerve chain, which explains why neuroblastomas are found from the neck down into the pelvis. In 90% to 95% of the children, catecholamines are identified in blood or urine samples.

Neuroblastomas may already be present prenatally; the most frequent prenatal location is in the adrenal glands. Most children are symptomatic with local symptoms resulting from the compression of functional structures by the tumor. Horner syndrome can be observed in cervical or mediastinal locations, and hypertonia may result from an encasement of the renal arteries. Neuroblastomas may occasionally be an incidental finding on plain-film radiographs. The tumor may be identified by the local mass effect or by intratumoral, disperse calcifications. Metastases are seen in up to 80% of children. The liver, bone marrow, skin, and lymph nodes may be involved. Bone metastases to the sphenoid bone and retrobulbar soft tissues with resulting orbital proptosis and ecchymosis may be characteristically present and referred to as so-called *raccoon eyes*. In addition, dural metastases may present with widened cranial sutures. Clinically, neuroblastomas may present with a paraneoplastic syndrome known as *opsoclonus-myoclonus syndrome* and is also described as *dancing eyes–dancing feet syndrome*. These children present with cerebellar ataxia and rapid eye movements. In up to 50% of children with this syndrome, a neuroblastoma is found. Neonatal neuroblastomas may show a spontaneous regression of both the primary tumor and the metastases by a maturation of the neuroblastoma cells into benign ganglioneuromas. Several biologic factors have been identified that may predict outcome. An increased lactate dehydrogenase (LDH) and ferritin levels, as well as an N-myc amplification, are related to a less-favorable prognosis. Final prognosis depends on the tumor stage, patient age, site of the primary tumor, and histologic factors. The cure rate for stages I and II neuroblastomas is currently 85% to 90%. In addition, neuroblastoma stage IVS (localized primary tumor as defined for stage I and II with dissemination limited to liver, skin, and/or bone) is also favorable.

Neuroblastomas are usually large on initial diagnosis. Imaging should determine the primary location (intraperitoneal versus retroperitoneal, adrenal versus extraadrenal) and distant disease. Findings suggestive of neuroblastoma are a tumor in a paravertebral location, spinal canal invasion, retroperitoneal vessel encasement, and displacement of the great vessels away from the spine. Midline extension, respectively, extension to or beyond the contralateral pedicle, differentiates stage II from III neuroblastomas. If a tumor surrounds 75% of the circumference of a major retroperitoneal vessel, then surgical resection is usually contraindicated. Intraspinal extension with acute cord compression should be treated with emergent decompressive laminectomy or radiotherapy.

Initial imaging usually includes a plain-film radiograph to search for calcifications and mass effect, followed by ultrasound examinations. Final staging should be performed either by contrast-enhanced computed tomography or preferably multiplanar magnetic resonance imaging, possibly combined with magnetic resonance angiography. Metaiodobenzylguanidine (MIBG) nuclear medicine studies are helpful in identifying the primary tumor and bone marrow involvement.

Differential diagnosis is wide. The most frequent adrenal mass in a neonate is a hemorrhage. These lesions will, however, show a characteristic evolution or regression on follow-up ultrasound. Adrenal carcinomas represent less than 1% of all adrenal neoplasms. Adrenal adenomas, aldosteronomas, and pheochromocytomas are very rare in children.

The presented case shows impressively how a stage 4S neuroblastoma can regress spontaneously without chemotherapy, radiotherapy, or surgery. The signal intensity of the liver recovered nearly completely, and the primary adrenal lesion disappeared.

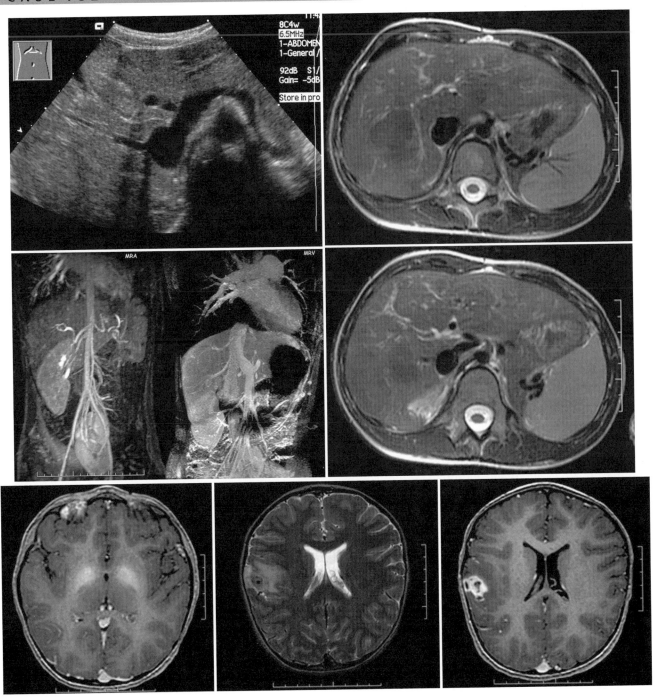

1. What are the imaging findings on ultrasonography (US), magnetic resonance imaging (MRI), magnetic resonance angiography (MRA), and magnetic resonance venography (MRV) in this 6-year-old girl with cyanosis and tachycardia?

2. What are the findings on a brain MRI?

3. What is the diagnosis?

4. How can the cerebral complication be explained?

Diagnosis: Congenital Absence of the Portal Vein (Abernethy Type Ib)

1. US shows anomalous drainage of the splenic vein into the inferior vena cava (IVC). MRI, MRA, and MRV studies reveal an absent portal vein, a patent hepatic artery, anomalous drainage of the splenic and superior mesenteric veins into the IVC, a left-sided pelvic kidney, and multiple focal hepatic nodules.

2. T1-hyperintensity of the lentiform nuclei, which indicates hepatic encephalopathy and a peripheral-enhancing septic embolus in the right temporal lobe.

3. Congenital absence of the portal vein (Abernethy type Ib) with a portosystemic shunt.

4. By a septic embolus into the brain as a result of multiple pulmonary arteriovenous shunts.

Reference

Niwa T, Aida N, Tachibana K, et al: Congenital absence of the portal vein: clinical and radiologic findings, *J Comput Assist Tomogr* 26(5):681–686, 2002.

Comment

The congenital absence of the portal vein is a rare malformation in which the mesenteric and splenic veins drain directly into the IVC, renal vein, or iliac vein. This congenital portosystemic shunt basically bypasses the liver. The liver has a normal arterial blood supply over the hepatic artery and drains into the IVC through the hepatic veins. The congenital absence of the portal vein is the result of the abnormal development of the portal venous system from the fourth through the tenth week of gestation. Portosystemic anomalies are classified in two groups: type I—the portal blood is completely diverted into the IVC as a result of an absent portal vein; and type II—the portal vein is intact, but portal blood is diverted into the IVC through a side-to-side extrahepatic communication. Type I is again subclassified into type Ia, in which the superior mesenteric and splenic veins do not join, and type Ib, in which the superior mesenteric and splenic veins join before draining into a systemic vein. Portosystemic shunting causes hypergalactosemia as a result of bypassing the liver. Increased blood galactose should raise the suggestion of a portal vein anomaly.

The congenital absence of the portal vein may be associated with other congenital anomalies including cardiac defects, biliary atresia, and polysplenia.

The portosystemic shunt with hyperammonemia may result in a portosystemic encephalopathy, frequently identified by an increased T1-weighted signal of the lentiform nuclei within the brain. In addition, the hyperammonemia may result in multiple arteriovenous shunts within the lungs. The cause remains unclear. As in this child, the arteriovenous shunts may present with cyanosis and tachycardia. In addition, this shunting is believed to increase the risk for septic emboli in, for example, the brain. After this child suffered from an episode with a seizure, a brain MRI revealed a septic embolus at the corticomedullary junction of the right temporal lobe.

Finally, the congenital absence of the portal vein may result in focal nodular hyperplasia of the liver. In addition, liver masses such as adenoma, hepatoblastoma, and hepatocellular carcinoma may exist.

US is usually the first-line imaging modality that reveals the congenital absence of the portal vein and anomalous drainage of the splenic and mesenteric veins. MRI is helpful in the exact delineation of the malformation and may rule out additional lesions. Chest CT or lung perfusion-ventilation scintigraphy should be considered to rule out pulmonary arteriovenous fistula. Treatment is usually symptomatic; if patients do not respond to medical therapy, then liver transplantation may be considered.

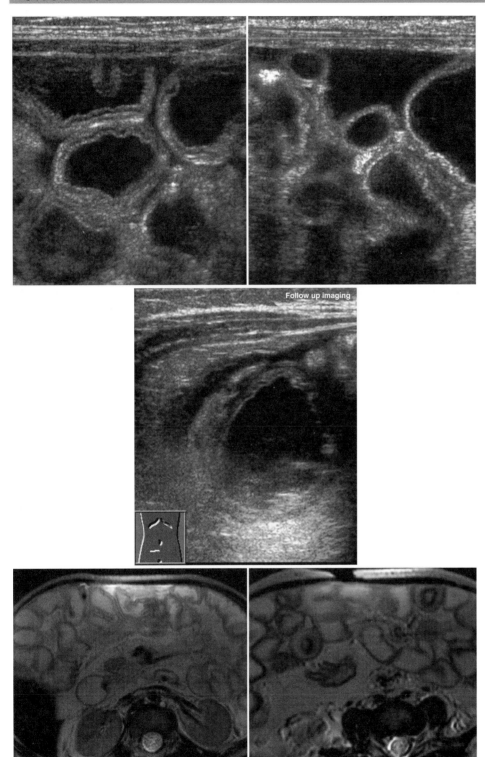

Follow up imaging

1. What are the imaging findings on ultrasonography (US) and magnetic resonance imaging (MRI) in this boy with bilateral lower limb edema?

2. What is the most likely diagnosis?

3. What are the differential diagnoses?

4. Which treatment was performed before the follow-up US was performed?

Diagnosis: Primary Intestinal Lymphangiectasia (Waldmann Disease)

1. Submucosal fluid collection along multiple small bowel loops, fluid within the bowel loops, and ascites.

2. Primary intestinal lymphangiectasia (PIL).

3. Secondary intestinal lymphangiectasia as a result of intestinal lymphoma, lymphenteric fistula, Whipple disease, Crohn disease, intestinal tuberculosis, or sarcoidosis.

4. A low-fat diet with medium-chain triglyceride supplementation.

Reference

Vignes S, Bellanger J: Primary intestinal lymphangiectasia (Waldmann's disease), *Orphanet J Rare Dis* 3:5, 2008.

Comment

PIL is a rare disorder first described in 1961 by Waldmann and colleagues (Waldmann disease) and is characterized by dilated submucosal lymph vessels along the small bowel. Consequently, lymph leaks into the intestinal lumen and into the peritoneal cavity and may result in a protein-losing enteropathy with hypoalbuminemia, hypogammaglobulinemia, and lymphopenia. The low-serum albumin and hypoproteinemia may present with bilateral lower limb edema, anasarca, pleural effusion, pericardial effusion, and chylous ascites. In addition, children may present with fatigue, abdominal pain, nausea, inability to gain weight (or even weight loss), growth retardation, and various symptoms resulting from malabsorption (e.g., vitamin deficiencies, hypocalcemia with resulting convulsions). PIL is generally diagnosed before the patient is 3 years of age. The cause remains unclear. High-resolution US examinations of the bowel, which will show submucosal, linear fluid collections that indicate intestinal lymphangiectasia combined with fluid within the bowel loops and ascites, can aid in determining the diagnosis. Magnetic resonance imaging (MRI) will reveal similar findings with T2-hyperintense submucosal fluid collections, dilated lymphatics within the villi, and a "halo or target sign." Diagnosis may be confirmed by intestinal biopsy. Treatment includes a low-fat diet with medium-chain triglyceride supplementation. The absence of fat in the diet limits the degree of intestinal lymphangiectasia. Consequently, intestinal MRI before and after maintaining a low-fat diet may show the dynamics of PIL. As presented in this patient, the degree of submucosal intestinal lymphangiectasia and chylous ascites decreased after 1 week on a fat-free diet (images not shown). PIL should be differentiated from secondary intestinal lymphangiectasia, which may result from intestinal lymphoma, lymphenteric fistula, Whipple disease, Crohn disease, intestinal tuberculosis, or sarcoidosis. The prognosis is favorable if the patients comply with a life-long low-fat diet.

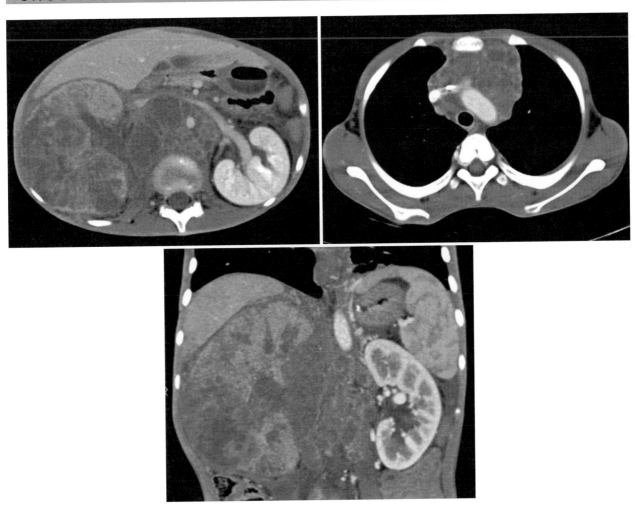

1. What can be seen in the imaging findings of this teenage patient?

2. What are the differential diagnoses?

3. If the patient has sickle cell disease, what is the likely cell type?

4. What is the prognosis of this condition?

Diagnosis: Renal Medullary Carcinoma

1. Multifocal mass in the right kidney, diffuse peritoneal and retroperitoneal masses, and inhomogeneous masses in the mediastinum.

2. Primary renal tumors such as renal cell carcinoma (clear cell) and its rare subtypes, Wilms tumor, clear cell sarcoma, rhabdoid tumor, and mesoblastic nephroma with widespread metastasis. Lymphoma not likely because only one kidney is involved.

3. Renal medullary carcinoma.

4. Almost always metastatic at diagnosis and is eventually fatal.

Reference

Prasad SR, Humphrey PA, Catena JR, et al: Common and uncommon histologic subtypes of renal cell carcinoma: imaging spectrum with pathologic correlation, *Radiographics* 26(6):1795–1806, 2006.

Cross-Reference

Blickman JG, Parker BR, Barnes PD: *Pediatric radiology— the requisites*, ed 3, Philadelphia, 2009, Mosby, pp 140–145.

Comments

Renal medullary carcinoma, also referred to as the seventh sickle cell nephropathy, is a very rare malignant neoplasm seen almost exclusively in patients with sickle cell hemoglobinopathy. It is believed to arise from the medullary collecting ducts and can be confused histologically with another rare type of renal cell carcinoma called *collecting duct carcinoma*. The association with sickle cell disease is helpful in making the proper diagnosis. Medullary carcinoma occurs in a younger population; age range is 10 to 40 years of age (the mean age is 22 years). Collecting duct carcinoma occurs between the ages of 13 and 83 years (the mean age is 55 years). Both tumors are aggressive and commonly metastatic at presentation. The mean duration of survival for patients diagnosed with medullary carcinoma is 15 weeks.

Grossly, the tumor appears as an infiltrative, heterogeneous kidney mass with a medullary epicenter when small. It may be multifocal within the kidney. Histological analysis shows poorly differentiated, mucin-producing eosinophilic cells in sheets with inflammatory, fibrous or edematous stroma. Sickled erythrocytes are found in most tumors.

The tumor is also heterogeneous in appearance by all imaging modalities. This heterogeneity is due to the presence of necrosis and hemorrhage in parts of the tumor. The tumor is hypovascular by angiogram. Spread is lymphatic and hematogenous; in addition to regional and distant lymph nodes, the liver and lung are often involved by metastasis.

The relationship between sickle cell disease and renal medullary carcinoma is not known. One theory is that this carcinoma arises from caliceal epithelium and patients with sickle cell disease have been shown to have epithelial proliferation of the terminal collecting ducts in the adjacent papillary mucosa. This proliferation of epithelial cells may predispose a patient to the development of the neoplasm.

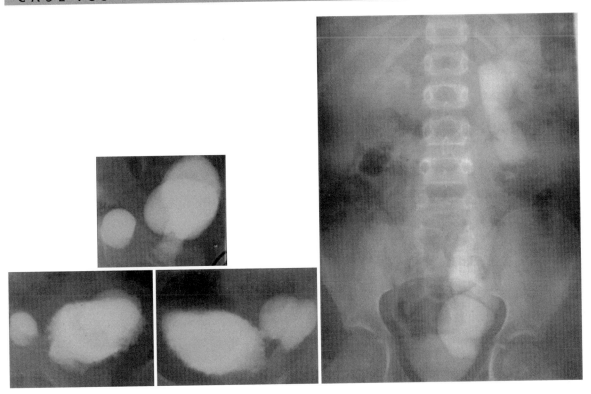

1. What can be seen on these postvoid images of a school-age boy from a voiding cystourethrogram (VCUG) and subsequent intravenous pyelogram (IVP)?

2. What is the diagnosis?

3. What is the cause of this abnormality?

4. What are some associated syndromes and conditions?

Diagnosis: Bladder Diverticulum

1. The findings include two diverticula, one rightward and the other leftward, both low in the bladder, and each considered a so-called *Hutch diverticulum*. The IVP shows evidence of a distal left ureteral obstruction.

2. Bladder diverticulum, an obstruction of the left ureter at the ureterovesical junction (UVJ), secondary to the Hutch diverticulum (paraureteral).

3. A weakness in the detrusor muscle with herniation of the bladder mucosa through the defect.

4. Menkes syndrome, Ehlers-Danlos syndrome, cutis laxa, and Williams syndrome are associated with congenital diverticulum.

Reference

Nguyen HT, Cilento BG Jr.: Bladder diverticula, urachal anomolies, and other uncommon anomalies of the bladder. In Gearhart JP, Rink RC, Mouriquand PD, editors: *Pediatric urology*, Philadelphia, 2001, Saunders, pp 565–568.

Cross-Reference

Blickman JG, Parker BR, Barnes PD: *Pediatric radiology—the requisites*, ed 3, Philadelphia, 2009, Mosby, pp 125–126.

Comments

Bladder diverticulum may be acquired or congenital. Acquired diverticula are usually associated with a trabeculated bladder and are multiple. They are usually the result of bladder outlet obstruction, infection, or iatrogenic causes such as a complication of ureteral reimplantation. Congenital diverticula are more likely solitary, occurring in an otherwise normal bladder, and more frequently found in boys. The diverticulum may be broad based or narrow necked, depending on the size of the bladder musculature defect. The congenital type often occurs near the trigone and may affect the nearby UVJ. They may contribute to the development of vesicoureteral reflux (only inevitable if the ureter inserts directly into the diverticulum). However, reflux associated with a paraureteric diverticulum may resolve spontaneously. In 5% of patients with paraureteric diverticula, ureteral obstruction develops, as in this patient. The diverticulum compresses the ureter, and inflammation or infection leads to fibrosis and scarring and ultimately obstruction. Large diverticula can be a source of urinary stasis and predispose the patient to urinary tract infection.

Detecting diverticula is sometimes challenging because of their dynamic quality and their elusive nature. On VCUG, they may be easier to see at the end of voiding. They are more difficult to visualize on bladder ultrasonography and are rarely shown by IVP.

Surgery is indicated if any of these complications occur.

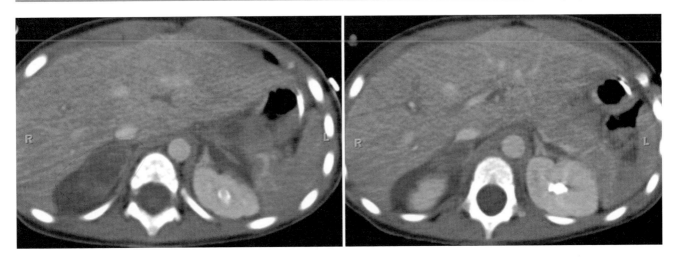

1. What are the findings on these two images of this infant?

2. What may be the cause?

3. Can this condition occur spontaneously?

4. What other imaging can be used to follow or further evaluate the process?

Diagnosis: Adrenal Hemorrhage

1. Low density in and around the enlarged right adrenal gland is demonstrated, as well as some fluid around the left adrenal gland.

2. Abdominal trauma with adrenal hemorrhage is a common cause. Adrenal neoplastic masses are usually not primarily hypodense on computed tomographic (CT) images; but neuroblastoma can be complicated by hemorrhage or have cystic components that may result in areas of hypodensity.

3. In a newborn, adrenal hemorrhage may be spontaneous; that is, related to birth or the stress of other perinatal illnesses.

4. If spontaneous hemorrhage is suggested, ultrasonography (US) is the best way to follow the lesion. If a concern for neoplasm exists, magnetic resonance imaging (MRI) allows for the detection of any significant solid component and definitive identification of blood and its by-products.

Reference

Westra SJ, Zaninovic AC, Hall TR, et al: Imaging of the adrenal gland in children, *Radiographics* 14(6): 1323–1340, 1994.

Cross-Reference

Blickman JG, Parker BR, Barnes PD: *Pediatric radiology— the requisites*, ed 3, Philadelphia, 2009, Mosby, pp 143–144.

Comments

The patient in this case was the victim of child abuse and had a fatal brain injury. Adrenal hemorrhage is an uncommon result of accidental and nonaccidental abdominal trauma. Typically, no significant sequelae of this injury are found, even in bilateral involvement. Adrenal function is normal. Right lobe hepatic or renal injury is frequently associated.

Adrenal hemorrhage in the newborn is usually asymptomatic but may result in a palpable mass, hypovolemic shock, anemia, and jaundice. Its cause is not known, but birth trauma, especially in a large infant, and serious illnesses, which include sepsis and hypoxia, have been proposed as causes. Adrenal hemorrhage is associated with renal vein thrombosis, especially on the left side.

The CT finding of ovoid hypodense material within the center of the adrenal gland and the retention of a roughly triangular-shaped gland are typical of traumatic adrenal hemorrhage.

Adrenal hemorrhage in the newborn is usually found with US and, in most cases, can be followed with US.

The amount of hemorrhage varies from small to so large that the gland itself is no longer visible, and the kidney is displaced inferiorly. Hemorrhage may be echogenic acutely and then it resolves in stages, first mixed in echogenicity and finally sonolucent as the blood clot liquefies. Calcification can be seen at the site of adrenal hemorrhage. This is a late development, and the mass has usually completely resolved by this time. If calcifications are seen in an adrenal mass in a neonate, neuroblastoma becomes more likely.

Although MRI may allow differentiation between a neoplasm and hemorrhage when other studies are inconclusive, it cannot reliably differentiate adrenal hemorrhage from a hemorrhagic tumor in all patients. MRI is most useful to confirm the presence and chronicity of hemorrhage associated with an adrenal mass. Determination of the age of the hemorrhage is especially useful when child abuse is suspected. Acute adrenal hemorrhage less than 7 days old is isointense or slightly low in signal on T1-weighted images and significantly low in signal on T2-weighted images as a result of intracellular deoxyhemoglobin. During the subacute phase (1 to 8 weeks), the clot begins to evolve. On T1-weighted images, a hyperintense rim signal is observed; if the hemorrhage is large, hyperintense T2-weighted signal is seen in the liquefying clot. In the chronic phase, both hemosiderin and calcification result in low signal on T1- and T2-weighted images.

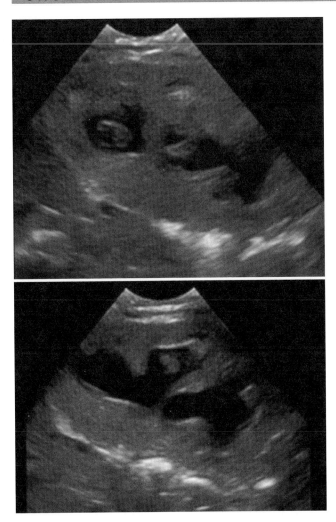

1. What are the findings in these images of a premature infant?

2. What are the differential diagnoses?

3. What tests are helpful in differentiating the causes of the finding?

4. Why are the kidneys vulnerable to fungal disease?

Diagnosis: Fungal Disease Kidneys

1. Several rounded echogenic nonshadowing masses in the dilated renal collecting system.

2. Fungal balls, blood clots, other formed debris in the infection, and nonshadowing stones.

3. Urinalysis and a urine culture.

4. In the premature infant, systemic candidiasis is a well-known entity. Because blood flow to the kidneys is up to 25% of the cardiac output, the organ is commonly infected.

Reference

Benjamin DK Jr, Fisher RG, McKinney RE Jr, et al: Candidal mycetoma in the neonatal kidney, *Pediatrics* 104:1126–1129, 1999.

Comments

Prematurity, low–birth weight, central venous access, the use of broad-spectrum antibiotics, intravenous lipids, and total parenteral nutrition are all risk factors for candidemia. A sustained and ongoing decline in the platelet count over several days is another common finding in candidemia. In the cited study, 33% of patients with candidemia and subsequent renal ultrasound examination had fungal balls or mycetomas. Not all of these patients had positive urine cultures. Ultrasound findings of fungal disease are nonspecific and include the presence of nonshadowing echogenic debris within the collecting system, fungal balls within a dilated collecting system, or echogenic focus in the region of the nondilated collecting system. No urinalysis abnormality is known to correlate with the presence of fungus by culture; however, the urinalysis may suggest other causes of the ultrasound findings. In the right clinical setting, the presence of suggestive findings on ultrasound examination is sufficient to begin the patient on antifungal therapy.

No long-term effect of kidney fungal disease on renal function is documented. Antifungal therapy may be stopped before the ultrasound findings have cleared because the imaging abnormalities may persist long after viable organisms are present. In fact, seeing no obvious improvement in the ultrasound long after the urine culture is negative is not unusual. Continuing therapy until the urine culture is negative, however, is important.

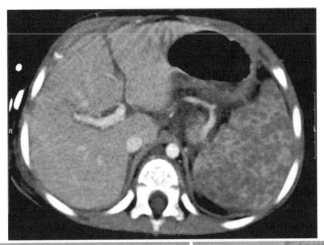

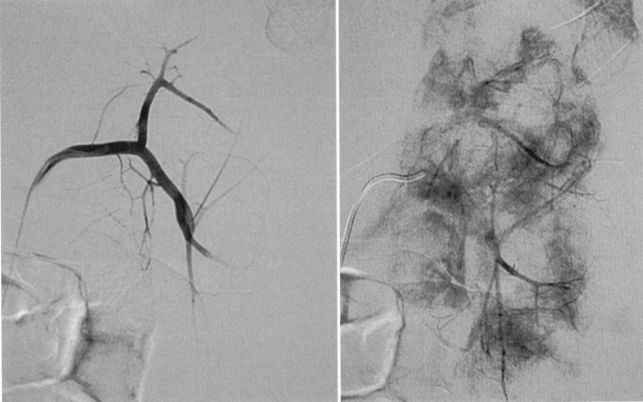

1. What are the imaging findings in this infant with skin lesions and thrombocytopenia? What is the likely diagnosis?

2. What is the most common type of tumor involved?

3. What is the typical clinical presentation?

4. What is the treatment?

Diagnosis: Kasabach-Merritt Syndrome

1. A contrast-enhanced computerized axial tomographic (CAT) scan and computed tomographic angiography (CTA) demonstrate a large vascular tumor of the spleen. The most likely diagnosis is Kasabach-Merritt syndrome (KMS), which is also known as hemangioma-thrombocytopenia syndrome. It consists of thrombocytopenia and coagulopathy secondary to a vascular tumor. The vascular lesion triggers intravascular coagulation with platelet trapping and activation and consumption of coagulation factors.

consumptive

2. Hemangioendothelioma is the most common vascular tumor involved with KMS.

3. Patients with KMS typically present with a reddish-brown skin lesion that evolves into a bulging mass found in the trunk, upper and lower extremities, retroperitoneum, and in the cervical and facial areas.

4. Treatment is typically surgical resection, if possible, or embolization of the vascular lesion with interventional radiology.

Reference

Blei F, Karp N, Rofsky N, et al: Successful multimodal therapy for kaposiform hemangioendothelioma complicated by Kasabach-Merritt phenomenon: case report and review of the literature, *Pediatr Hematol Oncol* 15(4):295–305, 1998.

Cross-Reference

Blickman JG, Parker BR, Barnes PD: *Pediatric radiology—the requisites*, ed 3, Philadelphia, 2009, Mosby, p 109.

Comment

KMS is a rare disease, usually seen in newborns or young infants, in which a vascular tumor leads to thrombocytopenia and coagulopathy. It is also known as hemangioma-thrombocytopenia syndrome. The vascular lesion triggers intravascular coagulation with platelet trapping and activation and consumption of coagulation factors. Males are affected more frequently than females.

KMS is usually caused by a hemangioendothelioma, especially the kaposiform type. Although these tumors are relatively common, they rarely cause KMS. The natural history of kaposiform hemangioendothelioma is that of slow regression, with the lesion leaving a reddish-brown discoloration. Large lesions do not become completely involuted. When these tumors are large or are growing rapidly, they can trap platelets, causing severe thrombocytopenia.

KMS may be lethal; the estimated overall mortality rate ranges from 10% to 37%. The typical patient initially presents with a reddish-brown skin lesion that evolves into a bulging mass. Tumors can be found in the trunk, upper and lower extremities, retroperitoneum, and in the cervical and facial areas. Generally, treatment of the underlying vascular tumor results in a resolution of KMS. If complete surgical resection is feasible, it provides a good opportunity for cure. If surgery is not possible, various other techniques can be used to control the tumor, especially embolization by interventional radiology.

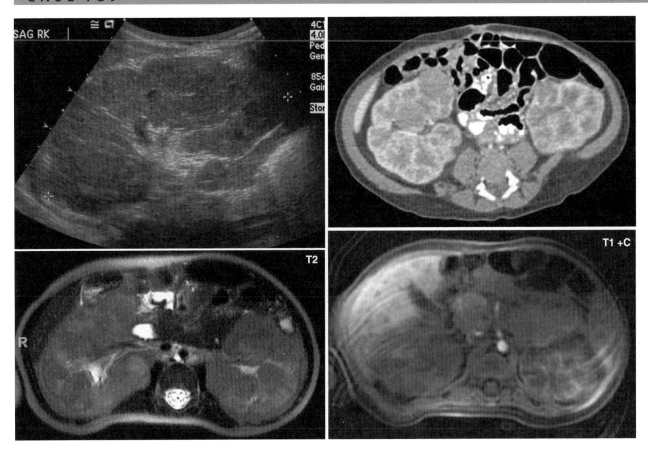

1. What are the imaging findings in this 1-year-old boy?

2. What is the diagnosis?

3. What are the differential diagnoses?

4. What is the cause?

Diagnosis: Beckwith-Wiedemann Syndrome

1. Findings include bilateral apparent enlargement of the kidneys, with multiple hypodense and hypointense, peripherally located, crescent-shaped renal masses, representing nephroblastomatosis. In addition, an enlargement of the pancreatic head is demonstrated. Radiographs of the lower extremities show an asymmetric overgrowth of the right lower extremity.

2. Beckwith-Wiedemann syndrome (BWS).

3. WAGR (**W**ilms tumor, **A**niridia, **G**enitourinary anomalies, and mental **R**etardation) syndrome, Perlman syndrome, Simpson-Golabi-Behmel syndrome, Sotos syndrome, glycogen storage disease, hyperpituitarism, omphalocele and gastroschisis, and persistent hyperinsulinemic hypoglycemia of infancy.

4. BWS is caused by alterations in the growth regulatory genes on chromosome region 11, position 15.5.

Reference
Cohen MM: Beckwith-Wiedemann syndrome: historical, clinicopathological, and etiopathogenetic perspectives, *Pediatr Dev Pathol* 8(3):287–304, 2005.

Cross-Reference
Blickman JG, Parker BR, Barnes PD: *Pediatric radiology—the requisites*, ed 3, Philadelphia, 2009, Mosby, p 113.

Comment
BWS is the most common and best-known congenital overgrowth syndrome characterized by exomphalos (anterior abdominal wall defect), macroglossia, gigantism, hemihypertrophy, and visceromegaly. In 1964 in Germany, Hans-Rudolf Wiedemann reported a familial form of omphalocele with macroglossia. In 1969, J. Bruce Beckwith of Loma Linda University in California described a similar series of patients. Originally, Professor Wiedemann coined the term *EMG syndrome* to describe the combination of congenital exomphalos, macroglossia, and gigantism. Over time, however, this constellation was renamed BWS.

The incidence is estimated to be approximately 1 in 13,700 births. Of the known cases, 85% are sporadic, and the remainder has autosomal dominant inheritance with variable expressivity and incomplete penetrance.

The clinical features are prenatal and postnatal overgrowth, macroglossia, anterior abdominal wall defects (most commonly, exomphalos), and neonatal hypoglycemia. Mental retardation and mild microcephaly are common. Strict maintenance of euglycemia reduces the risk of nervous tissue damage. Mandibular progratism,

organomegaly (most commonly nephromegaly), and hepatomegaly are seen. Skeletal age may be advanced, and metaphyseal widening and cortical thickening may be demonstrated. In addition, an increased risk of adrenal hemorrhage or hemorrhagic cysts and adrenal calcifications exists with BWS.

An increased risk of embryonal tumors is reported. Wilms tumor is the most common cancer in children with BWS, occurring in approximately 5% to 7% of all children with BWS. The second most common cancer occurring in patients with BWS is hepatoblastoma in those up to 1 year of age. Most children develop Wilms tumor before 4 years of age.

Tumor surveillance includes quarterly evaluation with abdominal ultrasound to the age of 8 years, as well as serum alpha-fetoprotein (AFP) to the age of 5 years. Screening for cancer is recommended in children with BWS, despite the observation that cancer does not develop in most children with BWS. Cancer develops in approximately 1 in 10 children with BWS; however, this risk is high enough to warrant cancer screening. The risk of cancer is dependent on age; the risk is higher in patients younger than 4 years of age. Intervals of 3 to 6 months are recommended for imaging. Longitudinal abdominal ultrasonography is the modality of choice, considering the lack of ionizing of radiation and short-time intervals for screening. In patients when the decision is difficult, contrast-enhanced magnetic resonance imaging or computed tomography can be performed. AFP levels are also measured to monitor for hepatoblastoma. Neuroblastoma, rhabdomyosarcoma, or adrenocortical carcinoma can also be seen. Fortunately, these cancers are rare in children with BWS, and screening for these has no proven benefit.

WAGR syndrome carries more than a 50% prevalence of Wilms tumor (compared with 5% in patients with BWS) and is differentiated from BWS because of its association with 11p13 deletion or mutation of the WT1 tumor–suppressor gene, aniridia, and genitourinary defects.

Prognosis depends on the expressivity of the gene and malignant transformation.

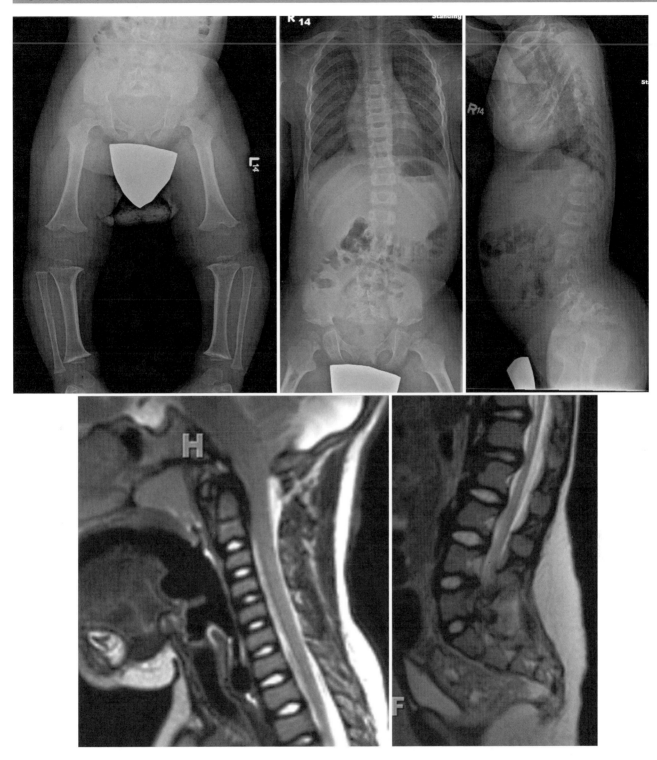

1. Based on the first, second, and third images, describe this image of skeletal dysplasia in a 3-year-old child.

2. Describe what the radiograph of the skull would show.

3. What two skeletal sites account for most of the neurologic morbidity in these patients (fourth and fifth images)?

CASE 190

Diagnosis: Achondroplasia

1. A shortening of all tubular bones with a disproportionate shortening of the proximal segments (rhizomelic micromelia), a decrease in the interpediculate distances from the thorax to the sacrum, a narrowing of the foramen magnum, and posterior vertebral scalloping.

2. A large calvarium with frontal bossing and a small skull base.

3. The lumbar spinal canal and the foramen magnum.

References

Spranger JW, Brill PW, Poznanski AK: *Bone dysplasias: an atlas of genetic disorders of skeletal development*, ed 2, New York, 2002, Oxford University Press, pp 83-89.

Taybi H, Lachman RS: *Radiology of syndromes, metabolic disorders, and skeletal dysplasias*, ed 4, St. Louis, 1996, Mosby, pp 749-755.

Cross-Reference

Blickman JG, Parker BR, Barnes PD: *Pediatric radiology—the requisites*, ed 3, Philadelphia, 2009, Mosby, pp 164-168 and 281-283.

Comment

Achondroplasia originates in a mutation of a gene that controls the fibroblast growth factor, resulting in deficient enchondral growth. It has autosomal dominant inheritance, but most cases are new mutations, born to unaffected parents. Because this anomaly is often diagnosed prenatally (short femurs seen on ultrasound), appropriate perinatal care can be provided and most infants survive. Therefore achondroplasia is one of the more frequently encountered forms of dwarfism in daily practice.

The result of the enchondral growth deficit is most evident in the skull, where the calvarium is normal to enlarged (membranous ossification) and the skull base is small (enchondral ossification). Initial problems are predominately respiratory as a result of the narrow nasal passages and small thorax. Cervicomedullary compression becomes apparent in childhood, whereas nerve root compression from osteophyte formation and disk herniation into the already-narrow spinal canal plague middle-aged patients.

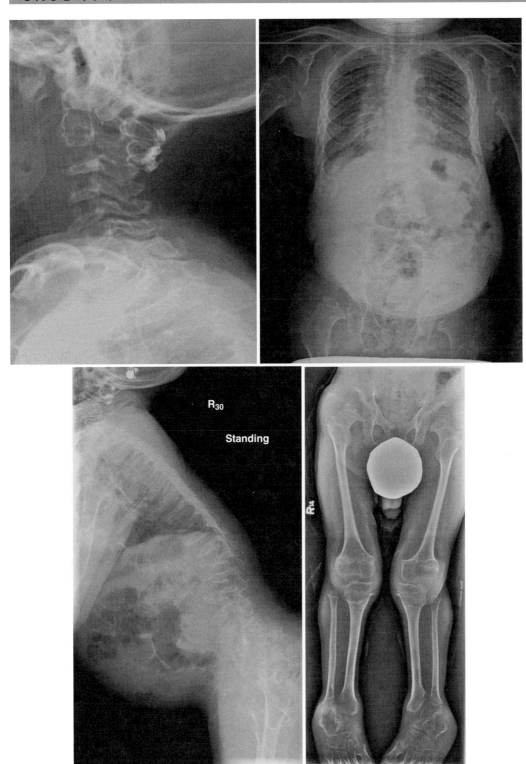

1. A 16-year-old male adolescent comes in for evaluation of scoliosis. What are the plain-film radiographic findings (first through fourth images)?

2. This group of bony findings is known as what?

3. The urine will test positive for what class of compounds?

4. What eponymous syndromes share some of these same bony changes?

Diagnosis: Dysostosis Multiplex—Mucopolysaccharidosis Type IV: Morquio Syndrome

1. Platyspondylia, thoracolumbar kyphosis, oarlike ribs, small dysplastic tarsal bones in a wedge-shape and V-shaped distortion of the distal tibia and fibula, short-thick elevated scapulae with poorly-formed glenoid fossae, aseptic necrosis of the femoral heads, a poorly formed acetabula, shortened limb bones with widened metaphyses, odontoid hypoplasia, and atlantoaxial instability (necessitating fusion).

2. Dysostosis multiplex.

3. The urine will test positive for mucopolysaccharides (keratan sulfate) in this case.

4. Morquio, Hunter, Hurler, Maroteaux-Lamy, Scheie, Sanfilippo, and Sly.

References

Spranger JW, Brill PW, Poznanski AK: *Bone dysplasias: an atlas of genetic disorders of skeletal development*, ed 2, New York, 2002, Oxford University Press, pp 261–262 and 281–286.

Taybi H, Lachman RS: *Radiology of syndromes, metabolic disorders, and skeletal dysplasias*, ed 4, Baltimore, 1996, Mosby, p 669 and 677–679.

Cross-Reference

Blickman JG, Parker BR, Barnes PD: *Pediatric radiology—the requisites*, ed 3, Philadelphia, 2009, Mosby, pp 167 and 282–283.

Comment

This spectrum of bony changes is also shared by other complex carbohydrate storage diseases (e.g., mucolipidosis, gangliosidosis, sialidosis, mannosidosis, galactosidosis, fucosidosis) which, though individually rare, combine in number to make dysostosis multiplex a more frequent occurrence. Other components of the pattern not illustrated here are macrocephaly with J-shaped sella, dysplastic carpal bones, and proximal tapering of metacarpals 2 through 5, resulting in a V shape with similar distortion of the distal radius and ulna. A great variability in the degree of expression of the bony changes among syndromes, within syndromes, and even in the same individual is affected by age. However, their basic commonality is distinctive; even describing it can set clinical testing in motion that can pinpoint a diagnosis.

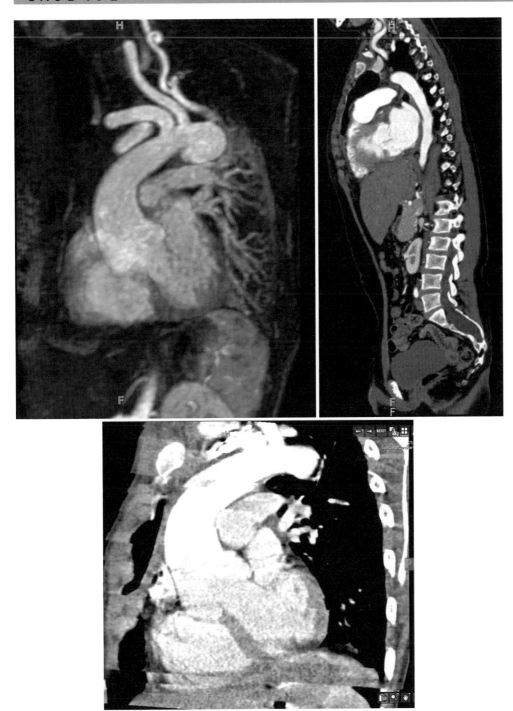

1. Five-year-old patient A had a magnetic resonance angiographic (MRA) scan obtained (first image). What were the findings?

2. A year later, he had a computed tomographic angiographic (CTA) scan obtained (second image). What has changed?

3. Patient B is 14 years old and carries the same diagnosis as Patient A. What additional features can be seen in the third image?

4. How early can this syndrome present?

Diagnosis: Loeys-Dietz Syndrome

1. MRA findings included a dilated aortic root (measuring 2.2 cm) and a very tortuous thoracic aorta.

2. Increased dilation (now 3.5 cm) and tortuosity.

3. Scoliosis, dural ectasia, and carotid tortuosity.

4. At birth.

References

Johnson PT, Chen JK, Loeys BL, et al: Loeys-Dietz syndrome: MDCT angiography findings, *AJR Am J Roentgenol* 189:W29–W35, 2007.

Yetman AT, Beroukhim RS, Ivy DD, et al: Importance of the clinical recognition of Loeys-Dietz syndrome in the neonatal period, *Pediatrics* 119(5):1199–1202, 2007.

Cross-Reference

Blickman JG, Parker BR, Barnes PD: *Pediatric radiology— the requisites*, ed 3, Philadelphia, 2009, Mosby, pp 281–283.

Comment

Loeys-Dietz syndrome (LDS) shares many phenotypic traits with other syndromes that affect the formation of bones, joints, and fibrous tissue. In the newborn period, these traits may take the form of *arthrogryposis*, a descriptive term for contracted, distorted joints. Other infants might have loose, hypermobile joints. Larsen, Beals, Ehlers-Danlos, and Marfan syndromes can all present this way, as can LDS. Similar to patients with either Marfan syndrome or the vascular subset of Ehlers-Danlos syndrome, patients with LDS show abnormal changes in the arterial walls, which lead to dilation. However, those with LDS exhibit fast, aggressive disease that encompasses the entire arterial tree, and the possibility of dissection or rupture at a very early age is quite high. Unlike the other two syndromes, however, patients with LDS progress well with surgery, which can significantly alter the course of their disease. A specific genetic mutation appears to be responsible (TGFβR2 [chromosome 3p22] or TGFβR1[chromosome 9q22]). Testing for this mutation should be performed in all patients in whom a vascular syndrome is suspected.

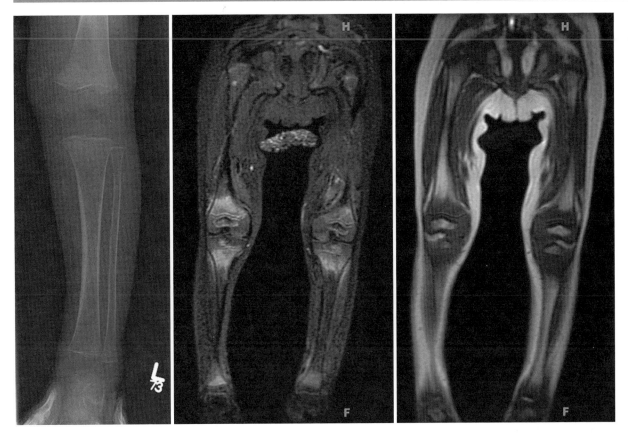

1. This 2-year-old boy refuses to walk. What are the plain-film radiographic findings in the left leg (first image)?

2. What differential diagnoses are suggested by these findings?

3. Oncologic concerns prompted a magnetic resonance image (MRI) (second image—coronal short T1-weighted inversion recovery [STIR] MRI; third image—T1-weighted MRI). What are the abnormal findings?

4. Medical history became available later that revealed, remarkably, a diet consisting solely of rice, milk, eggs, and ground chicken. What is the diagnosis?

Diagnosis: Scurvy

1. Osteopenia, prominent metaphyseal dense band with osteopenic metaphyseal band along the diaphyseal margin, and a dense ring around the margin of the epiphyses with central lucency.

2. Infiltrative process in the metaphysis (neuroblastoma, lymphoma, leukemia) and metabolic process (scurvy, early rickets).

3. Abnormal edema-like signal in metaphyses (low on T1-weighted MRI, high on STIR); *cloaking* periosteal signal over the distal femurs (high intensity on both images), and compatible with blood products.

4. Vitamin C deficiency.

Reference

Silverman FN, editor: *Caffey's pediatric x-ray diagnosis*, ed 8, Chicago, 1985, Yearbook Medical Publishers, pp 674–679.

Cross-Reference

Blickman JG, Parker BR, Barnes PD: *Pediatric radiology— the requisites*, ed 3, Philadelphia, 2009, Mosby, p 174.

Comment

The lack of vitamin C interferes with cellular activity in all parts of the body. In the bones, where mineralization is the result of both cellular action (of the osteoblasts and osteoclasts) and noncellular, diffusion-mediated calcium deposition and resorption, this results in characteristic radiographic findings. The zone of provisional calcification (ZPC) continues to become denser, because calcium is laid down in this region without cellular action and the resting cartilage no longer converts to proliferating cartilage on the physeal side. The zone thickens because it is not being converted to spongy bone on the diaphyseal side. The ZPC is even more conspicuous because the diaphyseal bone resorption continues, particularly in the region immediately adjacent on the diaphyseal side. This atrophic band is called the *scurvy line*. The ZPC widens horizontally because the osteoclasts that normally remodel it are inactive and form spurs. The spurs, the rest of the ZPC, and the scurvy line are all brittle and prone to fissuring and fracturing; the *corner sign,* another distinctive finding, is formed in this way. The epiphysis acts like a small metadiaphysis and undergoes the same changes. The ZPC forms a ring around the margin of the ossification center while the center demineralizes.

Scurvy denatures the intercellular "cement" that binds together the capillary endothelial cells, allowing bleeding to occur even though clotting factors are normal. This form of subperiosteal hemorrhage can cloak the long bones.

Because the amounts of vitamin C needed for health are so small, it takes 3 to 6 months of deprivation before symptoms are noted. When vitamin C is restored, the findings reverse: the bone remineralizes, the ZPC is remodeled, and growth resumes. Subperiosteal hematoma often calcifies dystrophically; only then is its true extent appreciated. The central portion of the thickened ZPC often remains intact and is visible as a transverse line as the bone grows away from it.

The last U.S. outbreak of scurvy occurred in the 1950s, when boiled-milk formulas became popular. Once it became evident that heating inactivated ascorbic acid, it was added back to the diet in other ways and the problem was eliminated. Currently, scurvy is seen mainly in underdeveloped countries or in refugee camps where the reliance on cereal crops or a monotonous diet devoid of fruits and vegetables exists, but new immigrants or temporary workers' families can be a source of new local cases.

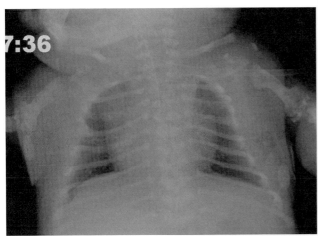
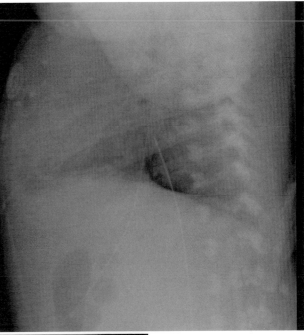
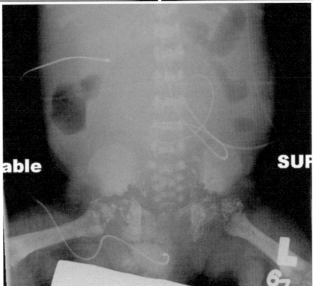

1. Describe the abnormalities seen in these studies of this newborn infant.

2. What type of bone dysplasia is this?

3. What type of inheritance is associated with this lesion?

4. Is this disease compatible with life?

Diagnosis: Chondrodysplasia Punctata

1. The abnormalities include stippled epiphyses in the proximal and distal humerus and in the proximal femur. The proximal extremities are short. The vertebral bodies are short in the anteroposterior diameter, and coronal clefts are seen. The lungs are small, and the stippled appearance of the sternum cartilage is also noted. A lower abdominal mass density is demonstrated.

2. Chondrodysplasia punctata is the type of dysplasia demonstrated in this study. Symmetric involvement is usually seen in the rhizomelic type.

3. Autosomal recessive.

4. Infants usually die within the first year of life.

Reference

Hertzberg BS, Kliewer MA, Decker M, et al: Antenatal ultrasonographic diagnosis of rhizomelic chondrodysplasia punctata, *J Ultrasound Med* 18:715-718, 1999.

Cross-Reference

Blickman JG, Parker BR, Barnes PD: *Pediatric radiology—the requisites*, ed 3, Philadelphia, 2009, Mosby, pp 165-166.

Comment

This patient has rhizomelic chondrodysplasia punctata (RCDP), which was diagnosed by fetal ultrasound examination. He had lung hypoplasia probably related to a long-standing urinary tract obstruction and oligohydramnios. The soft-tissue mass in the pelvis was found to be an enlarged bladder on ultrasound examination, possibly secondary to posterior urethral valves. No further imaging studies were obtained, and the patient died at 2 days of age. He was found to have typical molecular changes associated with this disorder of peroxisome biogenesis and the peroxin-7 gene.

RCDP is an autosomal recessive disease. Its manifestations include the aforementioned skeletal changes, as well as cerebellar atrophy, midface hypoplasia, cataracts, cervical canal stenosis, skin lesions, contractures, and severe development delay. The prognosis is poor; most of the affected children die before 10 years of age; some die in the neonatal period as in this patient. The finding of stippled epiphyses is not specific for RCDP and can be seen in other entities such as the Conradi-Hünermann syndrome and the brachytelephalangic types of chondrodysplasia.

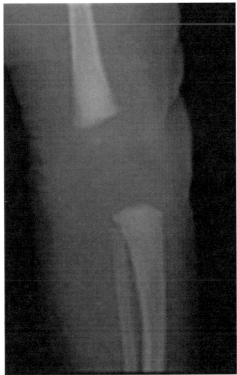

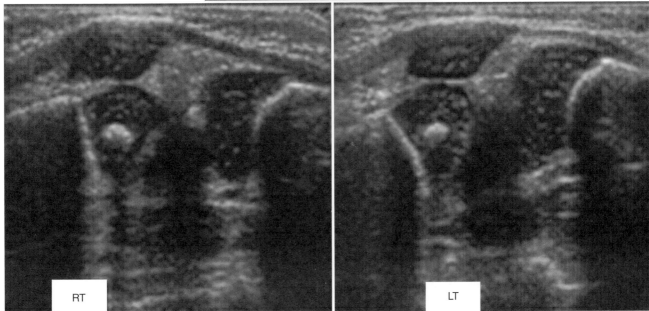

1. Which knee is abnormal?

2. Describe the ultrasound abnormality demonstrated in these sagittal images.

3. What is the appearance of the knee during the physical examination?

4. What is the treatment of this entity?

Diagnosis: Congenital Dislocation of the Knee

1. The left knee.

2. The tibia is anteriorly subluxated.

3. The knee is hyperextended. It may have limited flexion.

4. Nonsurgical casting or splinting.

Reference

Kamata N, Takahashi T, Nakatani K, et al: Ultrasonographic evaluation of congenital dislocation of the knee, *Skeletal Radiol* 31:539–542, 2002.

Laurence M: Genu recurvatum congenitum, *J Bone Joint Surg* (Br) 49:121–134, 1967.

Comments

Congenital dislocation of the knee (CDK) is uncommon and occurs 80 times less than developmental dysplasia of the hip. It is usually an isolated abnormality but may be associated with multiple dislocations such as arthrogryposis or syndromes like Larsen or Ehlers-Danlos syndrome. CDK was classified by Laurence in three clinical categories: (1) hyperextension (the knee hyperextends more than 15 degrees but fully flexes); (2) subluxation (the knee hyperextends more than 15 degrees, and some restriction of flexion is noted or it feels unstable); and (3) dislocation (the knee is unstable and extension/flexion is variable). When hyperextension is present without subluxation or dislocation, the abnormality is called *genu recurvatum*. Conservative management with traction and casting is the preferred treatment, but surgery may be necessary in the more severe deformities such as dislocation.

The cause of CDK is not known. In isolated cases, theories of the causes include intrauterine position involving breech presentation and oligohydramnios. Fibrosis and contracture of the quadriceps muscle is characteristic of CDK. In addition, tight anterior joint capsule, hypoplasia of the suprapatellar bursa, and abnormal anterior cruciate ligament have been described. Whether these are the causes or the results of the dislocation is not clear.

Radiographic findings show fixed hyperextension when the images are obtained without manipulation. The presence of subluxation or dislocation can be seen on the lateral view. Typically, the distal femoral epiphysis is small for the age of the patient and may not be ossified, even in the full-term newborn with this abnormality. In addition to subluxation, the distal femoral epiphysis is small in this patient. Ultrasound imaging shows the presence of subluxation or dislocation, and the quadriceps tendon can be evaluated. It may be thin with increased echogenicity, a sign thought to be secondary to fibrosis.

In this patient, not only is an obvious anterior subluxation of the tibia noted, but the quadriceps tendon is slightly thinner and more echogenic on the affected side (left) than on the normal side. This appearance will normalize in time.

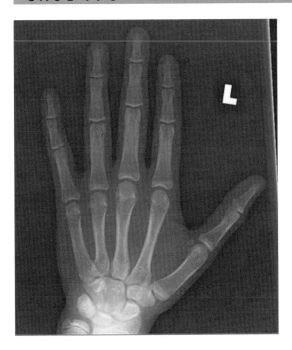

1. What are the imaging findings in this teenage girl?

2. What is the differential diagnosis?

3. In light of the findings in this patient, can sclerosis of the bones also be demonstrated?

4. What hormones are responsible for this process in renal osteodystrophy?

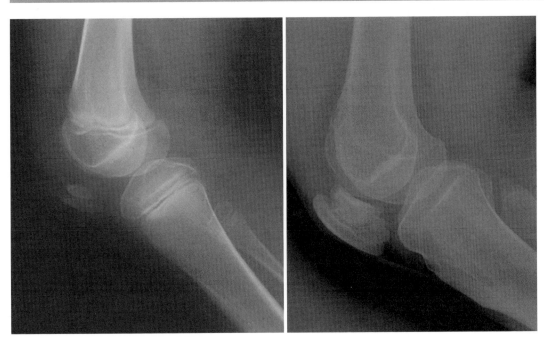

1. These two images show the same patient at age 7 and then at 20 years of age. What is the finding?

2. Do other types of this abnormality exist?

3. With what condition is this finding mostly associated?

4. Are any other associations found?

Diagnosis: Secondary Hyperparathyroidism

1. Subperiosteal resorption of the radial aspects of the middle phalanges of the second through fifth digits.

2. Primary, secondary, or tertiary hyperparathyroidism.

3. In some cases of secondary or tertiary hyperthyroidism, diffuse bony sclerosis is also seen. Metaphyseal sclerosis may be demonstrated in the primary form.

4. A deficiency of 1,25 dihydroxyvitamin D (1,25-[OH]2D), a metabolite of vitamin D formed in the kidney and parathyroid hormone (PTH).

Reference

Kuhn JP, Slovis TL, Haller JO, editors: *Caffey's pediatric diagnostic imaging*, ed 10, Philadelphia, 2004, Mosby, p 2245 and 2439–2441.

Cross-Reference

Blickman JG, Parker BR, Barnes PD: *Pediatric radiology—the requisites*, ed 3, Philadelphia, 2009, Mosby, p 173.

Comment

This patient with chronic renal insufficiency exhibits changes of secondary hyperparathyroidism. The subperiosteal resorption is a classic finding in this entity. The bony changes associated with renal disease are called *renal osteodystrophy*. Other radiographic features include osteopenia, patchy or generalized sclerosis, and findings of rickets, osteomalacia, and secondary hyperparathyroidism. In the spine, osteosclerosis is often more significant along the vertebral body endplates, which is referred to as a *rugger jersey spine*. Subperiosteal resorption not only occurs on the radial side of the middle phalanges but also in the distal tufts of the terminal phalanges and in the medial aspects of the proximal tibia, humerus, and femur. Generalized bone resorption may be present, and brown tumors may be seen. These tumors are secondary to the accumulation of fibrous tissue and giant cells replacing or expanding the bone. Brown tumors may lead to a pathologic fracture. The finding of osteosclerosis is associated with higher levels of PTH and alkaline phosphatase.

Primary hyperparathyroidism is caused by a parathyroid adenoma in most cases. Secondary hyperparathyroidism is most commonly caused by renal insufficiency, but intestinal malabsorption and vitamin D deficiency can also be causes. Tertiary hyperparathyroidism is the persistence of findings after renal transportation for renal failure, which is due to autonomic hyperfunction of the parathyroid glands.

Diagnosis: Double-Layer Patella

1. The patella has two components, one in front of the other.

2. Five types exist. This is a form of bipartite patella.

3. Multiple epiphyseal dysplasia (MED).

4. No other associations are found.

Reference

Rubenstein JD, Christakis MS: Case 95: fracture of double-layered patella in multiple epiphyseal dysplasia, *Radiology* 239:911–913, 2006.

Cross-Reference

Blickman JG, Parker BR, Barnes PD: *Pediatric radiology—the requisites*, ed 3, Philadelphia, 2009, Mosby, p 158.

Comment

Once thought to be specific for the diagnosis of autosomal recessive MED, it is now known that some patients with autosomal dominant disease also have this patellar abnormality called a *double-layer patella*. MED is a heterogeneous skeletal dysplasia best classified by its genetic basis. Mutations are found in genes responsible for coding cartilage oligomeric matrix protein, type IX collagen, and matrilin-3. A disturbance of endochondral ossification and hypoplasia of the epiphyseal cartilage of tubular bones cause the resulting chondrodysplasia; the vertebrae are usually normal. The epiphyseal abnormalities are bilateral, symmetric, and more significant in the lower extremities. Patients are usually of short stature, normal intelligence, and may have early osteoarthritis.

Patients with recessive MED may have a clubfoot deformity, brachydactyly, scoliosis, cleft palate, joint contracture and patellar subluxation, or dislocation related to the double-layer patella. Surgical treatments for the patella include resection of the posterior component and surgical fusion of the two segments.

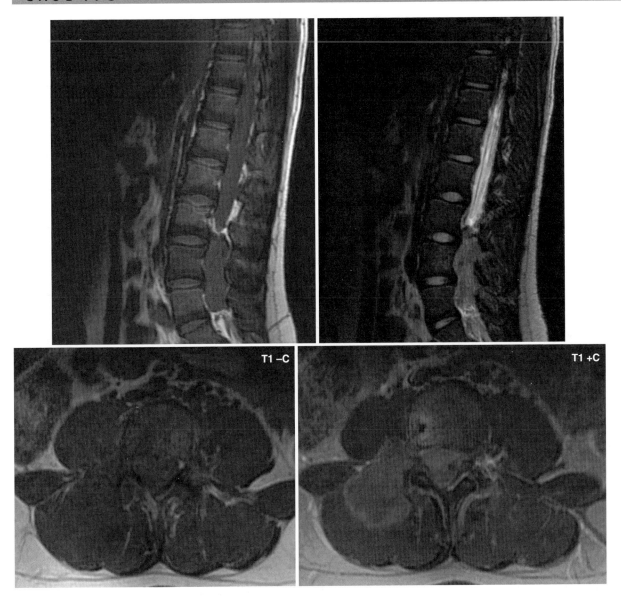

T1 −C

T1 +C

1. What are the imaging findings in this 10-year-old boy with back pain?

2. What is the classic radiographic presentation of this entity?

3. Is this entity closely related to primitive neuroectodermal tumor of the bone?

4. What are the differential diagnoses?

Diagnosis: Extraosseous Ewing Sarcoma

1. The findings include a large, lobular T1-weighted hypointense, T2-weighted heterogeneously hypointense, and heterogeneous-enhancing mass in the lumbosacral spinal canal and paraspinal soft tissues. It involves the right posterior spinal musculature, extending into the spinal canal of the spinal column, displacing the dura to the left, and enlarging the neural foramina. In addition, signal intensity changes, and expansion in the right lamina indicates bone marrow involvement in this level.

2. The classic presentation includes a central, diaphyseal, lytic, lamellated *onion-skin* or permeative periosteal reaction. Any part of the bone can be involved, and the onion-skin periosteal reaction is not a pathognomonic sign.

3. These findings are related to primitive neuroectodermal tumor.

4. Osteosarcoma, metastatic neuroblastoma, Langerhans cell histiocytosis (LCH), or rhabdomyosarcoma.

Reference

Weber KL, Sim FH: Ewing's sarcoma: presentation and management, *J Orthop Sci* 6:366–371, 2001.

Cross-Reference

Blickman JG, Parker BR, Barnes PD: *Pediatric radiology— the requisites*, ed 3, Philadelphia, 2009, Mosby, pp 186–187.

Comment

Ewing sarcoma is a small, blue, round-cell malignant bone tumor. It is the fourth most common malignancy of bone and the second most common primary malignant bone tumor in children after osteosarcoma, accounting for approximately 10% of primary malignant bone tumors. The peak incidence of Ewing sarcoma occurs during the second decade of life, with 80% of the tumors occurring in patients younger than 20 years of age. There is male preponderance, and this tumor most frequently develops in the long bones and flat bones such as in the pelvis and scapula. The most common presenting symptoms include pain, swelling, and a mass. Approximately 20% of the patients have fever, which may lead to the misdiagnosis of osteomyelitis.

Upper and lower extremities are the most commonly involved sites, followed by the pelvis, ribs, spine, and any place in the soft tissues in a decreasing order of frequency. Pelvis girdle or long tubular bone involvement make up approximately 70% to 75% of patients. A greater propensity exists for flat bones than for other primary bone malignancies. Metastatic disease presents with involvement of other bones or lung involvement and lymph nodes.

Involvement of the spine is quite rare and occurs in only 3.5% of patients with Ewing sarcoma. The most common location is the lumbosacral spine. These patients may exhibit neurologic deficits.

Radiographs are the initial modality of choice to visualize aggressive, lucent, ill-defined intramedullary lesion with cortical disruption. No ossified tumor matrix is demonstrated. Magnetic resonance imaging (MRI) is the best modality to visualize the local extent of disease. An associated soft-tissue mass may be disproportionately larger than the actual bone destruction. Computed tomography may be superior to MRI in showing the cortical bone destruction. MRI is preferred in follow-up imaging of local disease. Bone scintigraphy is used to evaluate for metastatic disease, and positron emission tomography is helpful in monitoring disease response.

Osteomyelitis is not a dominant differential diagnosis in the central presentation of Ewing sarcoma; however, in extremity involvement, osteomyelitis is an important consideration. Osteomyelitis more commonly presents in younger children and has a rapid rate of progression after the onset of symptoms. Osteosarcoma presents with osteoid tumor matrix in 90% of the patients. LCH also has an onset that can rapidly regress or disappear.

Chemotherapy and radiation therapy, followed by surgery for local control, is the general management plan in most patients. Poorer prognostic factors include larger tumor volume and pelvic location and metastatic disease.

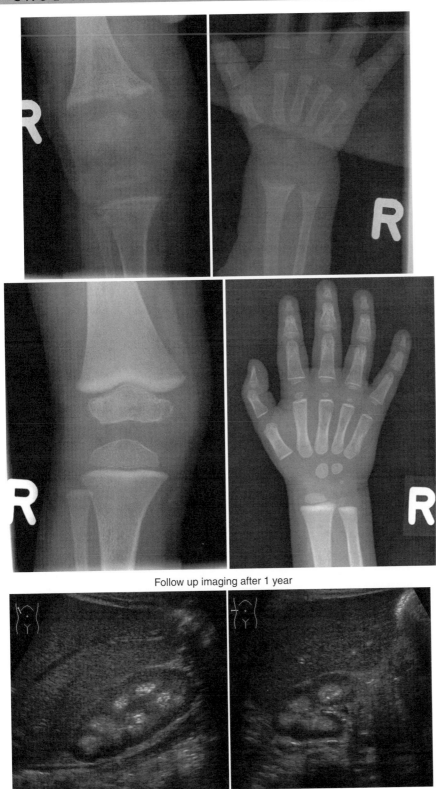

Follow up imaging after 1 year

1. What are the imaging findings?

2. What is the most likely diagnosis?

3. What appears to have occurred between both plain-film radiographs?

4. What may be the reason for the renal findings?

Diagnosis: Rickets in Hypophosphatasia

1. A widened growth plate, cupping and irregularity of all metaphyses, diffuse osteopenia, remineralization on follow-up imaging, and medullary nephrocalcinosis.

2. Rickets in hypophosphatasia.

3. This child has had successful phosphate replacement therapy and vitamin D supplementation.

4. Nephrocalcinosis may be the result as a consequence of vitamin D therapy.

Reference

Kottamasu SR: Metabolic bone diseases. In Kuhn JP, Slovis TL, Haller JO, editors: *Caffey's pediatric diagnostic imaging*, ed 10, Philadelphia, 2004, Elsevier, pp 2242-2268.

Cross-Reference

Blickman JG, Parker BR, Barnes PD: *Pediatric radiology— the requisites*, ed 3, Philadelphia, 2009, Mosby, pp 172-173.

Comment

Rickets is the result of an inadequate mineralization of osteoid and newly formed bone in a growing skeleton. Rickets may be the result of a variety of metabolic bone diseases. It is classified as a disorder of vitamin D metabolism, phosphate metabolism, or calcium metabolism. Vitamin D deficiency may have several causes including nutritional and deprivational etiologic origins. A dietary vitamin D deficiency can be the result of a strict vegetarian diet or a lack of exposure to sunlight. In addition, many diseases are associated with the development of rickets; these include hepatobiliary and gastrointestinal or renal disorders. Occasionally, rickets is the result of anticonvulsant therapy that accelerates the catabolism of active vitamin D levels. Chronic renal disease can cause renal osteodystrophy, which is a combination of rickets and secondary hyperparathyroidism.

Rickets as a result of hypophosphatasia is so-called vitamin D–resistant rickets caused by an excess excretion of phosphates in the proximal renal tubules. It is characterized by a low serum phosphate level and a low-to-normal serum calcium level. Treatment is primarily with phosphate replacement and vitamin D supplementation. Rickets as a result of hypophosphatasia is an X-linked dominant disorder.

Clinically, children present with bowleg deformities, as well as swelling of the wrists, knees, and ankles. The long bones have prominent or bulbous ends. The costochondral junction is frequently expanded, which may resemble a "rosary." Scoliosis and thoracic kyphosis are also seen. Most children have impaired growth.

Imaging findings are most prominent in areas of active, rapid growth. Consequently, the best single plain-film radiograph is of the knee that includes the metaphyseal ends of the femurs and tibias. Alternatively, the wrist can be examined.

The characteristic imaging findings include a widening and irregularity of the growth plate and metaphyses. The metaphyses typically show cupping. Diffuse osteopenia is seen, and the long bones are frequently bowed. Further metabolic work-up is necessary to determine the exact cause of the rickets. Occasionally, vitamin D supplementation can result in a medullary nephrocalcinosis, as noted in this patient. Follow-up imaging under treatment may show a remineralization of the metaphyses and a recovery of the osteopenia.

Differential diagnoses include leukemia and congenital syphilis.

T1 with contrast and fat sat

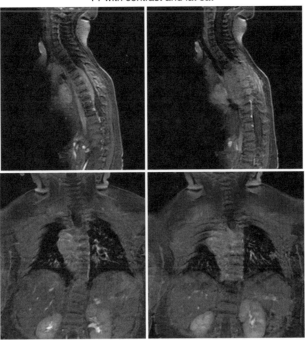

T2 with fat sat

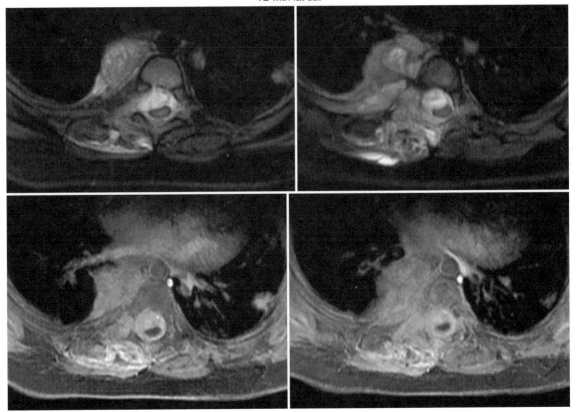

T1 with contrast and fat sat

1. What are the imaging findings in this 14-year-old boy with back pain?

2. What is the most likely diagnosis?

3. What other benign soft-tissue tumors should be considered possibilities?

4. What other malignant soft-tissue tumors should be considered?

Diagnosis: Desmoid Tumor-Aggressive Fibromatosis

1. Infiltrative, T2-hyperintense, strong-enhancing soft-tissue tumor in the paraspinal musculature.

2. Desmoid tumor of the paraspinal musculature (aggressive fibromatosis).

3. Hemangioma, hemangiopericytoma, and a peripheral nerve sheath tumor.

4. Rhabdomyosarcoma, fibrosarcoma, liposarcoma, lymphoma, and neuroblastoma.

Reference

McCarville MB, Hoffer FA, Adelman CS, et al: MRI and biologic behavior of desmoid tumors in children, *AJR Am J Roentgenol* 189(3):633–640, 2007.

Cross-Reference

Blickman JG, Parker BR, Barnes PD: *Pediatric radiology—the requisites*, ed 3, Philadelphia, 2009, Mosby, p 330.

Comment

Aggressive fibromatosis or desmoid-type fibromatosis is the most common type of fibromatosis in children. Desmoid-type fibromatosis of childhood refers to a proliferation of fibroblasts and myofibroblasts in musculoaponeurotic tissues (fascial sheaths and aponeuroses of striated muscles) that may act locally aggressive or "malignant" as a result of diffuse infiltrative growth. Desmoid-type fibromatosis is classified by the World Health Organization as a tumor of intermediate grade. Although a desmoid tumor does not metastasize, local infiltration and compression of adjacent functional structures including bone may result in significant complications. The optimal treatment is controversial; a multidisciplinary approach includes surgery, chemotherapy, and radiation therapy and is frequently mandatory. The goal of treatment is to provide local control while preserving function. Historically, surgery has been the primary treatment. However, achieving the wide margin that offers the best chance of avoiding recurrence is difficult because of the infiltrative nature. Unfortunately, local recurrence after surgical excision is frequent.

On magnetic resonance imaging (MRI), desmoid-type fibromatosis is usually T1-isointense or slightly hyperintense to muscle but may show intermediate- or high-signal intensity on T2-weighted imaging. Contrast enhancement is usually intense. Desmoid fibromatosis may infiltrate and displace adjacent structures. If located in the paraspinal musculature, tumor extension may be observed through the neuronal foramina into the spinal canal with significant compression of the spinal cord. Tumor margins may be sharp or ill-defined. Prediction of a surgical cleavage plane may be difficult. MRI is especially helpful in the preoperative planning by identifying tumor components that encircle neurovascular bundles. A baseline MRI is essential for follow-up imaging during and after treatment to differentiate between residual and recurrent tumor, as well as postoperative changes. Computed tomography may be useful to identify bony changes; MRI is, however, mandatory to determine the exact extension of the lesion.

A

Abernethy type Ib, 355*f*, 356
Achalasia, 45*f*, 46
Achondroplasia, 371*f*, 372
Acute brainstem ischemia, 107*f*, 108
Acute disseminated encephalomyelitis (ADEM), 107*f*, 108
Acute hippocampal injuries
after febrile seizure, 99*f*, 100
Acute ileocecal intussusception, 199*f*, 200
Acute lupus pneumonitis, 338
Acute osteomyelitis, 289*f*, 290
Acute pancreatitis, 197*f*, 198
Adrenal hemorrhages, 363*f*, 364
Agenesis
corpus callosum, 3*f*, 4
Aggressive fibromatosis, 389*f*, 390
Albers-Schönberg disease, 275*f*, 276
Alexander disease, 317*f*, 318
Alobar holoprosencephaly, 312
Ambiguous genitalia
and urogenital sinus, 231*f*, 232
American Association of Surgery of Trauma, 48, 50
Anal atresia
associated with acronym VACTERL, 298
Aneurysmal bone cysts (ABCs), 281*f*, 282
Aortic arch
double, 39*f*, 40
ductus arteriosus derived from, 156
and dysphagia lusoria, 157*f*, 158
Aorticopulmonary window, 150
Apert syndrome
choanal atresia associated with, 326
Aplasia
vagina and uterus, 245*f*, 246
Appendicitis, 159*f*, 160
Apple-peel intestinal atresia, 210
Arnold-Chiari II malformations, 103*f*, 104
Arthritis
juvenile rheumatoid arthritis (JRA), 273*f*, 274
Arthrogryposis, 376
Aspergillosis, 23*f*, 24
Aspirations
in left main bronchus, 35*f*, 36
and meconium aspiration syndrome, 133*f*, 134
Asplenia syndrome, 213*f*, 214
Atresia
anal, 298
apple-peel intestinal, 210
biliary, 161*f*, 162
choanal, 325*f*, 326
esophageal, 177*f*, 178, 298
jejunal, 207*f*, 208
pulmonary, 341*f*, 342
Atrial septal defects (ASDs), 150, 152
Atrioventricular (AV) canal, 149*f*, 150
"Aunt Minnie," 17*f*, 18
Autoimmune disorders
autoimmune thyroiditis, 11*f*, 12
Crohn disease (CD), 215*f*, 216
human immunodeficiency virus (HIV), 198, 270, 320
microscopic polyangiitis, 339*f*, 340
mixed connective tissue disorders (MCTDs), 287*f*, 288
systemic lupus erythematosus (SLE), 337*f*, 338

Autoimmune thyroiditis, 11*f*, 12
Autosomal dominant polycystic kidney disease (ADPKD), 233*f*, 234
Autosomal recessive disorders
chondrodysplasia punctata, 379*f*, 380
cystic fibrosis (CF), 17*f*, 18
muscle-eye-brain disease, 305*f*, 306
Shwachman-Diamond syndrome, 351*f*, 352
Avulsion fractures
and medial elbow dislocation, 85*f*, 86

B

Bacterial infections
causing Lemierre syndrome, 332
and neonatal pneumonia, 25*f*, 26
causing osteomyelitis, 290
pulmonary tuberculosis, 37*f*, 38
causing renal abscesses, 238
round pneumonia, 31*f*, 32
causing spondylodiscitis, 101*f*, 102
"Barking cough," 5*f*, 6
Beckwith-Wiedemann syndrome, 369*f*, 370
Bilateral cystic ovarian teratomas, 261*f*, 262
Bilateral inguinal hernias, 51*f*, 52
Biliary atresia, 161*f*, 162
Bilious emesis
and jejunal atresia, 207*f*, 208
and malrotation, 209*f*, 210
Bipartite patella, 384
Bladder
classic bladder exstrophy, 241*f*, 242
diverticulum, 361*f*, 362
ears, 227*f*, 228
neurogenic bladder, 61*f*, 62
Bladder diverticulum, 361*f*, 362
Bladder ears, 227*f*, 228
Bladder exstrophy, 241*f*, 242
Bochdalek hernias, 27*f*, 28
Bone tumors
Ewing sarcoma, 385*f*, 386
hereditary multiple exostosis (HME), 81*f*, 82
osteosarcoma, 293*f*, 294
Bones
aneurysmal bone cysts (ABCs), 281*f*, 282
brittle bone disease, 295*f*, 296
extraosseous Ewing sarcoma, 385*f*, 386
Langerhans cell histiocytosis (LCH), 285*f*, 286
manifestations of sickle cell anemia on, 279*f*, 280
osteogenesis imperfecta type II, 295*f*, 296
osteopetrosis, 275*f*, 276
osteosarcoma, 293*f*, 294
rickets in hypophosphatasia, 387*f*, 388
Bowels
malrotation, 209*f*, 210
Brain
and Alexander disease, 318
lissencephaly type I, 313*f*, 314
muscle-eye-brain disease (MEB), 305*f*, 306
Brainstem
and Alexander disease, 318
glioma, 112
lesions, 107*f*, 108
Brittle bone disease, 295*f*, 296
Bronchiolitis, 15*f*, 16

Note: Page numbers followed by *f* indicate figures.

Tuber cinereum hamartoma,
— at the hypothalamus b/w mamillary bodies and above pituitary stalk
— causes gelastic sz
— floor 3rd ventricle
— spectrum of grey matter heterotopia